Gastroenteritis: Clinical Assessment and Management

Gastroenteritis: Clinical Assessment and Management

Edited by Augustus Green

hayle medical
New York

Hayle Medical,
750 Third Avenue, 9th Floor,
New York, NY 10017, USA

Visit us on the World Wide Web at:
www.haylemedical.com

ISBN: 978-1-63241-607-0

The publisher's policy is to use permanent paper from mills that operate a sustainable forestry policy. Furthermore, the publisher ensures that the text paper and cover boards used have met acceptable environmental accreditation standards.

Printed in China.

Cataloging-in-Publication Data

Gastroenteritis : clinical assessment and management / edited by Augustus Green.
p. cm.
Includes bibliographical references and index.
ISBN 978-1-63241-607-0
1. Gastroenteritis. 2. Gastrointestinal system--Diseases. 3. Gastrointestinal system--Diseases--Diagnosis.
4. Gastrointestinal system--Diseases--Treatment. I. Green, Augustus.
RC840.G3 G37 2019
616.33--dc23

Table of Contents

Preface

The purpose of the book is to provide a glimpse into the dynamics and to present opinions and studies of some of the scientists engaged in the development of new ideas in the field from very different standpoints. This book will prove useful to students and researchers owing to its high content quality.

The inflammation of the gastrointestinal tract, which includes the stomach and small intestine, is known as gastroenteritis or infectious diarrhea. Vomiting, diarrhea, dehydration, lack of energy, fever and abdominal pain are some of its common symptoms. Viruses such as rotavirus, adenovirus and norovirus, and bacteria such as Campylobacter jejuni, Shigella and Escherichia coli are some of the causes of gastroenteritis. Assessment of the stool, serum glucose, electrolytes and kidney function are some common ways to diagnose gastroenteritis. Oral rehydration therapy and the intake of medicines like, metoclopramide, ondansetron and butylscopolamine are helpful. This book explores new techniques and their applications for the clinical assessment and management of gastroenteritis. It consists of contributions made by international experts. Those in search of information to further their knowledge will be greatly assisted by this book.

At the end, I would like to appreciate all the efforts made by the authors in completing their chapters professionally. I express my deepest gratitude to all of them for contributing to this book by sharing their valuable works. A special thanks to my family and friends for their constant support in this journey.

Editor

1

Pathogenicity of *Shigella* in Chickens

Run Shi[¶], Xia Yang[¶], Lu Chen*, Hong-tao Chang, Hong-ying Liu, Jun Zhao, Xin-wei Wang, Chuan-qing Wang

Collage of Animal Science and Veterinary Medicine, Henan Agricultural University, Zhengzhou, People's Republic of China

Abstract

Shigellosis in chickens was first reported in 2004. This study aimed to determine the pathogenicity of *Shigella* in chickens and the possibility of cross-infection between humans and chickens. The pathogenicity of *Shigella* in chickens was examined via infection of three-day-old SPF chickens with *Shigella* strain ZD02 isolated from a human patient. The virulence and invasiveness were examined by infection of the chicken intestines and primary chicken intestinal epithelial cells. The results showed *Shigella* can cause death via intraperitoneal injection in SPF chickens, but only induce depression via crop injection. Immunohistochemistry and transmission electron microscopy revealed the *Shigella* can invade the intestinal epithelia. Immunohistochemistry of the primary chicken intestinal epithelial cells infected with *Shigella* showed the bacteria were internalized into the epithelial cells. Electron microscopy also confirmed that *Shigella* invaded primary chicken intestinal epithelia and was encapsulated by phagosome-like membranes. Our data demonstrate that *Shigella* can invade primary chicken intestinal epithelial cells in vitro and chicken intestinal mucosa in vivo, resulting in pathogenicity and even death. The findings suggest *Shigella* isolated from human or chicken share similar pathogenicity as well as the possibility of human-poultry cross-infection, which is of public health significance.

Editor: David M. Ojcius, University of California Merced, United States of America

Funding: The project was supported by National Natural Science Foundation of China grant 30972187 (http://www.nsfc.gov.cn) and Specialized Research Fund for the Doctoral Program of Higher Education of China grants 20114105110031⁄4 http://www.cutech.edu.cn/cn). The funders had no role in study design, data collection and analysis, decision to publish, or preparation of the manuscript.

Competing Interests: The authors have declared that no competing interests exist.

* Email: chenluhau@hotmail.com

¶ These authors contributed equally to this work.

Introduction

Shigella is a genus of gram-negative, facultative anaerobic Enterobacteriaceae that includes *S. dysenteriae*, *S. flexneri*, *S. boydii*, and *S. sonnei*. *Shigella* species have highly evolved invasive systems that enable the bacteria to invade and multiply within the human intestinal epithelia, ultimately leading to severe inflammatory colitis called bacillary dysentery or shigellosis. Shigellosis remains a worldwide health concern. Statistics from 1966–1997 estimated that over 1.1 million deaths were caused by shigellosis each year worldwide, the vast majority (0.88 million) of which occurred in Asia [1]. Another report based on 1990–2009 statistics estimated that 125 million people in Asia were infected with *Shigella*, resulting in 14,000 deaths annually, most of which were children under 5 years of age [2].

The natural hosts of *Shigella* are conventionally humans and other primates. However, reports of *Shigella* infection in new hosts including monkeys, rabbits, calves, and piglets have emerged [3–6]. In 2004, our team first reported chicken shigellosis, characterized by bloody and purulent dysentery in chickens [7]. A serum epidemiological survey of poultry flocks in China with a history of dysentery showed that the seroprevalence of *Shigella* was 28.3–33.7%, suggesting that *Shigella* is an important etiology of chicken dysentery in China [8]. *Shigella* species isolated from human or chicken have identical biological and serological characteristics [9] and are highly genetically homogeneous, suggesting that *Shigella* isolated from chicken may be a descendant or a new subtype of *Shigella* isolated from human [10].

To determine the origin of *Shigella* isolated from chicken and its pathogenicity in humans and therefore identify potential cross-infection between humans and poultry, it is necessary to infect primates with *Shigella* isolated from chicken and study its pathogenicity. However, such animal models have not been established and would be extremely difficult to perform. In this study, specific pathogen-free (SPF) chickens and primary chicken intestinal epithelial cells were infected with *Shigella* isolated from human to investigate the pathogenicity and invasive capacity of *Shigella* in chickens, the origin of *Shigella* isolated from chicken, and the possibility of *Shigella* cross-infection between humans and poultry.

Materials and Methods

Ethics statement

This study was carried out in strict accordance with the Guidance Suggestions for the Care and Use of Laboratory Animals formulated by The Ministry of Science and Technology of the People's Republic of China. The protocol was approved by the Institutional Animal Care and Use Committee at The University of Henan Agriculture. All surgery was performed under sodium pentobarbital anesthesia, and all efforts were made to minimize suffering.

Culture of the *Shigella* strain ZD02

The *Shigella* strain ZD02 (identified as *S. flexneri* serotype 2a) [11] was isolated from stool from a male donor whose clinical

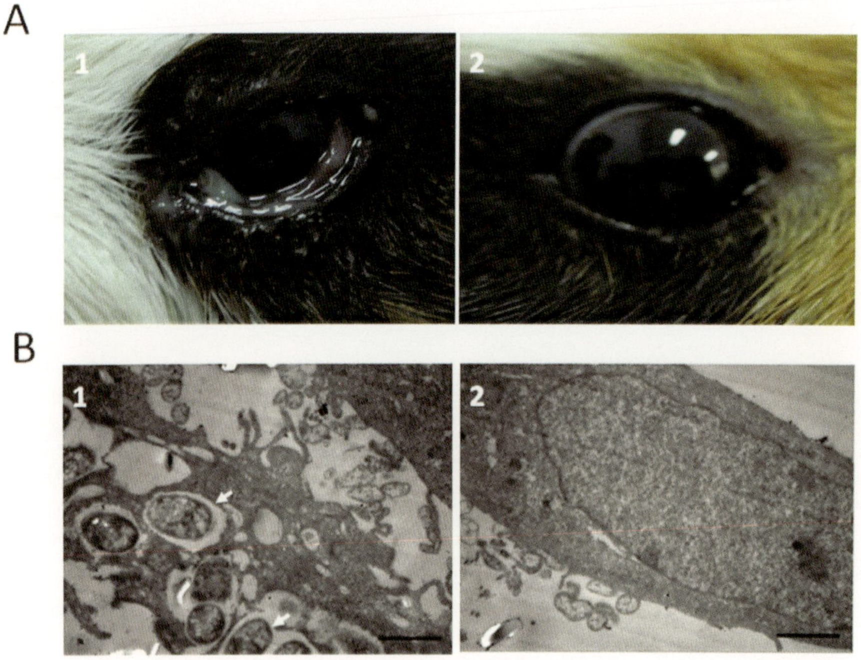

Figure 1. The virulence of the human *Shigella* strain ZD02 using the Sereny test and the HeLa cell invasiveness test. (A) Sereny test. Guinea pigs were infected with *Shigella* strain ZD02 via the cornea and conjunctiva. Corneal and conjunctiva inflammation were seen in infected eyes at 18 h post-inoculation (A1). Corneas and conjunctiva is normal in uninfected control eyes (A2). (B) HeLa cells infected with the *Shigella* strain ZD02. Transmission electron microscopy was used to detect the internalized bacteria within HeLa cells. Representative pictures are shown. The internalized bacteria (arrowheads) were detected at 2 h post-inoculation (B1). Control HeLa cells without infection (B2). Scale bars = 1 μm.

symptoms were diarrhea and bloody dysentery following informed consent. Written consent was obtained from subjects in accordance with approved ethics committee of medical research, First Affiliated Hospital of Zhengzhou University and HIPPA regulations. These bacteria were inoculated in Luria-Bertani (LB) broth and grown with shaking overnight at 37°C. Then the bacteria were subcultured into fresh LB broth at a volume ratio of 1:30 and cultured with shaking at 200 rpm for 3 h at 37°C. The cells were pelleted by centrifugation at 12,000×*g* for 5 min at 4°C and washed three times with phosphate-buffered saline (PBS, pH 7.4). The pellet was then resuspended in antibiotic-free culture medium.

Virulence determination of the *Shigella* strain ZD02

To determine its virulence and invasiveness on epithelial cell, the strain ZD02 was subjected to a keratoconjunctivity assay (Sereny test) and a HeLa cell invasiveness ability test. The Sereny test using guinea pigs was performed as described previously [12]. Female Hartley guinea pigs ranging in weight from 350 to 400 g were purchased from Zhengzhou University. Two guinea pigs were randomized for inoculation with ZD02, and one inoculated with LB broth as a control. Briefly, a 20-μL bacterial suspension at a density of 1.6×10^{10} CFU/mL was inoculated into the conjunctival sacs of guinea pigs anesthetized with an intraperitoneal injection of sodium pentobarbital (0.6 mg/10 gr). The areas surrounding the eyes were gently rubbed to distribute the medium evenly. Pathological changes in the guinea pig eyes were observed at 4 h, 24 h, 48 h, and 72 h. Abiding to the most stringent animal welfare standards [13], human endpoints were applied. The guinea pigs were euthanized using T61 intravenously at 72 h after the inoculation with the occurrence of signs of appetite loss, lethargy, and listlessness.

ZD02 cells were suspended in Dulbecco's Modified Eagle's Medium supplemented with Ham's F12 (DMEM/F12; Gibco, USA) and inoculated into HeLa cells at a ratio of 10:1 [14]. Two hours later, the HeLa cells were digested with trypsin and centrifuged. The pellet was fixed with 2.5% glutaraldehyde and the bacterial invasive capacity in HeLa cells was observed using transmission electron microscopy (TEM) (JEM-1400; Japan).

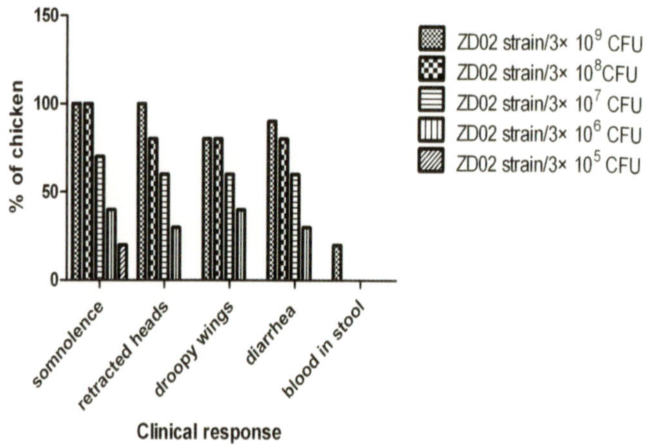

Figure 2. Clinical responses of chickens after intraperitoneal injection. Each bar denotes number of the clinical response/total in each experimental group after 12 h of intraperitoneal injection with *Shigella* strain ZD02.

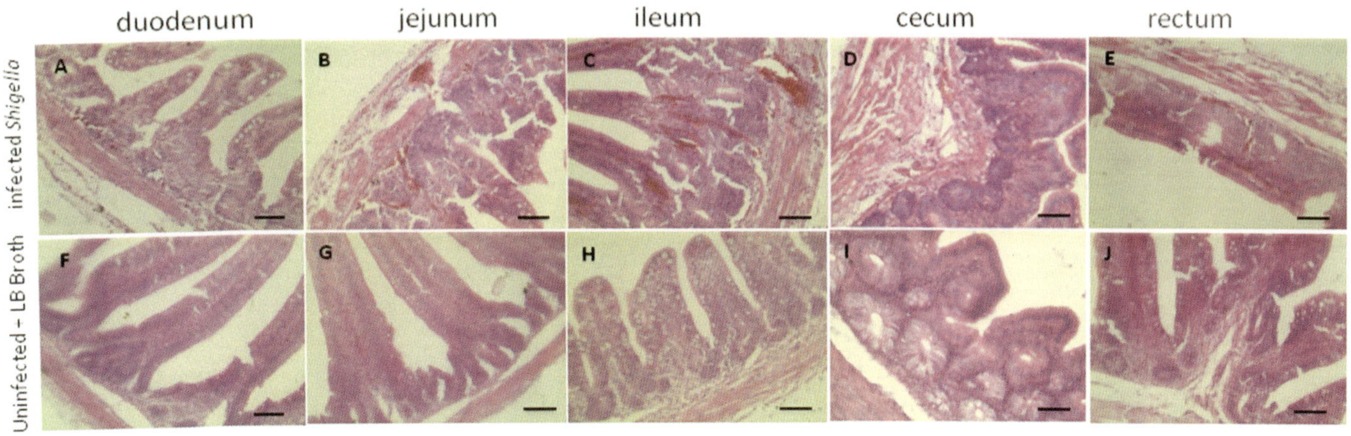

Figure 3. Histopathology of the intestine of one-day-old SPF chickens infected with the *Shigella* strain ZD02 via ligated intestinal loop. The duodenum, jejunum, ileum, and cecum from *Shigella*-infected chickens showed congestion, edema, and neutrophil infiltration (A–E, respectively). No significant pathological changes were noticed in the uninfected controls (F–J, respectively). The sections were stained with hematoxylin and eosin. Representative pictures are shown. Scale bars = 50 μm.

Pathogenicity of the *Shigella* strain ZD02 in three-day-old SPF chickens

Three-day-old SPF male chickens (license SYXK (Yu) 2011–0010, Sipafas Poultry, Jinan, China) were infected with the *Shigella* strain ZD02 via intraperitoneal or crop injection. Each infection route contained five subgroups of 10 chickens each. The bacterial suspension at a density of 6×10^9 CFU/mL was serially diluted into five concentrations at 10× intervals. Each animal was inoculated with a 0.5-mL bacterial suspension. Another 10 chickens inoculated with 0.5 mL of LB broth via either route as controls (Table S1). The clinical signs were observed every 6 h. After 48 h post-infection, some chickens showed non-transient hypothermia, appetite loss, severe distress and impending death. Abiding to the most stringent animal welfare standards, human endpoints were applied when animals were moribund and severely cachectic. The moribund chickens infected with the *Shigella* ZD02 were euthanized using T61 intravenously (0.3 ml/kg) (Intervet, Ukkel, Belgium). The median lethal dose (LD50) was calculated using the Reed-Muench method. The dead chickens were dissected for observation of the gross pathological changes. All of the surviving chickens infected with the *Shigella* ZD02 were euthanized using T61 intravenously at 120 h after the inoculation and dissected for observation as well.

Invasiveness of the *Shigella* strain ZD02 in chicken intestinal epithelial cells

Eight one-day-old SPF chickens were randomized for inoculation with ZD02. The animals were anesthetized with an intraperitoneal injection of sodium pentobarbital (0.6 mg/10 gr). Anesthesia was maintained with 1% isoflurane in conjunction with 1% pure oxygen using a semi-closed circuit. Intramuscular injection of fentanyl was used for pain management. Midline incisions were made in the chickens and the intestinal loops were created by ligation near the lower end of the muscular stomach and the rectum while preserving intestinal blood supply, as described previously [15]. The loops of the infection group were injected with 1 mL of the bacterial suspension containing 10^9 CFU/mL, while the controls received LB broth only. The intestines were covered with a piece of gauze wetted with normal saline to retain humidity. The chickens were maintained under anesthesia for 2 h, 6 h, 8 h, and 12 h. Afterwards, they were euthanized using T61 intravenously and the intestines were removed for examination. Histological samples were fixed for 48 h in 10% neutral buffered formalin, embedded in paraffin, and processed using standard techniques for haematoxylin and eosin or immunohistochemistry staining. Rabbit anti-*S. flexneri* immunoglobulin G (IgG) (1:200; Tianrun Biotech, China) was used as the primary antibody and goat anti-rabbit IgG labeled with horse-

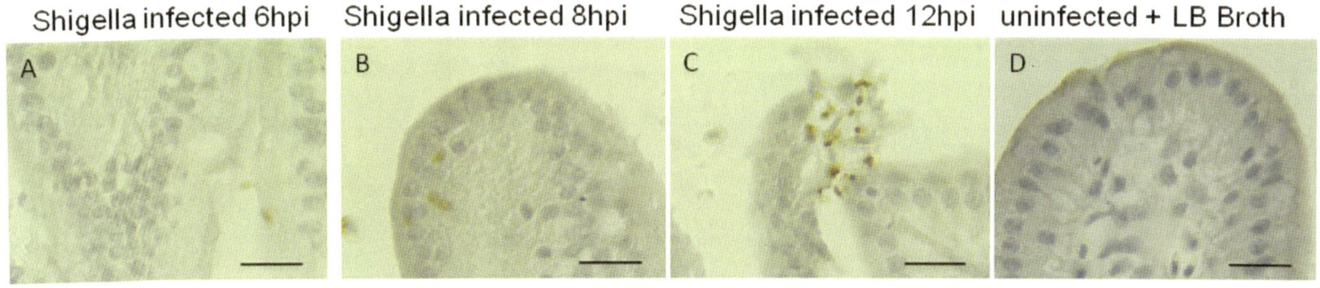

Figure 4. Immunohistochemistry of the jejunum of one-day-old SPF chickens infected with the *Shigella* strain ZD02 via ligated intestinal loop. Bacterial invasion (brown staining) was noticed in the epithelial cells 6 h (A) and 8 h (B) post-inoculation. The intestinal villus detached and the bacteria (brown staining) were released from the lysed epithelial cells (C). Intestinal villus of uninfected chicken was shown as control (D). Scale bars = 20 μm.

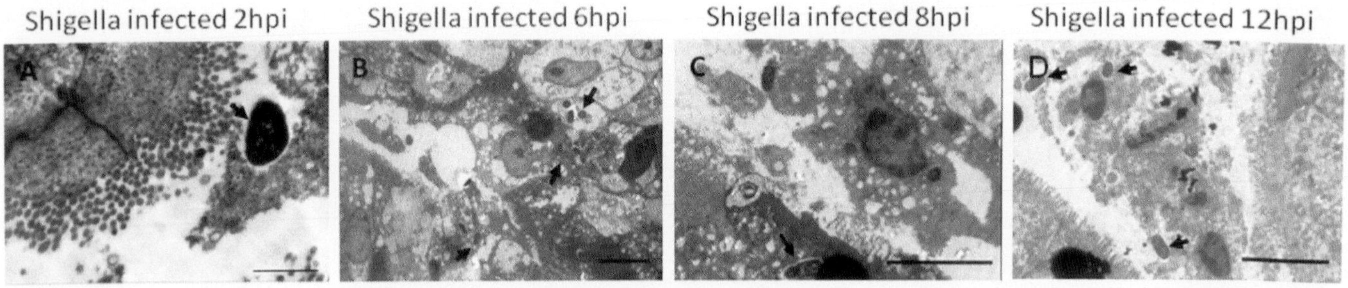

Figure 5. Transmission electron microscopy of the jejunum of one-day-old SPF chickens infected with the *Shigella* strain ZD02 via ligated intestinal loop. *Shigella* (arrowheads) were found near the epithelial cells at 2 h post-inoculation (A. Scale bar = 1 μm). Internalized bacteria (arrowheads) in the epithelial cells were found at 6 h (B. Scale bar = 5 μm) and 8 h (C. Scale bar = 5 μm). The epithelial cells started to lyse and release bacteria (arrowheads) at 12 h (D. Scale bar = 5 μm).

radish peroxidase (1:200; Bioss, China) was used as the secondary antibody in the immunohistochemical staining. The invasive capacity of the strain ZD02 within the intestinal epithelial cells was observed by TEM.

Invasiveness of the *Shigella* strain ZD02 in primary chicken intestinal epithelial cells

Primary chicken intestinal epithelial cells were prepared and cultured as described previously [16]. The cells were cultured in 6-well plates for 48 h and washed three times with PBS. A 200-μL aliquot of the bacterial suspension diluted with DMEM/F12 at a density of 3×10^7 CFU/mL was added to each cell and the plates were further incubated at 37°C under 5% CO_2 for 1 h, 2 h, 3 h, and 4 h. The cells were then collected and examined to determine the invasive rate of the strain ZD02 in chicken intestinal epithelial cells using immunohistochemistry. Rabbit anti-*S. flexneri* IgG (1:200, Tianrun Biotech) was used as the primary antibody and goat anti-rabbit IgG labeled with horseradish peroxidase (1:200, Bioss) was used as the secondary antibody. Ten fields were selected and observed for each well under light microscopy. The invasive rate was calculated as the number of infected cells/total cells ×100%. Scanning electron microscopy (SEM; S-4800; Hitachi, Japan) [17] and TEM (JEM-1400) were used to examine the interactions between the invaded bacteria and epithelial cells.

Results

Virulence of the *Shigella* strain ZD02

The infected guinea pigs developed edematous eyelids, congestive conjunctiva, cloudy corneas, and purulent discharge 18 h after infection with the *Shigella* strain ZD02 (Figure 1 A1). The clinical signs became exaggerated at 40 h. No significant changes were noticed in the control animals (Figure 1 A2). TEM showed that *Shigella* invaded the HeLa cells (Figure 1 B1). These results show that the human *Shigella* strain ZD02 is both invasive and virulent.

Chicken infected with the *Shigella* strain ZD02

In the intraperitoneal injection group, the chickens huddled together post-infection and demonstrated clinical signs including severe depression, weakness, somnolence, droopy wings, retracted heads, ruffled feathers, loss of appetite, and standing still with eyes closed at 6 h as well as diarrhea and pasting of vent feathers at 12 h (Figure S1 and Figure 2). Deaths occurred in subgroups I, II, and III at 48–96 h post-infection. There were not deaths in subgroups IV and V, or rather only depression and hypersomnia were observed. An additional file shows this in detail (Table S2). On postmortem examination, findings in chickens of the intraperitoneal injection group included: degeneration and yellow color of the liver; hemorrhage within the heart, lung, and spleen; intestinal edema; and fluid and gas accumulation within the cecum. The bacteria could be isolated from organs of dead chickens and stool or cloaca of infected chickens. The significant clinical signs and death weren't observed, and the bacteria could not be isolated from stool or cloaca in the crop injection groups. Clinical manifestations and dissection findings in the controls were normal. The LD_{50} of *Shigella* infection via intraperitoneal injection in the three-day-old chickens was 1.19×10^8 CFU.

Histopathology of SPF chickens infected with the *Shigella* strain ZD02 via ligated intestinal loop

One-day-old SPF chickens were infected with *Shigella* strain ZD02 via ligated intestinal loop. Various degrees of intestinal

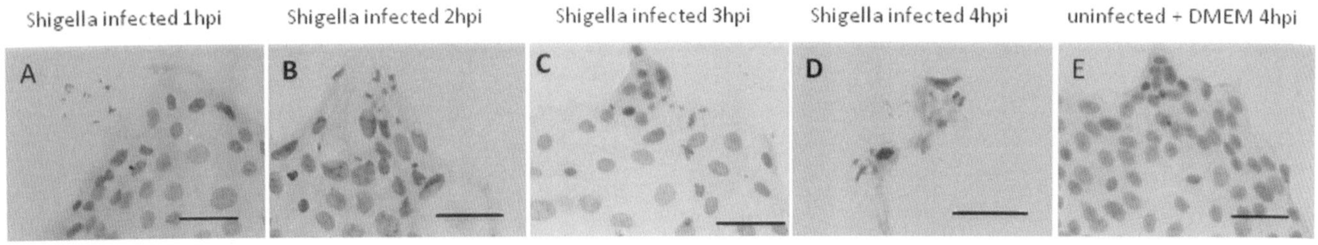

Figure 6. Immunohistochemistry of the primary chicken intestinal epithelial cells infected with the *Shigella* strain ZD02. Uninternalized bacteria (brown staining) were seen near the epithelial cells at 1 h post-inoculation (A). Internalized bacteria (brown staining) were found at 2 h (B) and 3 h (C). The lysed epithelial cells released bacteria (brown staining) at 4 h (D). Uninfected epithelial cells were shown as control (E). Scale bars = 20 μm.

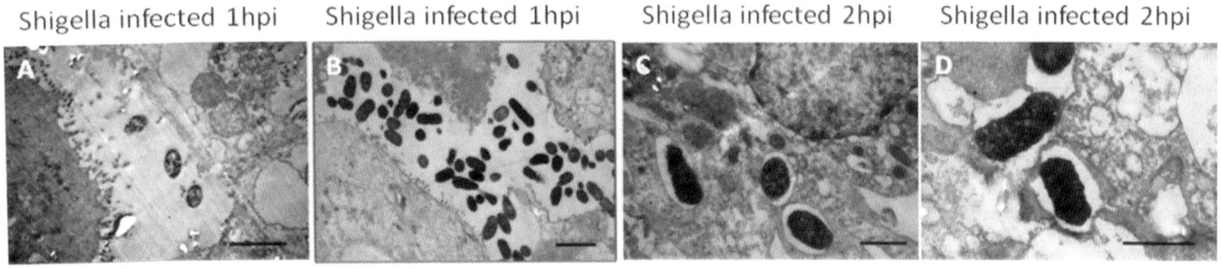

Figure 7. Transmission electron microscopy of the primary chicken intestinal epithelial cells infected with the *Shigella* strain ZD02. Uninternalized bacteria were seen near the epithelial cells at 1 h post-inoculation (A, B. Scale bars = 2 μm). The internalized bacteria were encapsulated with phagosome-like membranes (C, D. Scale bars = 1 μm).

hemorrhage and edema were noted in the infected chickens (Figure S2). At 12 h post-inoculation, severe congestion and edema were seen in the jejunum and ileum accompanied by neutrophil infiltration (Figure 3B, 3C). Neutrophil infiltration and mild congestion was seen in the duodenum as well (Figure 3A), while the cecum and rectum displayed only mild congestion (Figure 3D, 3E). Red blood cells, necrotic epithelial cells, cell debris, and protein-like materials were found in the intestinal cavity. No anomalies were found in the control chickens.

Invasiveness of the *Shigella* strain ZD02 within the chicken intestine

Immunohistochemistry studies of the chicken intestines infected with *Shigella* strain ZD02 via the ligated intestinal loop showed that the bacteria were not internalized within the epithelial cells of the jejunum and ileum at 2 h post-inoculation; nevertheless, it was noticed at 6–8 h (Figure 4A, 4B). Detached intestinal villi, necrotic epithelial cells, and released *Shigella* cells were noted at 12 h (Figure 4C). No internalized bacterial cells were noticed in the epithelial cells of the duodenum, cecum, or rectum. Electron microscopy showed that *Shigella* attached to the surfaces of the intestinal epithelial cells 2 h post-inoculation (Figure 5A), while internalized bacteria were found at 6 and 8 h (Figure 5B, 5C). Intestinal epithelial cells had lysed at 12 h and released the bacteria (Figure 5D). Only epithelial cells in the jejunum and ileum had internalized bacteria.

Invasiveness of the *Shigella* strain ZD02 in primary chicken intestinal epithelial cells

Primary chicken intestinal epithelial cells infected with the *Shigella* strain ZD02 were examined using immunohistochemistry, TEM, and SEM. The immunohistochemistry study showed that *Shigella* could invade the chicken epithelial cells as early as 2–3 h post-infection (Figure 6B, 6C) and the infected cells started to lyse and release the bacteria at 4 h (Figure 6D). The number of invading *Shigella* increased with infection time and the invasive rate reached up to 11.2±0.43% at 4 h. TEM showed that internalized bacteria within the chicken epithelial cells at 2 h were encapsulated by phagosome-like membranes (Figure 7C, 7D). SEM showed that the bacteria attached to the epithelial cell surfaces at 1 h (Figure 8A, 8B) and started becoming internalized the epithelial cells at 2 h (Figure 8C).

Discussion

Shigella is a pathogen with constrained hosts. However, its host range has showed to expand in recent years. The pathogenesis of *Shigella* is attributed to the organism's ability to invade, replicate and spread intercellularly within the colonic epithelium. Virulent *Shigella* can invade intestinal epithelial cells, causing dysentery and other intestinal clinical signs in hosts [18]. *Shigella* virulence can be usually assessed using the Sereny test [12], HeLa cell invasiveness test [14], and Congo red binding assay [19]. This study has demonstrated the virulence of the human *Shigella* strain ZD02 using the Sereny test and the HeLa cell invasiveness test.

Given that *Shigella* is tissue specific organism which always invade large intestine, we have ever infected chicken with *Shigella* strain ZD02 via the intrarectal route. Immunohistochemistry and electron microscopy showed that there wasn't any internalized bacterium in large intestine. The inoculation of *Shigella* in SPF chickens via intraperitoneal injection caused severe clinical signs and even death, suggesting that *Shigella* is pathogenic in chickens. In contrast, the inoculation of *Shigella* via crop injection caused depression merely. We speculate that *Shigella* can't reach the

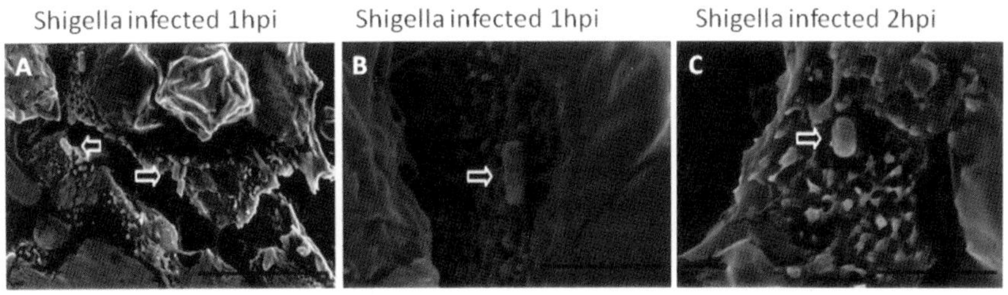

Figure 8. Scanning electron microscopy of the primary chicken intestinal epithelial cells infected with the *Shigella* strain ZD02. Uninternalized bacteria (arrowhead) were seen near the epithelial cells 1 h post-inoculation (A. Scale bar = 10 μm). Bacteria (arrowheads) attached to the surfaces of the epithelial cells at 1 h (B. Scale bar = 3 μm). Bacteria (arrowheads) were being internalized by the epithelial cells at 2 h (C. Scale bar = 3 μm).

intestines of chickens with normal immune function via crop injection "safely", therefore, no significant clinical signs were induced in this group. However, the specific mechanisms require further study.

Shigella can invade human epithelial cells, proliferate, and then spread, which is the critical process of its pathogenicity and the mechanism for its virulence [18]. Complex interactions are involved in the invasion of *Shigella* into the intestinal barrier, such as activating some signaling pathways to interrupt target cells, which plays an important role in its pathogenesis [20–22]. Therefore, the SPF chicken intestine and primary chicken epithelial cells were infected with *Shigella* strain ZD02 to investigate its invasiveness.

Multiple animal models of shigellosis have been established. Rabbani et al [23] infected the rabbit intestine *with Shigella* using the ligated ileal loop assay and found that it caused inflammation within the colon. Fernandez et al [24] established a mouse model of shigellosis by orally infecting four-day-old mice with *Shigella* and found similar pathological changes to those of human bacterial dysentery and inflammation. Martino et al [25] provided a streptomycin-treated murine model in which *Shigella* are able to reach their natural tissue target: colon. Shim et al [26] established a guinea pig model by inoculating *S. flexneri* 2α or 5α in the rectum. Jeong et al [27] established a piglet model of acute gastroenteritis with *Shigella* type I and found that piglets are highly sensitive to *Shigella* and demonstrate clinical signs such as acute diarrhea, anorexia, and dehydration. Barman et al [28] established a shigellosis in the guinea-pig model infected with *Shigella dysenteriae* into the cecocolic junction after ligation of the distal cecum without any preparatory treatment, which induced acute inflammation. Yang et al [29] established an adult mice model of Shigellosis by intraperitoneal infection. This study was the first to demonstrate that *Shigella* strain ZD02 can invade epithelial cells in the jejunum and ileum of one-day-old SPF chickens via ligated intestinal loop inoculation and cause severe congestion and edema. Therefore, *Shigella* can cause intestinal damage and disease after it invades the jejunum and ileum of chickens in some cases.

To further investigate the invasiveness of *Shigella* isolated from human in chickens, we infected isolated primary chicken epithelial cells with the strain ZD02. These cells became contaminated with fibroblastic cells and could not reach 100% confluence in 48-well plates. In addition, infected cell morphology was inconsistent among different wells. Therefore, the classical Gentamicin protection assay could not be used to determine the invasion rate of *Shigella* isolated from human within chicken intestinal epithelial cells. Instead, we used immunohistochemistry to determine the invasiveness of the strain ZD02 into cells and calculated the invasion rates. The results showed that *Shigella* isolated from human can invade the chicken intestinal epithelial cells. The invasion rate increased with infection time and reached 11.2±0.43% at 4 h post-inoculation, confirming the invasive capacity of *Shigella* in chicken intestinal epithelial cells.

Shigella is transmitted primarily via the fecal-oral route. This study showed that *Shigella* is pathogenic in chickens and invasive in chicken intestinal epithelial cells. However, *Shigella* could induce depression but didn't cause intestinal clinical signs such as diarrhea and blood dysentery via crop injection. We found that *Shigella* was less pathogenic in chickens via natural infection route than that in human because *Shigella* has difficulty in invading the chicken intestinal barrier and escaping immune clearance. *Shigella* can circumvent a host's innate immune system via versatile pathogenic mechanisms [18]. Similarly, adult mice are resistant to oral *Shigella* infection. However, intraperitoneal challenge with virulent *S. flexneri* 2a resulted in diarrhea and severe body weight loss in adult B6 mice. The bacteria could invade and colonize not only systemic tissues but also the serosa and lamina propria region of the large intestine [29]. *Shigella* in the peritoneal cavity which was injected into SPF chickens via intraperitoneal route attached and colonized in the serosa and muscle layer of the chicken intestine and entered the lamina propria region successfully, then caused death and other clinical symptoms. So, the intraperitoneal route may be also a promising entry site for *Shigella* which results in shigellosis–like symptoms in SPF chicken. Endogenous flora could protect the intestinal tissue from *Shigella* infection, so adult mice are resistant to oral *Shigella* infection. However, treatment of adult mice with streptomycin is a prerequisite for colonization of the intestinal tract by *Shigella*. The colon and eventually the cecum of the streptomycin-treated adult mice were the main targets for the invasion of *Shigella* [25]. Antibiotic usage is known to be rampant in the poultry industry which may cause enteric dysbacteriosis. We speculated that *Shigella* can cause disease if it invades the chicken intestines in the presence of immune suppression or enteric dysbacteriosis. Such cases usually happen in poultry production. In fact, this might be the reason for the occurrence of clinical chicken shigellosis in China.

Microbes have adapted many fascinating strategies to co-evolve with their hosts. There is a constant molecular interplay between host factors and invading pathogens. The microbes can obtain a range of host factors by horizontal gene transfer or rearrangement [30,31] as well as loss or deactivation of unimportant or even deleterious genes [32] to escape immune clearance, or even adapt [33] by switch [30] or jump [34,35] within a new host. We have ever tried to identify the origin of *Shigella* isolated from chicken by comparing the sequences of eight housekeeping genes (*thrB/thrC, trpC/trpB, purM/purN, mdh/argR*) between *Shigella* isolated from human and chicken previously. The results showed that *Shigella* isolated from human or chicken is highly homogeneous without uncertain evolutionary evidence [10].

We have previously detected the expression of receptors CD44 and α5β1 in chicken intestinal epithelial cells, which can serve as the basis for the invasion of intestinal epithelial cells and *Shigella* pathogenesis [36,37,38]. A variety of factors, such as human intervention, the stress-inducing breeding environment, co-infection of pathogens, and immune dysfunction, may confer the *Shigella* with invasiveness and pathogenicity within chickens without the apparent need for host-adapting evolution, resulting in human–poultry cross-infection.

In conclusion, *Shigella* can invade chicken intestinal epithelial cells in vitro and chicken intestinal mucosa in vivo. Meanwhile, receptors required for the entry of *Shigella* are detected in chicken intestinal epithelial cells [38]. Consequently, it is possible for *Shigella* to infect or even kill chickens under certain condition. The findings suggest that *Shigella* isolated from human or chicken have highly similar pathogenicity as well as the possibility of human–poultry cross-infection, which is of public health significance.

Supporting Information

Figure S1 The symptoms of SPF chickens infected with the *Shigella* strain ZD02 via intraperitoneal injection. The chickens showed depression (A), dysentery and pasting vent (B).

Figure S2 Gross pathology of the SPF chicken intestines infected with the *Shigella* strain ZD02 at 12 h post-inoculation. The intestine of chicken infected with *Shigella* ZD02 showed severe congestion and edema (upper panel). No significant pathological changes were noted in the uninfected controls (lower panel).

Table S1 Detailed information of chicken infected with *Shigella* strain ZD02 via intraperitoneal or crop injection.

Table S2 Detailed incidence and mortality of three-day-old SPF chickens infected with the *Shigella* strain ZD02 via intraperitoneal injection. The LD_{50} of *Shigella* infection via intraperitoneal injection in the three-day-old chickens was 1.19×10^{8} CFU using the Reed-Muench method.

Acknowledgments

We would like to thank Dr. Xuefang Liu (Research and test center, Henan University of Traditional Chinese Medicine) for the sample preparation and observation of electron microscopy. We are grateful to the animal care staff at Henan Agricultural University for their assistance in animal care and sample collection.

Author Contributions

Conceived and designed the experiments: LC. Performed the experiments: RS XY. Analyzed the data: RS XY. Contributed reagents/materials/analysis tools: RS XY. Wrote the paper: LC. Review the manuscript: RS XY LC HTC HYL JZ XWW CQW.

References

1. Kotloff KL, Winickoff JP, Ivanoff B, Clemens JD, Swerdlow DL, et al. (1999) Global burden of *Shigella* infections: implications for vaccine development and implementation of control strategies. B World Health Organ 77: 651–666.
2. Bardhan P, Faruque ASG, Naheed A, Sack DA (2010) Decreasing Shigellosis-related Deaths without *Shigella spp.*-specific Interventions, Asia. Emerg Infect Dis 16: 1718–1723.
3. Pan BJ, Wang WL, Xie YP, Wei ML, Luo ZF, et al. (2006) Detection, serology classification and drug susceptibility of *Shigella* from experimental monkeys. Guangxi Agri Sci 37: 331–332.
4. Jiang JJ, Wang PY, Pan GQ, Kang LC (2005) Isolation and Identification of Rabbits *Shigella* Dysenteriae in a Large Scale Warren. J Anhui Agri Sci 33: 1666–1667.
5. Priamukhima NS, Kilesso VA, Tikhomirov ED (1984) Animal carriers of *Shigella* and their possible epidemiological importance. Zh Mikrobiol Epidemiol Immunobiol 11:20–24.
6. Mattrelli AT, Routh PR, Dillman RC (1998) *Shigella* infection as observed in the experimentally inoculated domestic pig, *Sus scrofa domestica*.Microb Pathogenesis 25:189–196.
7. Xu LJ, Wang CQ, Hu GZ, Kang XT, Ren J, et al. (2004) Discovery on shigellosis of flock in china and studies on the pathogenic specialty. Chin J Prev Vet Med 26: 281–286.
8. Xu LJ, Wang CQ, Ma SF, Xue S, Zhao YL, et al. (2005) Serum Epidemiology Survey on *Shigella* Infection in the chicken. Chin J Vet Sci 25: 594–596.
9. Xu LJ, Zang WM, Kang XT, Hu GZ, Wang CQ, et al. (2004) Pathogen Identification of Shigellosis of Flock. Acta Veterinaria et Zootechnica Sinica 35: 362–366.
10. Yang X, Chen L, Xu LJ, Liu HY, Chang HT, et al. (2009) Molecular Identification and Evolvement Analysis of *Shigella boydii* strain hn03 Isolated from Chicken. Acta Veterinaria et Zootechnica Sinica 40: 402–408.
11. Shi R, Liu HY, Chen L, Yang X, Lv WQ, et al. (2013) Invasive Characteristics of Human Source S. flexneri on chicken Intestinal epithelial cells. Acta Veterinaria et Zootechnica Sinica 44: 95–101.
12. Murayama SY, Sakai T, Makino S, Kurata T, Sasakawa C, et al. (1986) The Use of Mice in the Sereny Test as a Virulence Assay of *Shigellae* and *Enteroinvasive Escherichia-Coli*. Infect Immun 51: 696–698.
13. Franco NH, Correia-Neves M, Olsson IAS (2012) How "Humane" Is Your Endpoint?-Refining the Science-Driven Approach for Termination of Animal Studies of Chronic Infection. PLoS Pathog 8(1): e1002399. doi:10.1371/journal.ppat.1002399
14. Niesel DW, Chambers CE, Stockman SL (1985) Quantitation of HeLa cell monolayer invasion by *Shigella* and Salmonella species. J Clin Microbial 22: 897–902.
15. Ingersoll MA, Moss JE, Weinrauch Y, Fisher PE, Groisman EA, et al. (2003) The ShiA protein encoded by the *Shigella* flexneri SHI-2 pathogenicity island attenuates inflammation. Cell Microbiol 5:797–807.
16. Athman R, Fernandez MI, Gounon P, Sansonetti PJ, Louvard D, et al. (2005) *Shigella* flexneri infection is dependent on villin in the mouse intestine and in primary cultures of intestinal epithelial cells. Cell Microbiol 7: 1109–1116.
17. Mounier J, Vasselon T, Hellio R, Lesourd M, Sansonetti PJ (1992) *Shigella* flexneri Enters Human Colonic Caco-2 Epithelial Cells through the Basolateral Pole. Infect Immun 60: 237–248.
18. Ashida H, Ogawa M, Mimuro H, Kobayashi T, Sanada T, et al. (2011) *Shigella* are versatile mucosal pathogens that circumvent the host innate immune system. Curr Opin Immunol 23:448–455.
19. Prakash R, Bharathi Raja S, Devaraj H, Devaraj SN (2011) Up-Regulation of MUC2 and IL-1b Expression in Human Colonic Epithelial Cells by *Shigella* and Its Interaction with Mucins. PLoS One 6: e27046. doi: 10.1371/journal.pone.0027046
20. Tran Van NG, Bourdet-Sicard R, Duménil G, Blocker A, Sansonetti PJ (2000) Bacterial signals and cell responses during *Shigella* entry into epithelial cells. Cell Microbiol 2: 187–193.
21. Ogawa M, Handa Y, Ashida H, Suzuki M, Sasakawa C (2008) The versatility of *Shigella* effectors. Nature 6: 11–16.
22. Rudel T (2012) To die or not to die: *Shigella* has an answer. Cell Host Microbe 11: 219–221.
23. Rabbani GH, Albert MJ, Rahman H, Islam M, Mahalanabis D, et al. (1995) Development of an improved animal model of Shigellosis in the adult rabbit by colonic infection with *Shigella* flexneri 2a. Infect Immun 63: 4350–4357.
24. Fernandez MI, Thuizat A, Pedron T, Neutra M, Phalipon A, et al. (2003) A newborn mouse model for the study of intestinal pathogenesis of shigellosis. Cell Microbiol 5: 481–491.
25. Martino MC, Rossi G, Martini I, Tattoli I, Chiavolini D, et al. (2005)Mucosal Lymphoid Infiltrate Dominates Colonic Pathological Changes in Murine Experiment Shigellosis. J Infect Dis 192:136–148.
26. Shim DH, Suzuki T, Chang SY, Park SM, Sansonetti PJ, et al. (2007) New animal model of Shigellosis in the guinea pig:its usefulness for protective efficacy studies. J Immunol 178: 2476–2482.
27. Jeong K, Zhang QS, Nunnari J, Nunnari J, Tzipori S (2010) A Piglet Model of Acute Gastroenteritis Induced by *Shigella* dysenteriae Type 1. J Infect Dis 201: 903–911.
28. Barman S, Saha DR, Ramamurthy T, Hemanta K (2011) Development of a new guinea-pig model of shigellosis. FEMS Immunol Med Mic 62: 304–314.
29. Yang JY, Lee SN, Chang SY, Ko HJ, Ryu S, et al. (2013) A Mouse Model of Shigellosis by Intraperitoneal Infection. J Infect Dis 209: 203–215.
30. Streicker DG, Altizera SM, Andrés VV, Rupprecht CE (2012) Variable evolutionary routes to host establishment across repeated rabies virus host shifts among bats. Proc Natl Acad Sci USA 109:19715–19720.
31. Kisiela DI, Chattopadhyay S, Libby SJ, Karlinsey JE, Fang FC, et al. (2012) Evolution of Salmonella enterica Virulence via Point Mutations in the Fimbrial Adhesin. PLoS Pathog 8: e1002733. doi:10.1371/journal.ppat.1002733
32. Delaney NF, Balenger S, Bonneaud C, Marx CJ, Hill GE, et al. (2012) Ultrafast Evolution and Loss of CRISPRs Following a Host Shift in a Novel Wildlife Pathogen, Mycoplasma gallisepticum. PLoS Genet 8: e1002511. doi:10.1371/journal.pgen.1002511
33. Toft C, Andersson SG (2010) Evolutionary microbial genomics: insights into bacterial host adaptation. Nat Rev Genet 11:465–475.
34. Bethan VL, Caitriona MG, Nouri LB, Zakoura LA, Weinertb ACM, et al.(2009)Recent human-to-poultry host jump, adaptation, and pandemic spread of Staphylococcus aureus. Proc Natl Acad Sci USA 106: 19545–19550.
35. Eppinger M, Baar C, Linz B, Raddatz G, Lanz C, et al. (2006) Who ate whom? Adaptive Helicobacter genomic changes that accompanied a host jump from early humans to large felines. PLoS Genet 2: e120. doi: 10.1371/journal.pgen.0020120
36. Lafont F, Tran Van NG, Hanada K, Sansonetti P, van der Goot FG (2002) Initial steps of *Shigella* infection depend on the cholesterol/sphingolipid raft-mediated CD44-IpaB interaction. EMBO J 21: 4449–4457.
37. Watarai M, Funato S, Sasakawa C (1996) Interaction of Ipa proteins of *Shigella* flexneri with alpha5beta1 integrin promotes entry of the bacteria into mammalian cells. J Exp Med 183:991–999.
38. Lv WQ, Shi R, Chen L, Zhang JL, Yang X, et al. (2013) Identification and temporal and spatial expression characteristic of CD44 in chicken intestine. Clin J Vet Sci 33: 53–63.

2

The Value of Body Weight Measurement to Assess Dehydration in Children

Isabelle Pruvost[1,3], François Dubos[1,2,3], Emmanuel Chazard[4], Valérie Hue[3], Alain Duhamel[1,2,4], Alain Martinot[1,2,3]*

1 Univ Lille Nord de France, UDSL, Lille, France, 2 EA2694, Public Health, Epidemiology and Quality of Care, Lille, France, 3 Paediatric Emergency and Infectious Diseases Unit, CHU Lille, Lille, France, 4 Department of Biostatistics, CHU Lille, Lille, France

Abstract

Dehydration secondary to gastroenteritis is one of the most common reasons for office visits and hospital admissions. The indicator most commonly used to estimate dehydration status is acute weight loss. Post-illness weight gain is considered as the gold-standard to determine the true level of dehydration and is widely used to estimate weight loss in research. To determine the value of post-illness weight gain as a gold standard for acute dehydration, we conducted a prospective cohort study in which 293 children, aged 1 month to 2 years, with acute diarrhea were followed for 7 days during a 3-year period. The main outcome measures were an accurate pre-illness weight (if available within 8 days before the diarrhea), post-illness weight, and theoretical weight (predicted from the child's individual growth chart). Post-illness weight was measured for 231 (79%) and both theoretical and post-illness weights were obtained for 111 (39%). Only 62 (21%) had an accurate pre-illness weight. The correlation between post-illness and theoretical weight was excellent (0.978), but bootstrapped linear regression analysis showed that post-illness weight underestimated theoretical weight by 0.48 kg (95% CI: 0.06–0.79, $p<0.02$). The mean difference in the fluid deficit calculated was 4.0% of body weight (95% CI: 3.2–4.7, $p<0.0001$). Theoretical weight overestimated accurate pre-illness weight by 0.21 kg (95% CI: 0.08–0.34, $p=0.002$). Post-illness weight underestimated pre-illness weight by 0.19 kg (95% CI: 0.03–0.36, $p=0.02$). The prevalence of 5% dehydration according to post-illness weight (21%) was significantly lower than the prevalence estimated by either theoretical weight (60%) or clinical assessment (66%, $p<0.0001$).These data suggest that post-illness weight is of little value as a gold standard to determine the true level of dehydration. The performance of dehydration signs or scales determined by using post-illness weight as a gold standard has to be reconsidered.

Editor: Lynette Kay Rogers, The Ohio State Unversity, United States of America

Funding: The study was supported by grants from Sanofi-Pasteur MSD pharmaceuticals, France. The funders had no role in study design, data collection and analysis, decision to publish, or preparation of the manuscript.

Competing Interests: The authors received funding from a commercial source (Sanofi-Pasteur MSD pharmaceuticals, France).

* E-mail: alain.martinot@chru-lille.fr

Introduction

Dehydration secondary to gastroenteritis is one of the most common reasons for office visits and hospital admissions in developed countries [1–3]. Among European children <3 years of age, incidence of diarrhea ranges from 0.5 to 1.9 episodes per child per year [4]. The management of acute diarrhea in children is largely based on clinical examination which allows assessment of hydration status. Underestimation of dehydration increases morbidity and mortality, while overestimation can result in inappropriate care and public expenditure. Dehydration is difficult to diagnose clinically [5]. Combinations of examination signs perform markedly better than any individual sign in predicting dehydration [6]. Many scores have been developed to estimate dehydration, but only one, the Clinical Dehydration Scale, has been validated to predict a longer length of Emergency Department (ED) stay and the need for intravenous fluid rehydration [7].

The development and validation of a dehydration scale requires the use of a gold standard. Weight loss is considered as the reference to diagnose dehydration in clinical practice and research [6]. Because the child's pre-illness weight is rarely known in the acute care setting, post-illness weight gain is widely used to estimate weight loss in research [5–13]. A systematic review found that the difference between post-illness (rehydration) weight and acute weight divided by post-illness weight was the best available gold standard to assess the percentage of volume lost [5]. This conclusion, however, was based on only one study, which demonstrated an excellent correlation between pre- and post-illness weight in only 19 children (for 17 of whom pre-illness weight was predicted from growth charts; only 2 had an accurate pre-illness weight) [6]. Other studies that subsequently applied this gold standard have not challenged its correlation with the theoretical weight determined from the growth charts. Moreover, the precise day used as the reference to determine stable post-illness weight was not validated and differed between studies [6–10].

The aim of this study was to estimate the value of post-illness weight gain prospectively as a gold standard for acute weight loss in a larger population. Additionally, we sought to study the concordance of the evaluation of 5% dehydration by post-illness weight (gold standard), "theoretical" weight, pre-illness weight, and clinical assessment.

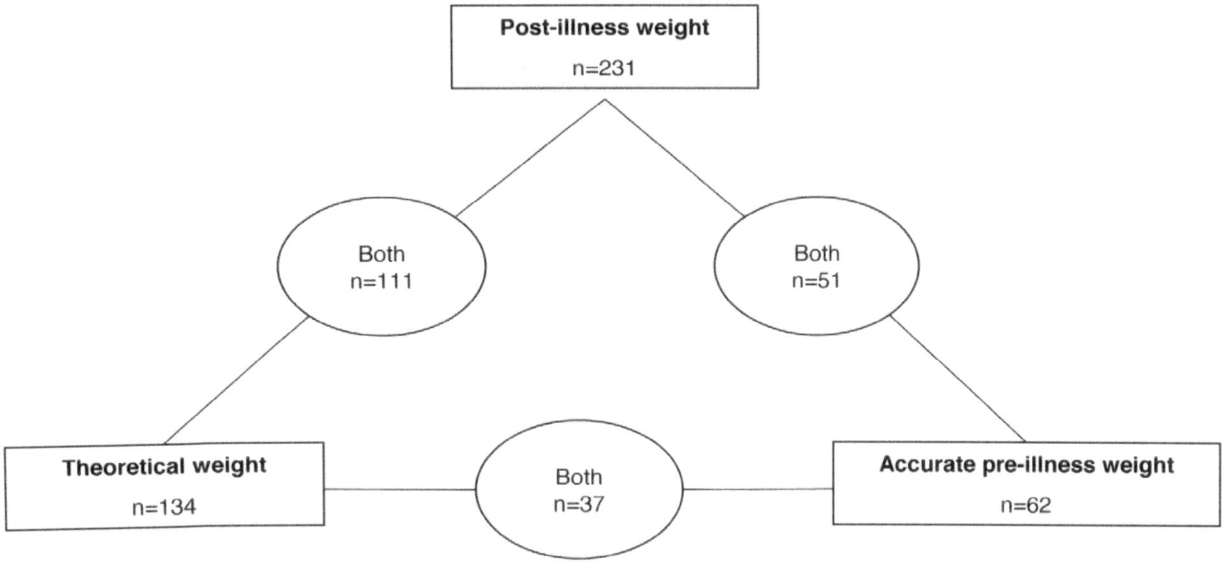

Figure 1. Distribution of children with acute diarrhea by available methods of measure of the weight (n = 293). Pre-illness weight: measured within 8 days before the ED visit. **Theoretical weight**: predicted from the child's individual growth chart. **Post-illness weight**: the first weight when two consecutive daily weight measurements differed by <1%, after diarrhea and vomiting had disappeared.

Methods

Ethics

The study protocol was approved by the French National Data Protection Authority (Commission Nationale Informatique et Libertés, CNIL) and the French National Institutional Review Board (Comité consultatif sur le traitement de l'information en matière de recherche dans le domaine de la santé, CCTIRS). Parents provided written informed consent before enrolment.

Study Population

This work was a prospective, observational, cohort study conducted from December 2005 through June 2009 at a tertiary care pediatric ED of a French university hospital with approximately 25,000 annual visits and 4,300 short-stay hospitalizations. This study followed all "STrengthening the Reporting of OBservational studies in Epidemiology" statements [14].

Children aged 1 to 24 months admitted to the ED with a chief complaint of acute diarrhea during the study period, whose parents agreed to study participation and to daily weight surveillance for 7 days following the ED visit, were included. For convenience reasons, recruitment took place during weekday working hours (8 am to 6 pm), to limit the number of investigators. Exclusion criteria were those concerning children with a fluid balance that could be modified by an underlying condition: a chronic disease (cardiac, gastrointestinal, or renal, diabetes mellitus, congenital adrenal hyperplasia, or cystic fibrosis), malnutrition or failure to thrive, and an ileostomy. We also excluded children living more than 30 kilometres away from the hospital, because of our inability to deliver an electronic scale to the home. Children were then treated by the ED staff, regardless of their participation in the study.

Definitions

Acute diarrhea was defined, ***according to the European Society of Pediatric Gastroenterology and Nutrition guidelines, as illness that started*** <7 days before admission and involved ≥3 soft and/or liquid stools within 24 hours [4]. To be considered accurate, pre-illness weight was defined as a weight of a baby undressed and without diapers, measured within 8 days before the ED visit and before any digestive complaint. No standardization was required for this weight [6].

Theoretical weight was defined as the non-sick baseline weight predicted on the date of the ED visit by extrapolation from the child's individual growth chart when available (part of French child health passports, which are portable paper records). This extrapolation was considered acceptable when at least three weight points were plotted over time to construct a growth curve and when that curve did not cross percentile lines (to detect any alterations from physiologic growth) [6]. Triage nurses weighed babies, undressed and without diapers, on an electronic scale (SECA, Germany, model 3767021094). This weight was defined as the admission weight. Post-illness weight was defined as the first weight with less than 1% of differences between two consecutive daily weight measurements, after diarrhea and vomiting had disappeared. Dehydration was defined as a fluid deficit of 5% or greater. It was calculated as (post-illness weight – admission weight)/(post-illness weight) x 100 for the "gold standard" method, or as (theoretical weight – admission weight)/(theoretical weight) x 100 or (pre-illness weight – admission weight)/(pre-illness weight) x 100. The presence of moderate or severe dehydration was also estimated by the physician, based on clinical assessment of the different signs of dehydration.

At the time of discharge from the ED, all included patients, whether admitted to the hospital or discharged home, were enrolled for a follow-up visit. Naked body weight was measured by parents on same regularly calibrated scale as at admission, and children were weighed daily at home in the morning on a similarly calibrated electronic scale, before the first meal, for seven days in a row. These weights were recorded daily on a questionnaire with the last day of diarrhea or vomiting.

Data Analysis

Data were entered into Epi-Data 2.1b software with check-in controls (Epidata Association, Odense, Denmark). Results were expressed as means, medians, and either standard deviations (SD)

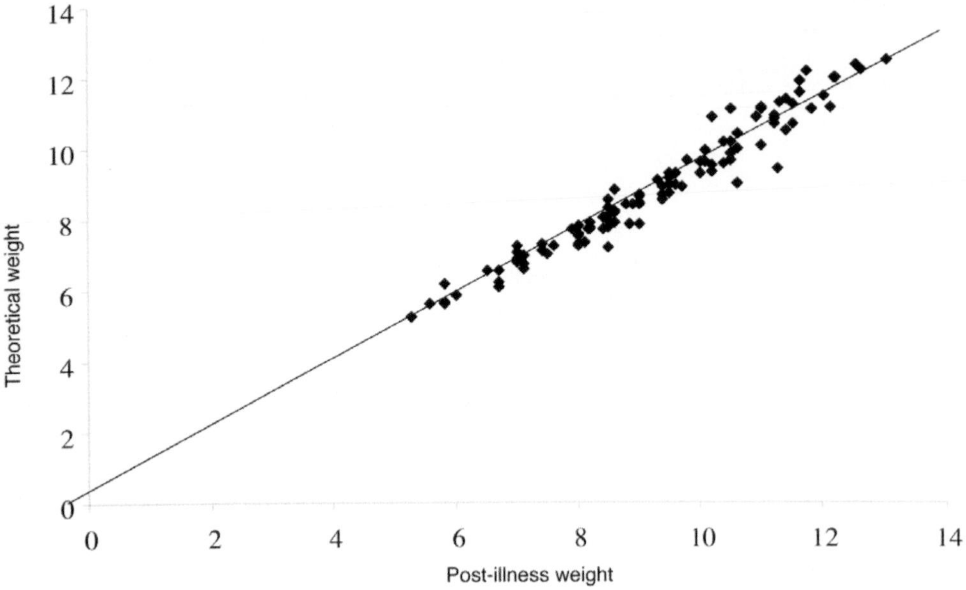

Figure 2. Correlation between theoreti cal and post-illness weight, assessed by Pearson Correlation (n = 111). Postillness weight = 0.978 x Theoretical weight ($p<10^{-6}$).

or interquartile ranges according to their distribution for continuous variables, and frequencies and percentages for categorical variables. The 95% confidence intervals (CIs) were calculated. The relationship between theoretical and post-illness weights was assessed by the Pearson correlation coefficient. A linear regression was performed to explain theoretical weight by post-illness weight. The CIs for the intercept and the regression coefficient were determined with the bootstrap method [15]. This method provides robust estimates for CIs without making any assumptions about the distribution of the characteristics. As a high correlation does not automatically imply that there is a good agreement between two methods, the agreement between these two weights was evaluated by Bland-Altman plots [16].

The correlation between the accurate pre-illness weight and each of the theoretical and the post-illness weights were investigated with a linear regression analysis and the intraclass correlation coefficient. These different weights were compared with a paired student's t-test and a linear regression analysis. All statistical analyses were performed with SAS software (SAS Institute, Cary, NC). A p value less than 0.05 was considered statistically significant.

Results

Patient Characteristics

A total of 293 children (median age: 12 months, mean: 11.5±6.2 SD, 57% boys) were included in the study for follow-up. Of those, 14% (n = 40) were admitted to the hospital, 30% (n = 88) stayed for a few hours in the observation unit for intravenous rehydration and 56% (n = 165) were directly discharged home from the ED. The median duration of diarrhea before admission was 3 days (IQR: 1–4), and 91% (n = 266) of the patients had vomiting. The mean weight at admission was 9.0 kg ±2.1 SD, 61% (n = 179) of the patients had a central temperature >38°C at home and 27% (n = 79) had no previous medical visit for this episode of diarrhea before admission.

Figure 1 describes the different subgroups based on available weight measurements. Of the 293 patients, 21% (n = 62) had been weighed within 8 days before the ED visit, before any digestive complaint. Theoretical weight could be measured for only 46% (n = 134) of the patients, because 41% (n = 119) of patients had been brought to the ED without child health passports, and 14% (n = 40) did not have valid growth charts to determine the theoretical weight as defined in the methods. Post-illness weight was measured for 79% (n = 231) of patients; 20% (n = 58) were excluded from the analysis, either because they did not return the weight questionnaire or were not weighed for 7 consecutive days, and 1% (n = 4) because they did not reach a stable weight within 8 days of ED visit.

Value of the Post-illness Weight Gain as a Gold Standard for Estimating Acute Weight Loss and Identifying Dehydration

Both post-illness and theoretical weights were obtained for 111 children (Figure 1). The mean age of this subgroup was 11.7 months ±5.9 SD, (median = 13.0). The correlation between post-illness and theoretical weight was excellent, with a Pearson correlation coefficient of 0.978 (Figure 2). The statistical assessment of concordance between these two weights measured by the intraclass correlation coefficient was also excellent (0.963). A linear regression analysis, to explain the theoretical weight by the post-illness weight was performed. With this method, the regression coefficient determined with the bootstrap method was 0.99 (95% CI: 0.95–1.04) and post-illness weight underestimated theoretical weight by 0.48 kg (95% CI: 0.06–0.79, p<0.02). Figure 3 shows the agreement between these two weights analyzed with a Bland-Altman plot that showed a pretty scattered distribution. Mean theoretical weight was 9.26 kg ±1.91 SD, while the mean post-illness weight was 8.88 kg ±1.87 SD. The mean difference between these two weights was 0.38 kg (95% CI: 0.30–0.45, p<0.0001). The mean difference between the fluid deficit calculated from the theoretical weight and that based on post-illness weight was 4.0% of body weight (95% CI: 3.2–4.7%, p<0.0001).

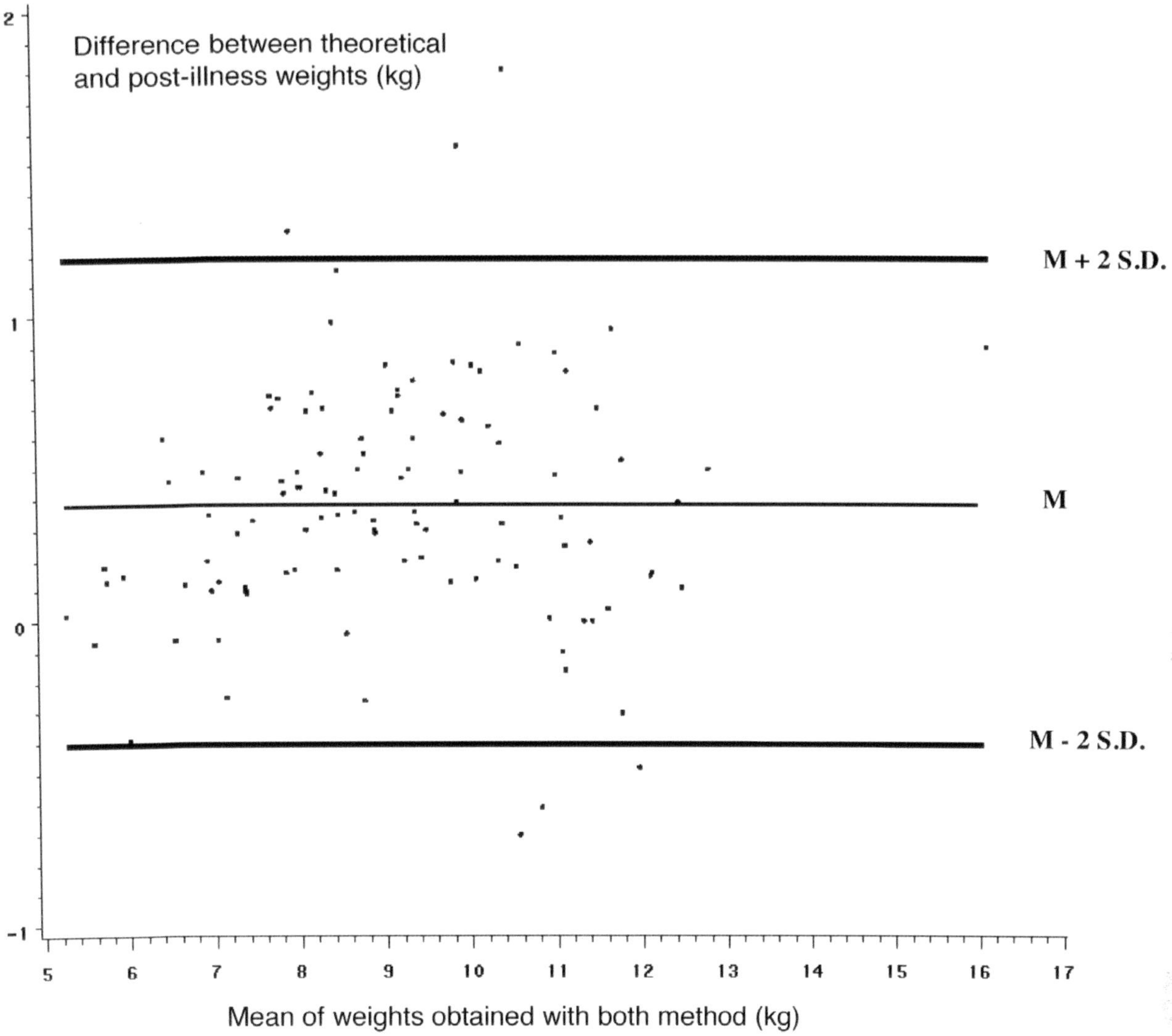

Figure 3. Agreement between theoretical and post-illness weight, analysed with a Bland-Altman plot, n = 111. M: mean, SD: Standard Deviation. Mean difference, which is the best guess as to the "correct" result. 95% limits of agreement. When the agreement between two measures is high, the mean difference between these two measures is close to 0. The 95% limits of agreement permit visual judgement of how well two methods of measurement agree. The smaller the range between these two limits the better the agreement is.

The prevalence of 5% dehydration determined by post-illness weight was 21% versus 60% by theoretical weight ($p<0.001$). The prevalence of moderate or severe dehydration by clinical assessment was 66%, also significantly different from the prevalence determined by post-illness weight ($p<0.001$).

Value of the Accurate Pre-illness Weight

Both post-illness and accurate pre-illness weights were obtained for 51 children (17%) (Figure 1) who did not differ significantly from others in terms of age (mean: 11.9±6.1 SD vs. 13.4±6.3 SD; $p = 0.1$), post-illness weight (mean: 8.9±1.9 SD vs. 9.1±2.0 SD; $p = 0.4$), and theoretical weight (mean: 9.0±1.9 SD vs. 9.7±2.1 SD; $p = 0.1$). There was an excellent correlation between post-illness and pre-illness weight, with a Pearson correlation coefficient of 0.979 ($p<0.0001$). Post-illness weight underestimated pre-illness weight by 0.19 kg (95% CI: 0.03–0.36, $p = 0.02$).

Both accurate and theoretical pre-illness weights were obtained for only 37 children (13%) (Figure 1). These children did not differ significantly from others in terms of age (mean: 12.0±6.2 SD vs. 13.3±5.8 SD; $p = 0.2$), post-illness weight (mean: 8.8±1.9 SD vs. 9.3±2.2 SD; $p = 0.2$), and theoretical weight (mean: 9.1±1.9 SD vs. 9.5±2.2 SD; $p = 0.3$). There was an excellent correlation between theoretical and accurate pre-illness weight, with a Pearson correlation coefficient of 0.985. Theoretical weight overestimated accurate pre-illness weight by 0.21 kg (95% CI: 0.08–0.34, $p = 0.002$).

Discussion

In our study, post-illness weight gain was not a gold standard for estimating acute weight loss and identifying dehydration in children with acute gastroenteritis. The mean absolute difference between fluid deficit calculated from the theoretical weight and that calculated from the post-illness weight was 4% of body weight (95% CI: 3.2–4.7, $p<0.0001$). As shown by the Bland-Altman plot, the agreement between these two weights was poor and post-illness weight underestimated dehydration. The prevalence of 5% dehydration according to post-illness weight was significantly lower than the prevalence estimated by either theoretical weight or by the physician's clinical assessment.

Gorelick et al. showed an excellent correlation between weight measured after treatment for children with acute gastroenteritis and their pre-illness "well" weight [6]. There was however a small positive intercept of the regression line, which suggests a slight bias towards an underestimation of pre-illness weight by post-illness weight, but without either a statistically significant or a clinically meaningful difference in dehydration between the two methods of measurement (0.67%). The differences between our results and those obtained using this so-called gold standard may stem from the methods used to determine final weight and from the very small number of patients to validate this standard (n = 19) [6]. Our study, which included more than five times more patients (n = 111) and applied the bootstrap method to obtain robust estimations for the confidence intervals, did not confirm that the post-illness weight is an appropriate gold standard for evaluating 5% dehydration in children with acute gastroenteritis. Mackenzie et al. [10] also found that post-illness weight overestimated dehydration by a mean of 3.2%, perhaps because objective clinical signs of dehydration tend to appear when fluid deficit is less than 5%. Underestimation of dehydration by post-illness weight might be due in part to weight loss from catabolism and nutritional loss, not yet offset at the end of diarrhea.

Our method of determining post-illness weight (two consecutive daily weight measurements that differed by <1%, after diarrhea and vomiting had disappeared) resulted in a smaller margin of error than in other studies, where post-treatment weights were considered stable if they agreed to within ±2% at two consecutive but not daily measures [6,11,13]. The precise day used as reference to determine the stable rehydrated weight has not yet been validated and differs between studies [6–10]. Indeed Mackenzie et al. defined post-illness weight as the naked weight at 24 or 48 hours after admission, with no clinical signs of dehydration and biochemical results back to normal [10]. Others weighed patients at follow up visits every 48–72 hours until a "stable weight" was reached. Patients not fully rehydrated within 2 weeks of the ED visit were excluded from the research [13]. Most studies have also used additional assessments to reinforce their choice of a true post-illness weight [5]. For example, Teach et al. [17] used the weight at normalization of examination findings with low urine specific gravity. Incorporating other assessments not based on weight into the gold standard could theoretically bias the results. Steiner et al. showed that varying the date of the final rehydration weight could introduce distortions [5]. For example, if it is obtained too early, children may still be dehydrated or may be overhydrated because of aggressive intravenous fluid administration.

Our study has limitations. Because significant dehydration is uncommon among children with gastroenteritis in industrialized countries, the number of children with dehydration in this study was relatively small and thus led to less precise estimates. However, the use of bootstrap methods limited imprecision. Another limitation was that we did not provide any standardization for "pre-illness weight" because it was measured before inclusion. Weights during well child care are sometimes not naked weight, which could overestimate pre-illness weight. The determination of acute weight loss by the theoretical weight, extrapolated from growth charts, most probably leads to bias, as children's growth is irregular. Overestimation of dehydration by theoretical weight might also be partially due to the relative imprecision of growth charts. Furthermore, theoretical weight could only be measured for 49% of the patients in our study. Finally, the use of body weight to determine the percentage of dehydration might also be criticized: 70% of the body is made of water, and acute weight loss is mainly due to acute water loss. But the same weight loss could over- or underestimates water loss because of variations in the digestive water retention or because the child was weighed before or after passing stool, vomiting, or just after feeding. All of these could produce a difference of up to 100 or 200 g, which represents roughly up to 3% of a 6-kg child.

The current study's findings suggest that post-illness weight gain is not a gold standard in research for estimating acute weight loss and identifying dehydration in children aged 1 to 24 months with acute gastroenteritis. Post-illness weight depends on rehydration and also on nutritional status with large individual variations between these two components. Thus this figure does not permit to estimate fluid loss based on post-illness weight. The results of many previous studies that provided diagnostic value of dehydration signs or scales based on this so-called "post-illness weight" gold standard have to be reconsidered. Future studies should focus on evaluating only children with accurate recent pre-illness weight for research purpose, although its availability (21% of our patients weighed in the 8 days before the ED visit and before any digestive disturbances) and reliability limit its use in current practice.

Author Contributions

Conceived and designed the experiments: IP FD AM. Performed the experiments: IP FD VH AM. Analyzed the data: IP EC AD. Contributed reagents/materials/analysis tools: IP FD AD AM. Wrote the paper: IP FD EC VH AD AM.

References

1. Parashar UD, Hummelman EG, Bresee JS, Miller MA, Glass RI (2003) Global illness and deaths caused by rotavirus disease in children. Emerg Infect Dis 9: 565–72.
2. Soriano-Gabarro M, Mrukowicz J, Vesikari T, Verstraeten T (2006) Burden of rotavirus disease in European Union Countries. Pediatr Infect Dis J 25: S7–S11.
3. Glass RI, Lew JF, Gangarosa RE, LeBaron CW, Ho MS (1991) Estimates of morbidity and mortality rates for diarrheal diseases in American children. J Pediatr 118: S27–33.
4. Guarino A, Albano F, Ashkenazi S, Gendrel D, Hoekstra JH, et al. (2008) European Society for Paediatric Gastroenterology, Hepatology, and Nutrition/European Society for Paediatric Infectious Diseases evidence-based guidelines for the management of acute gastroenteritis in children in Europe. J Pediatr Gastroenterol Nutr 46: S81–122.
5. Steiner MJ, De Walt DA, Byerley JS (2004) Is this child dehydrated? JAMA 291: 2746–54.
6. Gorelick MH, Shaw KN, Murphy KO (1997) Validity and reliability of clinical signs in the diagnosis of dehydration in children. Pediatrics 99: 99–106.
7. Friedman JN, Goldman RD, Srivastava R, Parkin PC (2004) Development of a clinical dehydration scale for use in children between 1 and 36 months of age. J Pediatr 145: 201–7.
8. Vega RM, Avner JR (1997) A prospective study of the usefulness of clinical and laboratory parameters for predicting percentage of dehydration in children. Pediatr Emerg Care 13: 179–82.
9. Duggan C, Refat M, Hashem M, Wolff M, Fayad I, et al. (1996) How valid are clinical signs of dehydration in infants? J Pediatr Gastroenterol Nutr 22: 56–61.
10. Mackenzie A, Barnes G, Shann F (1989) Clinical signs of dehydration in children. Lancet 2: 605–7.
11. Saavedra JM, Harris GD, Li S, Finberg L (1991) Capillary refilling (skin turgor) in the assessment of dehydration. Am J Dis Child 145: 296–8.
12. Yilmaz K, Karaböcüoglu M, Citak A, Uzel N (2002) Evaluation of laboratory tests in dehydrated children with acute gastroenteritis. J Paediatr Child Health 38: 226–8.
13. Porter SC, Fleisher GR, Kohane IS, Mandl KD (2003) The value of parental report for diagnosis and management of dehydration in the emergency department. Ann Emerg Med 41: 196–205.
14. von Elm E, Altman DG, Egger M, Pocock SJ, Gøtzsche PC, Vandenbroucke JP, et al. (2007). The Strengthening the Reporting of Observational Studies in Epidemiology (STROBE) statement: guidelines for reporting observational studies. PLoS Med 4: e296.

15. Carpenter J, Bithell J (2000). Bootstrap confidence intervals: when, which, what? A practical guide for medical statisticians. Stat Med 19: 1141–64.
16. Bland JM, Altman DG (1986) Statistical methods for assessing agreement between two methods of clinical measurement. Lancet 1: 307–10.
17. Teach SJ, Yates EW, Feld LG (1997) Laboratory predictors of fluid deficit in acutely dehydrated children. Clin Pediatr (Phila) 36: 395–400.

Comparison of Age-Stratified Seroprevalence of Antibodies against Norovirus GII in India and the United Kingdom

Vipin Kumar Menon[1], Santosh George[1], Farah Aladin[2], Sameena Nawaz[2], Rajiv Sarkar[1], Ben Lopman[3], James J. Gray[4], Miren Iturriza Gomara[5], Gagandeep Kang[1]*

1 Department of Gastrointestinal Sciences, Christian Medical College, Vellore, India, **2** Virus Reference Department, Centre for Infection, Health Protection Agency, London, United Kingdom, **3** Division of Viral Diseases, National Center for Immunization and Respiratory Diseases, Centers for Disease Control and Prevention, Atlanta, Georgia, United States of America, **4** Norfolk and Norwich University Hospital Specialist Virology Centre, Microbiology Department, NRP Innovation Centre, Norwich, United Kingdom, **5** Department of Clinical Infection, Microbiology and Immunology, Institute of Infection and Global Health, University of Liverpool, Liverpool, United Kingdom

Abstract

Noroviruses are a common cause of gastroenteritis worldwide, but outbreaks appear to be more common in industrialized countries than in developing countries, possibly reflecting differences in exposure and immunity. In this study, age-stratified sera from India and UK populations were analysed for the presence of norovirus-genogroup II specific IgG by a time resolved immunofluorescence assay and relative levels of antibodies in the two populations were compared. Antibody levels were higher among all age groups in India than in UK and increased with age in India, whereas in the UK, levels of antibody decreased in adulthood. These results indicate different patterns of exposure to noroviruses in the two countries.

Editor: D. William Cameron, University of Ottawa, Canada

Funding: This study was funded by British Council, with grant number SA08-040. The funders had no role in study design, data collection and analysis, decision to publish, or preparation of the manuscript.

Competing Interests: The authors have declared that no competing interests exist.

* E-mail: gkang@cmcvellore.ac.in

Introduction

Noroviruses (NoV) are a major cause of sporadic gastroenteritis worldwide, as well as of outbreaks in hospitals and semi-closed communities such as residential and nursing homes [1–2]. Transmission is mainly via the fecal-oral route, through person-to-person contact or through contaminated food, water or the environment [3]. Infection elicits incomplete and short lived immunity, and previous studies with volunteers demonstrated that although pre-existing serum antibodies to NoV do not protect from re-infection, antibody levels to NoV are associated with protection after repeated exposure [4]. Seroprevalence studies have demonstrated that NoV infections are ubiquitous and infections occur early in life with prevalence reaching >95% in adults [5–7].

Reports of NoV prevalence in India are primarily from hospital and community based studies of sporadic acute gastroenteritis [8–11] and only one outbreak in a semi-closed setting has been reported [12].

This study examined the levels of human NoV-specific antibodies in age-stratified sera from India and UK populations as a measure of exposure to NoV infections in the two populations throughout life and demonstrated a difference which may, at least in part, explain the low incidence of NoV outbreaks in India in comparison to the UK.

Materials and Methods

Ethics Statement

The study was approved by the Institutional Review Boards of the Christian Medical College, Vellore, India. Prior to enrollment, written informed consent was obtained from the parents or legal guardians of eligible children.

Study Area and Population

In India, 1044 sera included sera collected in a probability proportional to size cluster survey conducted in Vellore from August 1999 to February 2000 [13] (samples from 0–40 years), and sera from the Biochemistry laboratory and the Community Health and Development Hospital, Vellore from residents in geographic areas of the serosurvey (sera from >40 years of age). The studies were approved by the Institutional Review Board of the Christian Medical College, Vellore. In the UK, 1034 sera collected in 2000 or 2005 from the HPA Seroepidemiology Programme (http://www.hpa.org.uk/webw/HPAweb&Page&HPAwebAutoListName/Page/1158313434390?p = 1158313434390) were used. Sera from both cohorts were distributed in 5 age groups (Table 1).

Time Resolved Fluorescence Immunoassay (TRFIA)

Detection of human NoV-specific serum IgG was done by Time Resolved Fluorescence Immunoassay (TRFIA), which incorporates lanthanide labels that confer high sensitivity and a wider dynamic range than ELISA assays [14], and hence allows quantitation without the need for inclusion of a dilution series. Human NoV virus like particles (VLPs) were produced from an epidemic strain GII.4v2 [15], circulating in the UK during 2002 and later detected worldwide, the viral protein 1 (VP1) has 94%

Table 1. Summary of sera tested.

Age Group	India Cohort	UK Cohort
<6 months	83	47
7 m–5 y	170	160
10–15 y	237	207
20–30 y	189	207
40–45 y	158	206
50–60 y	207	207
Total	1044	1034

amino acid homology to the predominant Indian strain. The VLPs were used at a concentration of 2 μg/ml in 0.05 M carbonate/bicarbonate buffer, pH 9.6 to coat 96-well high-binding microwell plates (Costar, Corning, N.Y.), overnight at 4°C. Plates were washed 5 times with DELFIA wash buffer (PerkinElmer, UK) and 100 μl of serum diluted 1:100 in DELFIA assay buffer (PerkinElmer, UK) was loaded per test well. Each plate included a standard curve of 8 serial two-fold dilution of a positive serum sample starting at 1:100, a blank (no serum) and positive control and a negative control (goat serum). The plates were incubated in a humid chamber for 2 h at 37°C and then washed 5 times. A total of 100 μl of europium (Eu) labelled anti-human IgG conjugate (PerkinElmer, UK) diluted 1:500 in DELFIA buffer was added to each well using a multi-channel pipette, followed by incubation for 1 h at 37°C and washing as before. A total of 150 μl of DELFIA enhancement solution (PerkinElmer, UK) was added to each well and plates were incubated in the dark at room temperature for 15 min with gentle rotation. Plates were read using a DELFIA 1234 reader (PerkinElmer, UK) and data analyzed using Multicalc software, version 4.0 (Wallac Oy, Finland). The distribution of the Eu counts was normalized by performing a natural log transformation. The plate-to-plate variability between the assays was eliminated by standardizing the slope and intercept across all experimental runs of the log-transformed europium counts, against a reference plate. Data were further analysed using STATA 10.0 for Windows (STATA Corp., TX, USA), using student's t-test and ANOVA, as appropriate.

Results and Discussion

Using a cut-off of +3SD above the mean of negative controls, the prevalence of human NoV-specific antibody in both cohorts was high, 99.5% and 99.4% in the India and the UK cohort, respectively. With a higher arbitrary Eu count cut-off of 7000, 4% of samples from UK and 1.6% samples from India were below this cut-off, mainly in the 0–5 year age group, with younger children within the group having fewer antibodies. The high prevalence found in this study, particularly for the UK cohort, when compared to previous studies may be due to the use of a more sensitive assay and also the choice of antigen, which used the recently widely circulating GII.4 strain, although a subset of sera were evaluated with a GII.4 VLP made with a pre-2002 strain also showed complete cross-reactivity (data not shown). Other studies have shown that the antibodies detected in human NoV-specific

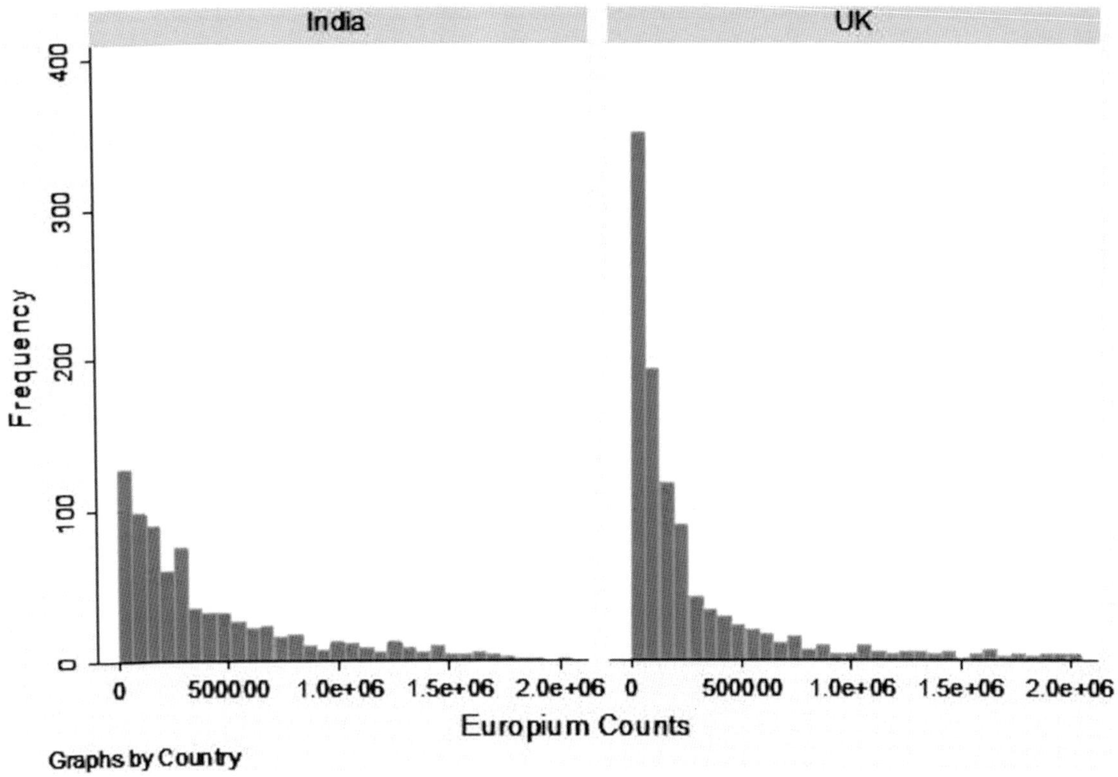

Figure 1. Distribution of Europium counts obtained with sera from the India and UK sera cohorts. The europium counts were log transformed for a normal distribution. The first plate from India was the reference category and a slope and intercept was calculated for all other plates from both India and the UK. The slope and the intercept values were used to standardize the log-transformed europium counts across experimental runs. Standardized log-transformed values were then used for all analyses.

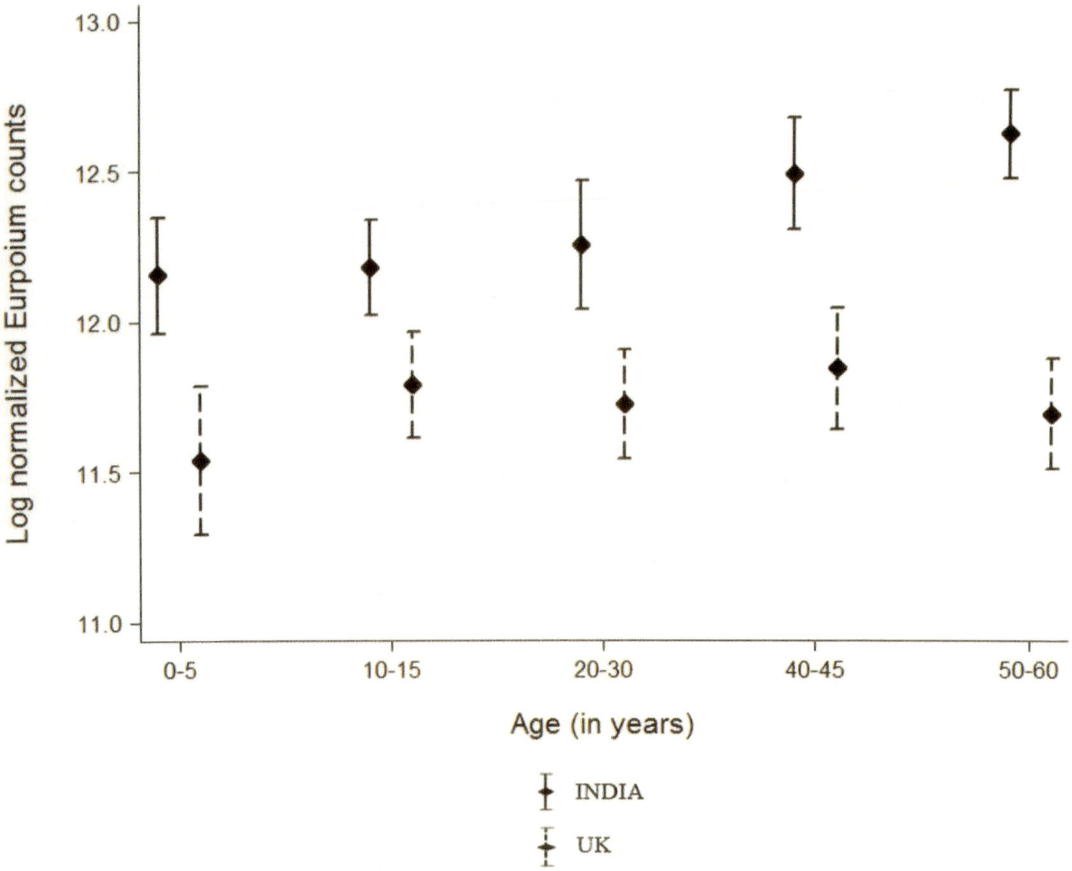

Figure 2. Distribution of log normalized Europium counts among the different age strata in India and the UK. The dots in the center represent the mean Europium counts for that age group whereas the horizontal error bars represent +2 standard deviations. Europium counts were measured by time resolved immunofluresecence assay.

EIA are largely cross-reactive across different NoV genotypes [16–19]. Studies examining seroprevalence to GII NoVs reported overall seropositivity of 91.2%, 74.1% 87% and 96.5% in Italy, France, Japan and South Africa, respectively [20–23] using conventional ELISAs. A study from China showed that the seropositivity increased from 70% among one year olds to 98% among 8–9 year old children for human norovirus GII and from 65% in the one year olds to 100% among the 8–9 year old children for human norovirus GI [24].

Although the proportion of seropositives to human NoV antibody was comparable in the two populations, the levels of antibodies as represented by the distribution of Eu counts were markedly different (Figure 1). Due to the lack of a standard serum for quatification of human NoV-specific antibodies, the results are presented as relative quantitation of antibody levels between the two cohorts rather than absolute quantification.

For the comparative analysis between the two cohorts, exclusion of the negative samples did not alter the results, and data shown includes the complete cohorts. Sera from India showed significantly higher levels of norovirus-specific IgG than the sera from UK across all 5 age groups (Fig. 2). The Indian panel showed a steady rise in human NoV-specific antibody levels with age, reaching the highest levels in the age group of 50–60 years of age (Fig. 2). In the UK panel, the antibody levels was lowest among the 0–5 year old children with a mean (SD) log normalized Eu count of 11.5 (1.8), increasing to 11.8 (1.3) in 10–15 years age group; the differences were not statistically significant ($P = 0.264$). Among the Indian samples, antibody levels were significantly different across age groups, with higher levels among the 50–60 year age group [Mean (SD) 12.6 (1.1)] in comparison to the younger age groups 0–5 [Mean (SD) 12.2(1.5), $P = 0.003$] and 10–15 year age groups [Mean (SD) 12.2(1.5), $P<0.001$]. No significant difference was observed (at $p = 0.003$ level, after Bonferroni correction) for any of the other age groups (Fig. 2). The antibody levels were comparable between males and females for all age groups except the 20–30 year olds. In this age group the antibody levels were higher in females (12.1, 1.4) than in males (11.8, 1.4, $P = 0.016$). Although not statistically significant, this relationship held true for both India [12.4 (1.5) vs. 12.0 (1.5), $P = 0.102$] and UK [11.8 (1.3) vs. 11.6 (1.3), $P = 0.188$] panels (data not shown).

The results show higher levels of human NoV-specific antibodies in the population in India compared to the UK, with the widest difference between the two populations in the youngest and the oldest age groups analysed. These findings suggest more constant exposure to noroviruses across all age groups in India when compared to the UK. A number of factors are known to play a role in the increased prevalence of some infectious diseases in developing countries. These include poor hygiene and sanitation, less access to healthcare, overcrowding as well as socio-cultural differences wherein people in India live in larger family units when compared to developed countries [25–28]. Norovirus infections, similar to rotavirus infections, are endemic in infants and children. Recently it has been demonstrated that in India, first rotavirus infections occur earlier than in the middle and high-income countries, and that number of reinfections is higher [29] and that seroprevalence of rotavirus group A antibodies is 100% in the same age-stratified population as evaluated here [30]. The same pattern could be expected for human norovirus infections, which would be consistent with the data presented here and with other studies from developing countries [23–24,31]. In the UK, the peak of human norovirus-specific antibody levels in the 5–10 year olds is likely to reflect increased opportunities for infection through contact with other children. Indeed, in Europe, social contact rates are highest in school age children [32]. The lower human norovirus–specific antibody levels in the >50 years old could also correlate with the increased susceptibility in this age group that translates into the high frequency of norovirus outbreaks that are seen each winter in the UK, particularly among elderly patients in hospitals and residential care institutions. In addition to the social contact across all ages, it is likely that in India there are also greater opportunities for food, water and environmental transmission of noroviruses, contributing to greater and steady exposure and boosting of immunity. This may result in reinfections being mostly subclinical, and outbreaks being rare in this population in contrast to the high incidence of outbreaks involving adults and the elderly in the UK and other high income countries.

Author Contributions

Conceived and designed the experiments: JJG MIG GK BL. Performed the experiments: VKM SG SN FA. Analyzed the data: RS VKM SG SN MIG FA. Contributed reagents/materials/analysis tools: BL MIG GK. Wrote the paper: VKM MIG GK.

References

1. Blanton LH, Adams SM, Beard RS, Wei G, Bulens SN, et al. (2006) Molecular and epidemiologic trends of caliciviruses associated with outbreaks of acute gastroenteritis in the United States, 2000–2004. J Infect Dis 193: 413–421.
2. Vipond IB, Caul EO, Hirst D, Carmen B, Curry A, et al. (2004) National epidemic of Lordsdale Norovirus in the UK. J Clin Virol 30: 243–247.
3. Atmar RL (2010) Noroviruses - State of the Art. Food Environ Virol 2: 117–126.
4. Johnson PC, Mathewson JJ, DuPont HL, Greenberg HB (1990) Multiple-challenge study of host susceptibility to Norwalk gastroenteritis in US adults. J Infect Dis 161: 18–21.
5. Gray JJ, Jiang X, Morgan-Capner P, Desselberger U, Estes MK (1993) Prevalence of antibodies to Norwalk virus in England: detection by enzyme-linked immunosorbent assay using baculovirus-expressed Norwalk virus capsid antigen. J Clin Microbiol 31: 1022–1025.
6. O'Ryan ML, Vial PA, Mamani N, Jiang X, Estes MK, et al. (1998) Seroprevalence of Norwalk virus and Mexico virus in Chilean individuals: assessment of independent risk factors for antibody acquisition. Clin Infect Dis 27: 789–795.
7. Cubitt WD, Green KY, Payment P (1998) Prevalence of antibodies to the Hawaii strain of human calicivirus as measured by a recombinant protein based immunoassay. J Med Virol 54: 135–139.
8. Chhabra P, Chitambar SD (2008) Norovirus genotype IIb associated acute gastroenteritis in India. J Clin Virol 42: 429–432.
9. Chhabra P, Dhongade RK, Kalrao VR, Bavdekar AR, Chitambar SD (2009) Epidemiological, clinical, and molecular features of norovirus infections in western India. J Med Virol 81: 922–932.
10. Nayak MK, Chatterjee D, Nataraju SM, Pativada M, Mitra U, et al. (2009) A new variant of Norovirus GII.4/2007 and inter-genotype recombinant strains of NVGII causing acute watery diarrhoea among children in Kolkata, India. J Clin Virol 45: 223–229.
11. Monica B, Ramani S, Banerjee I, Primrose B, Iturriza-Gomara M, et al. (2007) Human caliciviruses in symptomatic and asymptomatic infections in children in Vellore, South India. J Med Virol 79: 544–551.
12. Girish R, Broor S, Dar L, Ghosh D (2002) Foodborne outbreak caused by a Norwalk-like virus in India. J Med Virol 67: 603–607.
13. Kang G, Samuel R, Vijayakumar TS, Selvi S, Sridharan G, et al. (2005) Community prevalence of antibodies to human immunodeficiency virus in rural and urban Vellore, Tamil Nadu. Natl Med J India 18: 15–17.
14. Smith DR, Rossi CA, Kijek TM, Henchal EA, Ludwig GV (2001) Comparison of dissociation-enhanced lanthanide fluorescent immunoassays to enzyme-linked immunosorbent assays for detection of staphylococcal enterotoxin B, Yersinia pestis-specific F1 antigen, and Venezuelan equine encephalitis virus. Clin Diagn Lab Immunol 8: 1070–1075.
15. Allen DJ, Noad R, Samuel D, Gray JJ, Roy P, et al. (2009) Characterisation of a GII-4 norovirus variant-specific surface-exposed site involved in antibody binding. Virol J 6: 150.
16. Cannon JL, Lindesmith LC, Donaldson EF, Saxe L, Baric RS, et al. (2009) Herd immunity to GII.4 noroviruses is supported by outbreak patient sera. J Virol 83: 5363–5374.
17. Green KY, Lew JF, Jiang X, Kapikian AZ, Estes MK (1993) Comparison of the reactivities of baculovirus-expressed recombinant Norwalk virus capsid antigen with those of the native Norwalk virus antigen in serologic assays and some epidemiologic observations. J Clin Microbiol 31: 2185–2191.
18. Parker S, Cubitt D, Jiang JX, Estes M (1993) Efficacy of a recombinant Norwalk virus protein enzyme immunoassay for the diagnosis of infections with Norwalk virus and other human "candidate" caliciviruses. J Med Virol 41: 179–184.
19. Widdowson MA, Rockx B, Schepp R, van der Poel WH, Vinje J, et al. (2005) Detection of serum antibodies to bovine norovirus in veterinarians and the general population in the Netherlands. J Med Virol 76: 119–128.
20. Pelosi E, Lambden PR, Caul EO, Liu B, Dingle K, et al. (1999) The seroepidemiology of genogroup 1 and genogroup 2 Norwalk-like viruses in Italy. J Med Virol 58: 93–99.
21. Nicollier-Jamot B, Pico V, Pothier P, Kohli E (2003) Molecular cloning, expression, self-assembly, antigenicity, and seroepidemiology of a genogroup II norovirus isolated in France. J Clin Microbiol 41: 3901–3904.
22. Honma S, Nakata S, Numata K, Kogawa K, Yamashita T, et al. (1998) Epidemiological study of prevalence of genogroup II human calicivirus (Mexico virus) infections in Japan and Southeast Asia as determined by enzyme-linked immunosorbent assays. J Clin Microbiol 36: 2481–2484.
23. Smit TK, Steele AD, Peenze I, Jiang X, Estes MK (1997) Study of Norwalk virus and Mexico virus infections at Ga-Rankuwa Hospital, Ga-Rankuwa, South Africa. J Clin Microbiol 35: 2381–2385.
24. Jing Y, Qian Y, Huo Y, Wang LP, Jiang X (2000) Seroprevalence against Norwalk-like human caliciviruses in beijing, China. J Med Virol 60: 97–101.
25. Dai YC, Nie J, Zhang XF, Li ZF, Bai Y, et al. (2004) Seroprevalence of antibodies against noroviruses among students in a Chinese military medical university. J Clin Microbiol 42: 4615–4619.
26. Parashar UD, Li JF, Cama R, DeZalia M, Monroe SS, et al. (2004) Human caliciviruses as a cause of severe gastroenteritis in Peruvian children. J Infect Dis 190: 1088–1092.
27. Koopmans M (2008) Progress in understanding norovirus epidemiology. Curr Opin Infect Dis 21: 544–552.
28. Garcia C, DuPont HL, Long KZ, Santos JI, Ko G (2006) Asymptomatic norovirus infection in Mexican children. J Clin Microbiol 44: 2997–3000.
29. Gladstone BP, Ramani S, Mukhopadhya I, Muliyil J, Sarkar R, et al. (2011) Protective effect of natural rotavirus infection in an Indian birth cohort. N Engl J Med 365: 337–346.
30. Mukhopadhya I, Anbu D, Iturriza-Gomara M, Gray JJ, Brown DW, et al. (2010) Anti-VP6 IgG antibodies against group A and group C rotaviruses in South India. Epidemiology and Infection 138: 442–447.
31. Smit TK, Bos P, Peenze I, Jiang X, Estes MK, et al. (1999) Seroepidemiological study of genogroup I and II calicivirus infections in South and southern Africa. J Med Virol 59: 227–231.
32. Mossong J, Hens N, Jit M, Beutels P, Auranen K, et al. (2008) Social contacts and mixing patterns relevant to the spread of infectious diseases. PLoS Med 5: e74.

4

The *Shigella* Type Three Secretion System Effector OspG Directly and Specifically Binds to Host Ubiquitin for Activation

Yan Zhou[1,2], Na Dong[2], Liyan Hu[2], Feng Shao[2*]

1 College of Life Sciences, Beijing Normal University, Beijing, China, 2 National Institute of Biological Sciences, Beijing, China

Abstract

The genus *Shigella* infects human gut epithelial cells to cause diarrhea and gastrointestinal disorders. Like many other Gram-negative bacterial pathogens, the virulence of *Shigella spp.* relies on a conserved type three secretion system that delivers a handful of effector proteins into host cells to manipulate various host cell physiology. However, many of the *Shigella* type III effectors remain functionally uncharacterized. Here we observe that OspG, one of the *Shigella* effectors, interacted with ubiquitin conjugates and poly-ubiquitin chains of either K48 or K63 linkage in eukaryotic host cells. Purified OspG protein formed a stable complex with ubiquitin but showed no interactions with other ubiquitin-like proteins. OspG binding to ubiquitin required the carboxyl terminal helical region in OspG and the canonical I44-centered hydrophobic surface in ubiquitin. OspG and OspG-homologous effectors, NleH1/2 from *enteropathogenic E coli* (EPEC), contain sub-domains I-VII of eukaryotic serine/threonine kinase. GST-tagged OspG and NleH1/2 could undergo autophosphorylation, the former of which was significantly stimulated by ubiquitin binding. Ubiquitin binding was also required for OspG functioning in attenuating host NF-κB signaling. Our data illustrate a new mechanism that bacterial pathogen like *Shigella* exploits ubiquitin binding to activate its secreted virulence effector for its functioning in host eukaryotic cells.

Editor: Yousef Abu Kwaik, University of Louisville, United States of America

Funding: This research was supported by the National Basic Research Program of China (973 Programs 2010CB835400 and 2012CB518700) to FS. The funders had no role in study design, data collection and analysis, decision to publish, or preparation of the manuscript.

Competing Interests: The authors have declared that no competing interests exist.

* E-mail: shaofeng@nibs.ac.cn

Introduction

Shigella spp. are Gram-negative bacterial pathogens whose infection causes a spectrum of symptoms ranging from watery diarrhea to severe dysentery [1]. *Shigella* harbors a 220-kb virulence plasmid that is essential for successful infection [2]. This plasmid encodes a specialized protein secretion apparatus called the type three secretion system as well as more than a dozen of type III-secreted effector proteins. Like in many other Gram-negative bacterial pathogens, effector secreted by *Shigella* type III secretion system function to facilitate infection, bacterial survival and replication [3]. Studies in the past 20 years have shown that type III secreted effectors can target multiple host cellular processes such as innate immunity, actin cytoskeleton dynamics and membrane trafficking [3,4]. In *Shigella* infection, the OspF effector functions as a novel MAPK phosphothreonine lyase to irreversibly inactivate mitogen-activated protein kinase (MAPK) [5] and downregulate host inflammatory responses [6,7]. IpgB1/2 are guanine-nucleotide exchange factors (GEFs) and preferentially activate small GTPase Rac1 and RhoA, respectively, to promote *Shigella* invasion of host epithelial cells [8,9,10]. The VirA effector is a novel TBC-like GTPase-activating protein (GAP), which inactivates host Rab1 and contributes to *Shigella* escape from host autophagy [11]. Expression of these *Shigella* effectors is under sophisticated genetic regulation by temperature and contact host cell contact. However, little is known about the regulation of effector biochemical activities.

Protein ubiquitination critically controls nearly all aspects of eukaryotic cellular processes including cell cycle progression, gene transcription, various signal transduction pathways [12]. Ubiquitination involves a three-enzyme cascade composed of ubiquitin-activating enzyme, ubiquitin-conjugating enzyme and ubiquitin ligase. In the third step, ubiquitin ligase catalyzes ubiquitin transfer from the ubiquitin-conjugating enzyme onto a lysine side chain in the substrate or another ubiquitin linked through an isopeptide bond linkage. The latter generates either free ubiquitin chains or ubiquitin chains attached to a substrate protein. Ubiquitin conjugation onto one of the seven lysines in another ubiquitin results in formation of ubiquitin chains with different linkages that often confer different fates on the substrate protein [13]. The ubiquitin system is frequently hijacked by bacterial pathogens [14,15], and bacterial type III effectors can even directly deamidate ubiquitin to paralyze its chain formation activity [16]. In the case of *Shigella* infection, the OspI effector deamidates an ubiquitin-conjugating enzyme Ubc13 that is dedicated to form K63-linked ubiquitin chains to dampen host NF-κB-mediated inflammatory response [17]. *Shigella* also harbors a group of effectors called IpaHs that define a third class of ubiquitin ligases structurally distinct from eukaryotic HECT- and RING-domain ubiquitin ligases [18,19,20]. IpaHs have also been implicated in tuning the host inflammatory responses [21].

OspG is another *Shigella* type III effector. OspG was firstly identified from the supernatant of *Shigella flexneri* Δ*ipaBCDA* strain that secretes effectors constitutively [22]. Expression of OspG is induced only after activation of the type three secretion apparatus, suggesting its function at a later stage during *Shigella* infection [23]. OspG shares sequence similarity to mammalian serine/threonine protein kinase and may interfere with innate immune responses by targeting host ubiquitin-conjugating enzyme [24]. However, the biochemical mechanism and regulation of OspG function remains largely unknown.

In this work, we discover that OspG binds to free ubiquitin, poly-ubiquitin chains as well as ubiquitin-conjugated proteins with high affinity and specificity. We further demonstrate that OspG binding to ubiquitin is mediated by the canonical I44-centered hydrophobic surface in ubiquitin and requires a unique carboxyl terminal helix in OspG. Ubiquitin binding significantly stimulates the kinase activity of OspG, shown by evidently increased autophosphorylation and intrinsic ATP hydrolysis activity. Ubiquitin binding is also required for OspG functioning in attenuating host innate immune NF-κB signaling. Our data provide the first example that bacterial effectors can make use of interaction with host ubiquitin to activate itself.

Results

OspG Directly Binds to Polyubiquitin Conjugates

To search for possible OspG-interacting proteins related to ubiquitination, purified GST-tagged OspG protein (GST-OspG) was immobilized onto glutathione beads and incubated with lysates of intact 293T cells or 293T cells pretreated with the proteasome inhibitor MG132. Proteins retained on the beads were then subjected to reducing SDS-PAGE and anti-ubiquitin (P4D1) Western blotting analysis. Unexpectedly, we found that GST-OspG, but not GST alone, could efficiently pull down a large amount of polyubiquitinated proteins from intact 293T cell lysates, as shown by the heavy smear signals recognized by the anti-ubiquitin antibody (Fig. 1A). When cells were pretreated with MG132 to increase the level of polyubiquitinated proteins, the amounts of polyubiquitinated species precipitated by GST-OspG were also significantly increased and such effects were not observed with pulldown assays performed with GST protein alone (Fig. 1A). These data suggest that OspG can specifically bind to polyubiquitinated proteins in eukaryotic host cells.

As mentioned earlier, polyubiquitin chains with different linkages are associated with different functions. K48-linked ubiquitin chain is established in signaling conjugated substrates for proteasomal degradation while the other prevalent K63 ubiquitin chain regulates the function or activity of the target substrate. To examine whether OspG prefers to bind ubiquitin chains with a particular linkage, His6-tagged ubiquitin chains (Ub2-4) of either K48 or K63 linkage were incubated with GST or GST-OspG. Consistent with the increased precipitation of polyubiquitinated proteins by GST-OspG from MG132-treated cells, GST-OspG, but not GST alone, was found to be efficiently precipitated by K48-linked ubiquitin chains (Fig. 1B). Notably, K63-linked ubiquitin chains (Ub2-7) could also specifically pull down GST-OspG with efficiency comparable to that observed K48 ubiquitin chains (Fig. 1C). These data demonstrate that OspG can directly bind polyubiquitin chains of either K48 or K63 linkage and further indicate that OspG may modulate host ubiquitin signaling that is not limited to proteasomal degradation.

OspG Directly Binds to Ubiquitin, but not Other Ubiquitin-like Proteins

One interpretation accounting for OspG binding to both K48- and K63-linked ubiquitin chains is that OspG may bind to the monomer form of free ubiquitin, which was missed in the previous cell-lysate pulldown assay because free ubiquitin ran out of the 12% SDS-PAGE gel used in that assay. To this end, samples of GST-OspG pulldown performed with 293T cell lysates were re-examined by Western blotting analysis using 4–20% gradient gel. As shown in Fig. 1D, GST-OspG did precipitate free ubiquitin more efficiently than the polyubiquitin-conjugated proteins. As a control, no binding between ubiquitin and GST alone was observed in this assay.

To confirm the direct interaction between OspG and ubiquitin, purified His6- OspG was used to pull down recombinant GST and GST-ubiquitin. Only GST-ubiquitin was precipitated by His6-OspG and the binding appeared to be highly robust (Fig. 2A). In eukaryotes, there are a large number of ubiquitin-binding modules that confer diverse regulations of ubiquitin signaling. Most of these ubiquitin-binding proteins recognize a critical conserved region on ubiquitin, the I44-centered hydrophobic patch [25,26]. Interestingly, when I44 of ubiquitin was mutated into Ala, precipitation of this mutant form of ubiquitin by OspG was not observed (Fig. 2A). This result indicates that OspG, similar to most ubiquitin-binding modules in the host, also recognizes the canonical I44 surface of ubiquitin to achieve high-affinity interaction.

Ubiquitin-like proteins (UBL proteins), such as SUMO and LC3, share a three-dimensional structural fold with ubiquitin. These UBLs can be conjugated onto target proteins through a similar enzymatic cascade, which critically regulates many cellular processes, including transcription, DNA repair, signal transduction, autophagy and cell-cycle control [27,28]. To test whether OspG can interact with other UBLs, His6-OspG was used to pull down GST-SUMO1 and GST-LC3, but no interaction was observed. This result suggests that OspG selectively binds to ubiquitin among the UBL-family members (Fig. 2A).

The interaction between OspG and ubiquitin was further tested by elution on a gel filtration column. Purified OspG (23.6 kDa) and ubiquitin (12.1 kDa), when loaded onto the column separately, were eluted at the volume corresponding to the molecular weight of their monomeric forms (Fig. 2B). When OspG was mixed with excess ubiquitin and the mixtures were loaded onto the same column, a complex species eluted earlier than OspG and ubiquitin alone appeared (Fig. 2B). The ~ 10.5 ml elution volume of this species corresponds to roughly ~ 50 kDa for a globular protein, suggesting a possible 1:1 stoichiometry for OspG and ubiquitin binding. Further SDS-PAGE analysis of each fraction confirmed the co-elution of OspG and ubiquitin as well as the roughly estimated 1:1 OspG-ubiquitin complex (Fig. 2C).

Both the Carboxyl Terminus and the Kinase-like Domain of OspG are Required for Ubiquitin Binding

OspG is a small-size protein with only 196 amino acids and its sequence from residue 24 to 160 exhibits confident similarities to sub-domains I to VII of eukaryotic serine/threonine kinase (Fig. 3A and Fig. 4). The extreme carboxyl terminus (residues 161–196), predicted to form an α helix, does not show any sequence similarity to known proteins. The fact that no classical ubiquitin-binding domains or motifs could be identified in OspG indicates a novel ubiquitin-binding mode and also promoted us to further investigate its ubiquitin binding mechanism. Truncation of the amino terminal 21 residues preceding the putative kinase domain did not affect OspG binding to ubiquitin in the *in vitro* pulldown assay (Fig. 3B). Notably, removal of the extreme carboxyl terminal 26 residues in OspG completely abolished its interaction with ubiquitin (Fig. 3C), suggesting that the carboxyl terminal region following the kinase-like domain in OspG is essential for ubiquitin

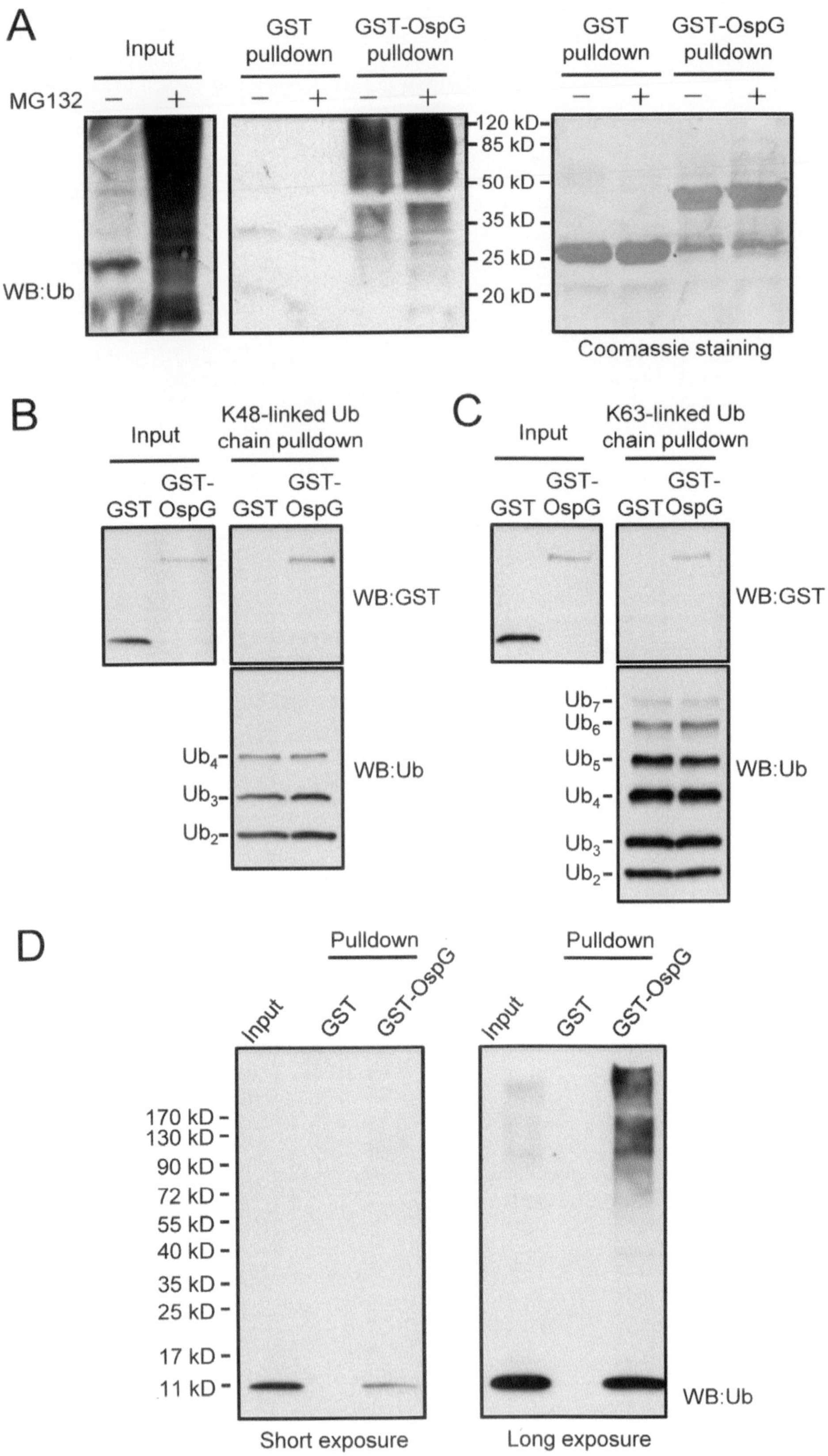

Figure 1. High-affinity binding between OspG and ubiquitin conjugates, poly-ubiquitin chains and free ubiquitin. (**A**) Pulldown of ubiquitin-conjugated proteins by purified GST-OspG. Glutathione-Sepharose beads coated with GST-OspG or GST alone were incubated with lysates of intact 293T cells or MG132- treated 293T cells. Proteins retained on the beads were eluted with SDS loading buffer and separated onto12% SDS-PAGE gels. Shown on the left are anti-ubiquitin immunoblots and on the right are Coomassie blue staining of GST or GST-OspG proteins present on

the beads. (**B** and **C**) Pulldown of OpsG by K48- or K63-linked poly-ubiquitin chains. Ni-NTA Sepharose beads coated with His6-ubiquitin chains with indicated linkages were incubated with GST or GST-OspG. Proteins retained on the beads were subjected to SDS-PAGE and anti-GST immunoblotting analysis. (**D**) Pulldown of free ubiquitin by GST-OspG. GST or GST-OspG proteins were immobilized onto Glutathione Sepharose beads and the beads were then incubated with lysates of 293T cells. The interacting proteins eluted from the beads were resolved by 4–20% gradient SDS-PAGE gel and analyzed by anti-ubiquitin immunoblotting.

binding. Mutation of two leucine residues (L190D/L191D) in this region abolishedOspG binding to ubiquitin (Fig. 3C), suggesting the importance of these two residues. Furthermore, when the carboxyl terminal 26, 31, or 35 residues were artificially fused to GST protein and the fusion proteins were assayed for co-precipitation by ubiquitin, none of the three chimeric proteins were capable of binding to ubiquitin (Fig. 3D). These data suggest that the carboxyl terminal helical region in OspG is essential but not sufficient for mediating specific interaction with ubiquitin and the kinase-like domain is also involved in ubiquitin binding.

We also tested OspG and ubiquitin interaction in eukaryotic host cells. Transient expression of OspG into 293T cells could efficiently co-immunoprecipitate endogenous ubiquitin (Fig. 3E). In contrast, mutation of the carboxyl-terminal two leucine residues (L190D/L191D) in OspG abolished the interaction in this transfection assay (Fig. 3E). To confirm this interaction during *Shigella* infection, an *ospG* deletion strain of *S. flexneri* was constructed. A Flag-tagged OspG was transformed into the deletion strain and infection was then performed. As shown in Fig. 3F, Flag-OspG expressed in the bacteria could co-immunoprecipitate endogenous ubiquitin from infected 293T cells, and importantly the L190D/L191D mutant was also defective in interacting with ubiquitin in this infection assay. As another control, OspG expressed in the type III secretion deficient Δ*mxiH* strain did not co-immunoprecipitate ubiquitin from infected 293T cells (Fig. 3F). These data demonstrate the type III-delivered OspG can bind to host ubiquitin and the interaction also requires the carboxyl terminal helical region in OspG.

OspG and OspG-like Effectors are a Type of Atypical Serine/threonine Kinases

OspG shows sequence similarity to eukaryotic protein serine/threonine kinase [24]. A typical serine/threonine kinase domain can be divided into eleven sub-domains (I-VI, VIIA, VIIB, VIII-XI) [29,30]. Aligning the sequence of OspG to the kinase domain of a prototypical eukaryotic serine/threonine kinase JNK3 shows that residues from 24 to 160 of OspG are homologous to JNK3 kinase sub-domains I-VII (Fig. 4). The predicted secondary structures of OspG can also be aligned well to those of JNK3 sub-domains I-VII, and all the catalytically important residues within these domains are maintained in OspG (Fig. 4). However, OspG apparently lacks the kinase sub-domains VIII–XI (Fig. 4). The sub-domain VIII is the activation loop whose conformational change usually stimulates the kinase activity upon serine/threonine phosphorylation of this loop by an upstream kinase or itself [29]. The sub-domains IX and X are generally required for maintaining the overall structural integrity [29]. Thus, OspG appears to be a half kinase with all necessary catalytic residues.

Given that no physiological substrates of OspG have been reported, we performed the kinase assay by using a generic artificial substrate myelin basic protein (MBP) and examined both MBP phosphorylation and OspG autophosphorylation either in the absence or presence of ubiquitin. While no MBP phosphorylation was detected, phosphorylation of GST-OspG by itself was observed (Fig. 5A), which confirms the observation made in the previous study [24]. Given that the autophosphorylation signal is rather weak, we further purified MBP-OspG and His6-OspG and assayed their autophosphorylation activity. Interestingly, no autophosphorylation occurred on MBP-OspG and His6-OspG (data not shown). Through mass spectrometry analysis, the autophosphorylation site of GST-OspG was mapped to a serine residue located in the linker region between the GST and OspG (Fig. S1A). This observation not only explains why no "autophosphorylation" occurred on MBP-OspG and His6-OspG, but also indicates that the observed "autophosphorylation" of GST-OspG differs from the classical kinase autophosphorylation that usually occurs on the activation loop. To confirm the kinase activity of OspG, we then assayed two other commercially available artificial substrates, casein from bovine milk and histone from calf thymus. While no phosphorylation of casein was observed, an evident phosphorylation signal was detected in the crude histone extract (Fig. S1B). Taken together, these data provide definitive experimental evidences for the kinase activity of recombinant OspG protein.

OspG has homologous effector proteins in other bacterial pathogens, including NleH1/2 in EPEC and enterohaemorrhagic *E. coli* (EHEC), and NleH in the mouse pathogen *Citrobacter rodentium*, which are all closely related diarrheagenic pathogens. OspG and NleHs share evident sequence similarities within the kinase domain (also sub-domains I-VII only) (Fig. S2A). In addition, NleH1/2 bears an extended N-terminal region that lacks the similarity to OspG. GST-NleH1 and GST-NleH2 could also phosphorylate themselves (Fig. S2B), similarly to that observed with GST-OspG. However, when the catalytic lysine residue important for ATP binding was mutated to alanine, no autophosphorylation of GST-NleH1/2 could be detected [31] (Fig. S2B). These results confirm that OspG and OspG-like bacterial effectors harbor serine/threonine kinase activity *in vitro*.

Ubiquitin Binding Stimulates the Kinase Activity of OspG

OspG binds to free ubiquitin, poly-ubiquitin chains and even ubiquitin-conjugated proteins. It is intuitively difficult to imagine that the function of OspG is to target host ubiquitin signaling as we hypothesized originally. Given that several type III effectors require binding to abundant host factors for their own activation, we then hypothesize that OspG may use ubiquitin binding to modulate its own biochemical activity, i.e. the kinase activity. Most notably, addition of ubiquitin into the phosphorylation reaction drastically promoted GST-OspG autophosphorylation (Fig. 5A) as well as phosphorylation of the crude histone extract (Fig. S1B). This ubiquitin-stimulated auto-phosphorylation was completely abolished when the serine residue in the linker region was mutated into alanine (Fig. 5B), suggesting a similar nature of autophosphorylation upon ubiquitin stimulation. Lys-53 of OspG is the predicted catalytic residue that anchors and orients the ATP, and Asp-138 is the potential catalytic residue to accept the proton from the attacking hydroxyl group. When these two residues were individually mutated toAla, autophosphorylation of GST-OspG was undetectable even in the presence of ubiquitin (Fig. 5C). This excludes the possibility that phosphorylation of GST-OspG comes from a contamination activity. In contrast to wild-type ubiquitin, ubiquitin I44A mutant or other UBL proteins did not stimulate the autophosphorylation of GST-OspG (Fig. 5D), which is consistent with their deficient binding to OspG. Similarly to ubiquitin, both

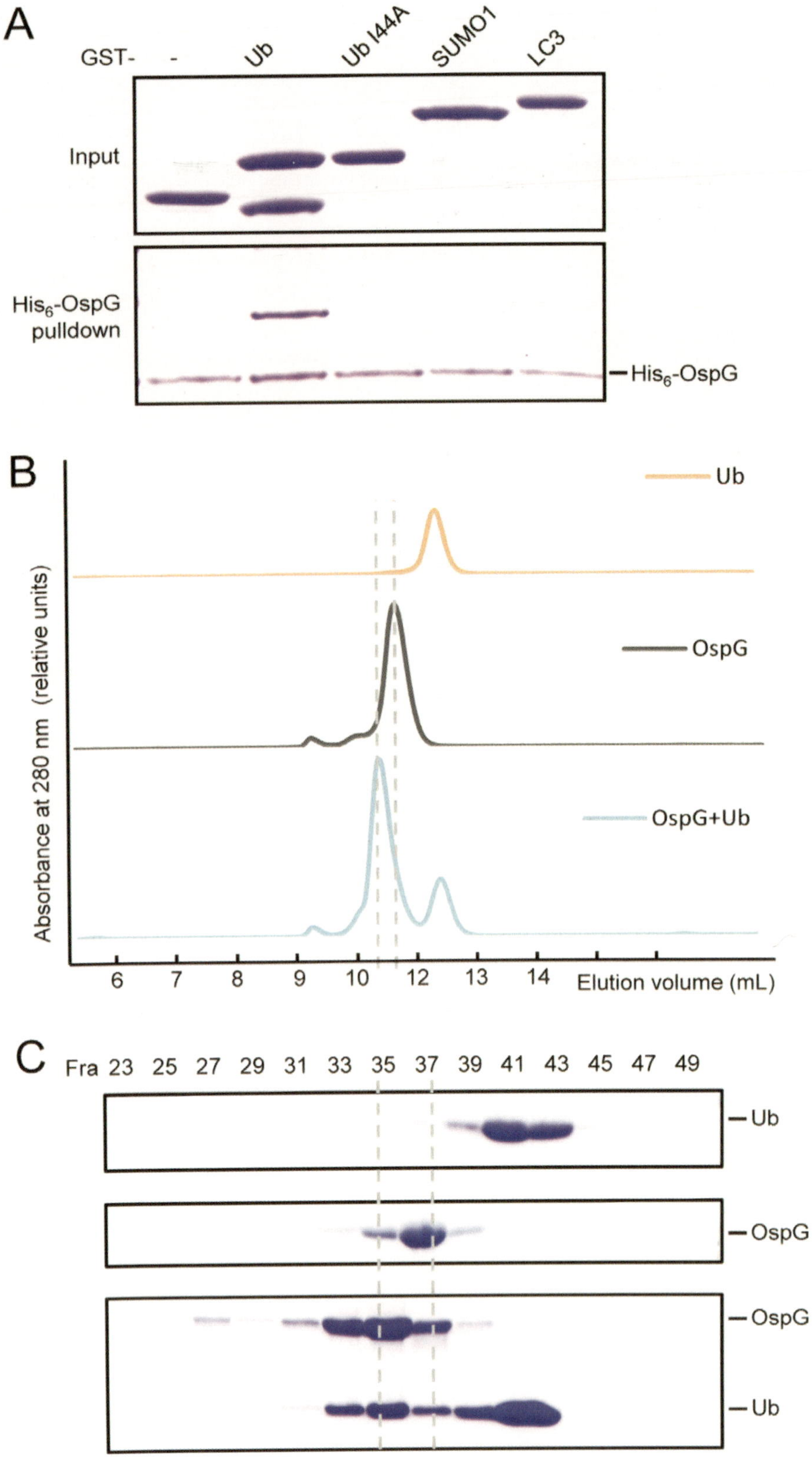

Figure 2. OspG directly and specifically binds to free ubiquitin. (**A**) Pulldown of free ubiquitin by OspG. His6-OspG was immobilized onto Ni-NTA beads and the beads were then incubated with GST, GST-ubiquitin, GST-ubiquitin I44A mutant, GST-LC3 or GST-SUMO1. Bound proteins were eluted from the beads and resolved on the SDS-PAGE gel followed by Coomassie blue staining. (**B** and **C**) Complex formation of ubiquitin and OspG on the gel filtration column. Purified Flag-His6-ubiquitin and His6-OspG proteins were subjected to Superdex-75 gel filtration chromatography individually or after being mixed together. Shown in (B) are the chromatograms. Aliquots of indicated fractions were resolved on the SDS-PAGE gel stained with Coomassie blue in (C).

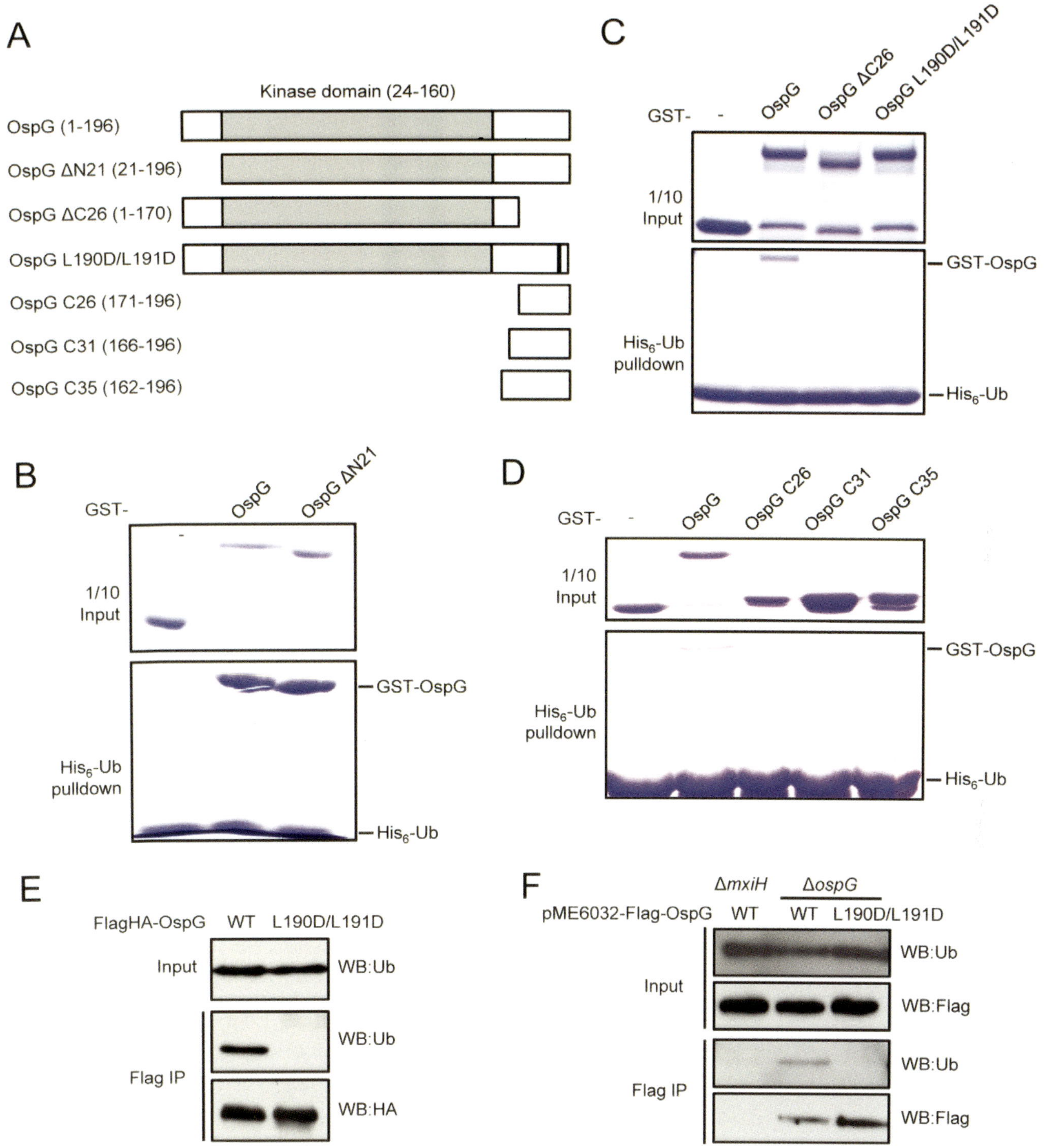

Figure 3. The carboxyl terminus of OspG is required for interaction with ubiquitin. (**A**) Schematic presentation of OspG truncations assayed in (B-D). The gray box donates the region that shows sequence similarity to eukaryotic serine/threonine kinase sub-domains I-VII. (**B**, **C** and **D**) Pulldown assays of the binding between ubiquitin and various OspG truncation proteins. Ni-NTA Sepharose beads coated with His6-ubiquitin were incubated with GST, GST-OspG or indicated GST-OspG truncation proteins. Proteins retained on the beads were eluted and then subjected to SDS-PAGE and Coomassie blue staining analysis. (**E**) Coimmunoprecipitation assay of OspG (WT or L190D/L191D mutant) and ubiquitin interaction in transfected HEK 293T cells. Shown are immunoblots of anti-Flag immunoprecipitates (Flag IP) and total cell lysates (Input). (**F**) Assay of OspG and ubiquitin interaction during *Shigella* infection. HEK 293T cells were infected with indicated *Shigella* deletion/complementation strains. Lysates of infected cell were subjected to anti-Flag immunoprecipitation. Δ*mxiH* is a type III secretion deficient strain; pME6032 is a rescue plasmid for expressing Flag-OspG (wild-type or L190D/L191D mutant) in the bacteria. Shown are immunoblots of anti-Flag immunoprecipitates (Flag IP) and total cell lysates (Input).

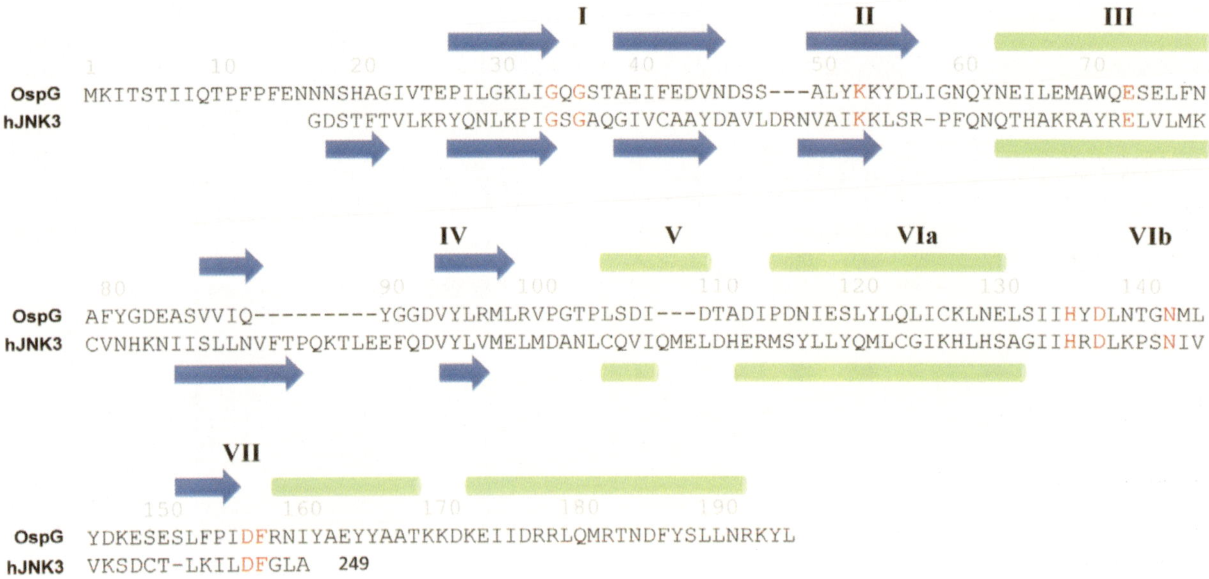

Figure 4. Secondary structure-based sequence alignment of OspG with human JNK3. The protein names are indicated at the left of the alignment. The key residues in the kinase domain are colored in red. Predicted secondary structures of OspG are shown on top of the OspG sequence. Secondary structures determined from crystal structure of JNK3 are shown underneath the sequence of JNK3 in the alignment. Green ovals are α helices and blue arrows are β strands. The sub-domains are labeled with Roman numerals.

K48-linked and K63-linked ubiquitin chains also promoted the autophosphorylation of GST-OspG (Fig. 5E). Deletion of the carboxyl terminal 26 residues from OspG that resulted in a defective ubiquitin binding severely attenuated the phosphorylation of GST-OspG (Fig. 5F). Similarly, autophosphorylation of GST-OspG L190D/L191D double mutant was not responsive to ubiquitin stimulation (Fig. 5F). Moreover, ubiquitin addition did not promote the autophosphorylation of GST-NleH1/2 (Fig. S2B), which is consistent with their lack of a carboxyl terminal sequence required for ubiquitin binding in OspG (Fig. S2A). In all above kinase assays, phosphorylation of ubiquitin was never observed (Fig. 5A). These data strongly support the hypothesis that ubiquitin is not a target of OspG but instead regulates the kinase activity of OspG.

Some kinases have been demonstrated to have intrinsic ATPase activity [32,33,34,35]. When His6-OspG was incubated with ATP and the phosphate release was detected by molybdate dye/phosphate complex formation, OspG exhibited intrinsic ATPase activity, which was also significantly increased by addition of ubiquitin (Fig. 5G). As expected, ubiquitin alone did not promote phosphate release from ATP. This again confirms our hypothesis that ubiquitin binding functions to stimulate the biochemical activity of OspG when it is translocated into host cells.

Ubiquitin Binding is Required for the Function of OspG in Attenuating Host NF-κB Signaling during Infection

Ubiquitin or ubiquitin-chain decoration of intracellular bacteria has been proposed as a signal that triggers autophagy-mediated host defense. To probe the functional consequence of OspG ubiquitin binding and activation of its kinase activity during *Shigella* infection, we first checked whether OspG plays a role in ubiquitin-chain formation surrounding intracellular *Shigella*. Using an antibody specific for polyubiquitinated proteins (FK1), we were able to detect some polyubiquitin signals around a portion of intracellular *S. flexneri* in infected HeLa cells, but this effect was not affected by deletion of *ospG* from the bacteria (Fig. 6A). This suggests that OspG does not play a role in recruitment or generation of polyubiquitinated proteins around *S. flexneri* during infection. Previous study suggests that OspG may interfere with the innate immune NF-κB signaling in *S. flexneri*-infected host cells [24].\ Confirming this observation, TNFα treatment induced a more rapid degradation of IκBα inhibitory protein in HeLa cells infected with the Δ*ospG* strain compared with that in wild-type strain (Fig. 6B). While re-expression of wild-type OspG in the deletion strain restored the inhibition of TNFα-induced IκBα degradation, the ubiquitin binding-deficient L190D/L191D mutant of OspG failed to complement the deletion strain in blocking IκBα degradation (Fig. 6B). These results suggest that OspG requires binding to host ubiquitin to exert its function in suppressing host innate immune signaling, which is likely through activation of its kinase activity.

Discussion

In summary, we have discovered that *Shigella* type III effector OspG directly and specifically interacts with host ubiquitin through the I44 hydrophobic patch on the ubiquitin surface. OspG also binds to poly-ubiquitin chains and ubiquitin-conjugated proteins. Binding to ubiquitin stimulates the kinase and intrinsic ATP hydrolysis activity of OspG, which, as an atypical kinase, exhibits sequence similarity to eukaryotic serine/threonine kinase sub-domains I-VII. Our data suggest a novel mechanism of activating a bacterial virulence effector by the host ubiquitin system. Our data also demonstrate that OspG and OspG-like effectors, NleHs from EPEC/EHEC, are atypical kinases and do exhibit *in vitro* kinase activity. It is important for future studies to identify the host target or kinase substrate of OspG, which shall advance our understanding of OspG binding to ubiquitin as well as its functional role in *Shigella* pathogenesis. *Shigella* secrets the IpaH family of ubiquitin ligase effectors and the OspI effector that targets host Ubc13 for deamidation. Therefore, ubiquitin binding and activation of OspG provides an additional layer of complexity to the interplay between *Shigella* and the eukaryotic ubiquitin

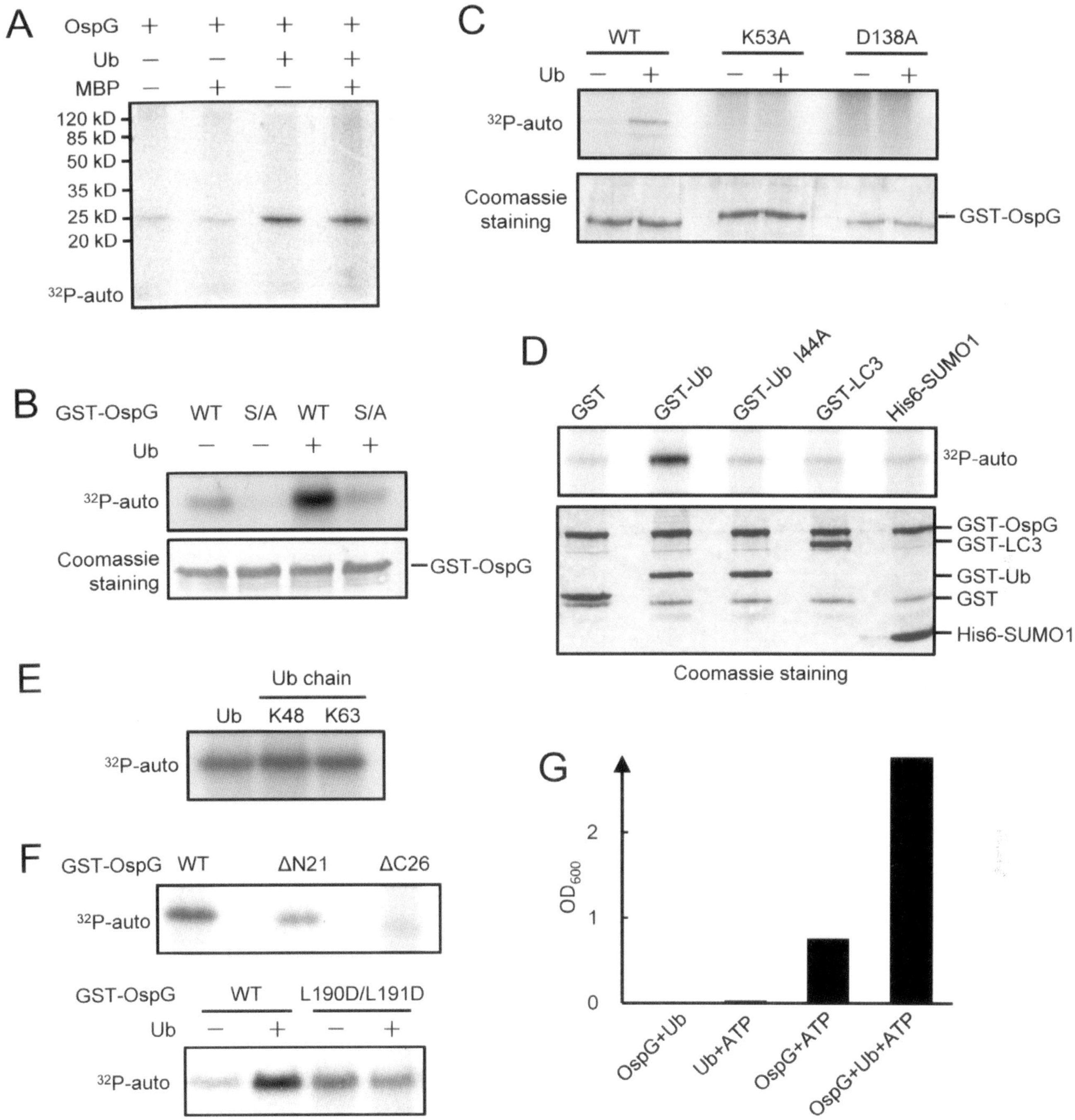

Figure 5. Ubiquitin binding stimulates the autophosphorylation and ATP hydrolysis activity of OspG. (**A**) Kinase assay of OspG in the presence or absence of ubiquitin. Purified OspG protein was incubated with [γ-P^{32}] ATP with or without the addition of ubiquitin into the reaction. Myelin basic protein (MBP) was included as the possible artificial substrate. Incorporation of phosphate into the protein was examined by autoradiography of the reaction mixtures resolved on the SDS-PAGE gel as shown. (**B**) Effects of mutation in the autophosphorylation site of GST-OspG. The autophosphorylated serine residue in the linker region of GST-OspG was mutated into alanine and the mutant protein (S/A) was subjected to the kinase assay in the presence or absence of ubiquitin as described in (A). (**C**) Effects of mutations in the putative catalytic residues on ubiquitin stimulation of OspG kinase activity. Wild-type or indicated mutant GST-OspG (K53A and D138A) proteins were used for the autophosphorylation assay in the presence or absence of ubiquitin. Autophosphorylation of OspG is shown by autoradiography in the upper panel. Coomassie blue staining of GST-OspG proteins are shown in the lower panel. (**D**) Autophosphorylation assay of GST-OspG in the presence of GST-tagged ubiquitin, ubiquitin I44A, LC3 or SUMO1. (**E**) Autophosphorylation assay of GST-OspG in the presence of free ubiquitin, K48- or K63-linked poly-ubiquitin chains. (**F**) Autophosphorylation assay of GST-OspG, GST-OspG ΔN23, GST-OspG ΔC26 or GST-OspG L190D/L191D mutant. The assays were all performed in the presence of ubiquitin. (**G**) ATP hydrolysis assay of OspG and effects of addition of ubiquitin. His6-OspG and ubiquitin were incubated together with or without ATP supplementation. Release of the phosphate following the reaction was detected by measuring the phospho-molybdate complex formation on a spectrometer (absorbance at 600 nm).

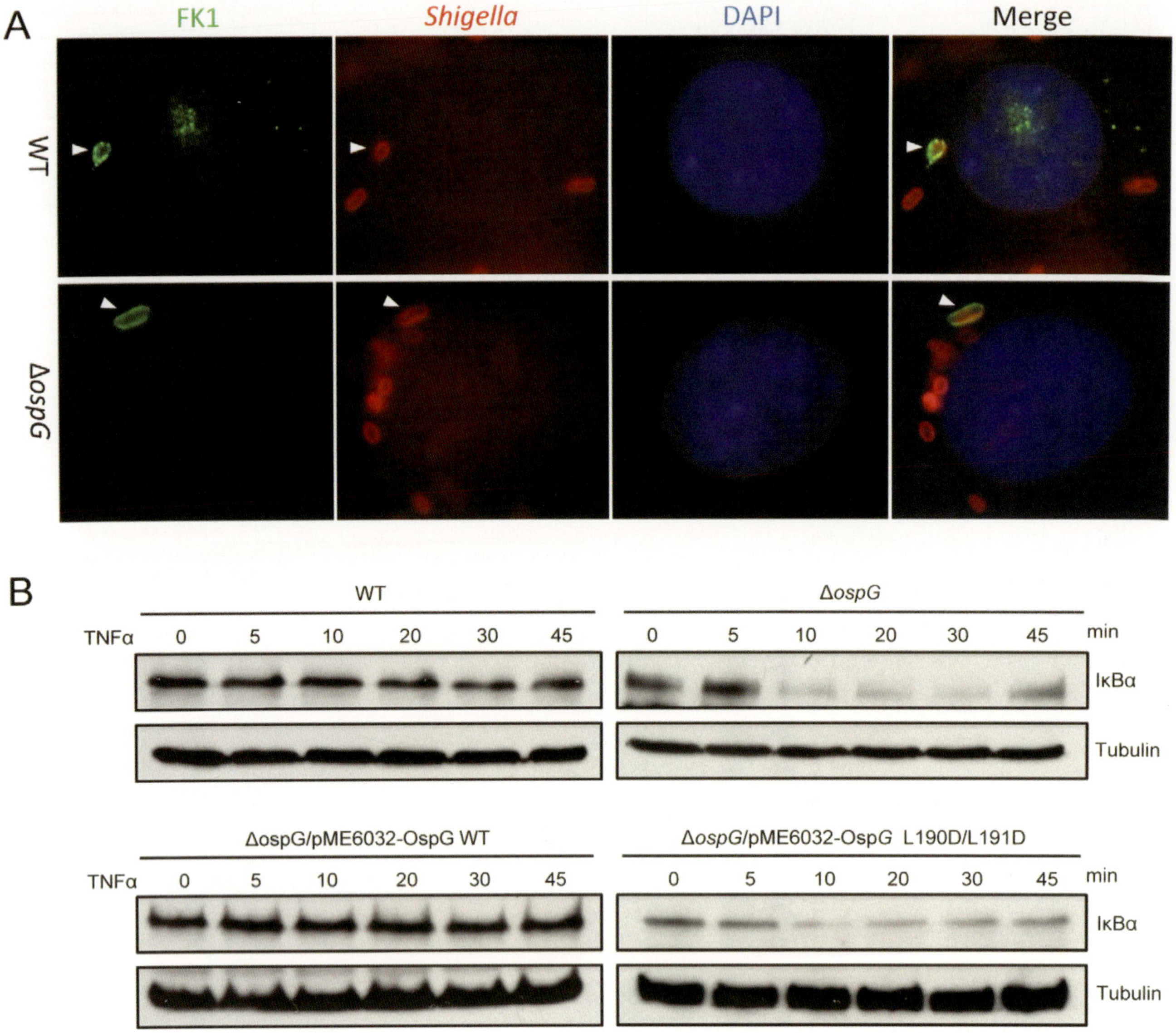

Figure 6. Ubiquitin binding of OspG is required for inhibiting host NF-κB signaling during *Shigella* infection. (**A**) The role of OspG in recruitment of ubiquitin to intracellular *Shigella*. HeLa cells were infected with wild type (WT) or Δ*ospG* mutant *S. flexneri* strain. Polyubiquitinated proteins stained by the FK1 antibody (green), intracellular bacteria stained by anti-*Shigella* antibody (red) and DAPI-stained nuclei (blue) were visualized by fluorescence microscopy. (**B**) The role of OspG ubiquitin binding activity in inhibiting NF-κB activation in *Shigella*-infected cells. HeLa cells were infected with indicated *S. flexneri* strains. Infected cells were treated with TNFα to stimulate NF-κB pathway activation. Lysates of infected cell collected at indicated time points after the stimulation were subjected to anti-IκBα and anti-tubulin immunoblotting analyses.

system, regardless of whether the substrate of OspG kinase is related to the ubiquitin system or not.

The activity of bacterial virulence effectors is often under tight and sophisticated regulation, through which the bacteria can manipulate host processes efficiently and effectively. Turning on the biochemical activity of bacterial type III effectors by binding to host factors have been shown for several other effectors in recent studies. The canonical *Yersinia* serine/threonine kinase effector YpkA has a low or undetectable kinase activity in the bacteria, which is significantly stimulated by actin binding to its extreme carboxyl terminal region [36]. Another type III effector AvrRpt2 from plant pathogen *Pseudomonas syringae* binds to plant cyclophilin protein to turn on its cysteine protease activity [37]. An extensively studied *Yersinia* type III effector YopJ harbors an O-acetyltransferase activity that is promoted by host small molecule inositol hexakisphosphate (IP6) [38]. All these effectors appear to bind to a rather abundant host factor for activation, and this feature also applies to OspG as ubiquitin is one of the most abundant proteins in eukaryotic cells. A general assumption for host activation of bacterial virulence factors is that bacteria, in this way, can prevent effector activities that might be harmful to themselves. This could be the case for the three characterized effectors mentioned above. However, due to the fact that OspG lacks the kinase activation loop as well as the kinase sub-domains VIII–XI, it is also possible that requiring of binding to a host factor for OspG activation might result from the intrinsic structural property of OspG and OspG-like atypical kinase effectors. This further predicts the presence of other distinct host factors that are required for activation of OspG-like NleHs effectors from EPEC/EHEC.

Materials and Methods

Plasmids and Reagents

OspG gene was PCR amplified from the *Shigella flexneri* 2a strain 301. For recombinant expression in *E. coli*, OspG was constructed into pGEX-6P-2 and pET21a vectors. cDNAs for ubiquitin, SUMO1 and LC3 were also subcloned into pGEX-6p-2 to generate GST fusion proteins. Point mutations were generated by the QuikChange site-directed mutagenesis kit (Stratagene). All of the plasmids were verified by DNA sequencing. His6-tagged poly-ubiquitin chains (K48-linked and K63-linked) were purchased from Boston Biochem. Anti-GST (sc-138) and anti-ubiquitin (P4D1, sc-8017) antibodies were from Santa Cruz Biotechnology. Artificial kinase substrates casein from bovine milk and histone from calf thymus were both purchased from Sigma.

Protein Expression and Purification

All recombinant proteins were expressed and purified from *E. coli* BL21 (DE3) strain. Protein expression was induced at room temperature (RT) with 0.4 mM isopropyl-b-D-thiogalactopyranoside (IPTG) for 12 hours when OD_{600} reached 0.6. Cells were harvested and re-suspended in the lysis buffer containing 25 mM HEPES (pH 7.4) and 150 mM NaCl. Cells were lysed by sonication, and the debris was pelleted at 16,000 rpm for 60 minutes. The supernatant was then applied to the corresponding resins for affinity purification. The GST fusion protein was purified by using glutathione-Sepharose resin (GE Healthcare). The His6-tagged fusion protein was purified by using Ni-NTA resin (Qiagen).The resins were washed with the lysis buffer and then eluted with glutathione or immidazole-containing buffer. Eluted proteins were dialyzed against the lysis buffer, concentrated and stored in 20% glycerol at −20°C. Concentrations of purified recombinant proteins were determined by Coomassie blue staining of SDS-PAGE gels using the BSA standards.

Cell Culture and Immunoprecipitation

HEK 293T cells obtained from ATCC were grown in DMEM (Hyclone) supplemented with 10% fetal bovine serum (Gibco) and 2 mM L-glutamine (Hyclone) at 37°C in a 5% CO_2 incubator. To prepare the cell extracts, approximately 1×10^7 cells were washed once with PBS and re-suspended in 1 ml of the lysis buffer (25 mM HEPES, pH 7.4,150 mM NaCl,1 mM DTT, and 1% Triton X-100). The cell lysates were placed on ice for 15 minute and then spun at 13,000 rpm for 15 minute to collect the supernatant. To block proteasomal degradation, cells were treated with 5 μM MG132 for 3 hours prior to lysis. For immunoprecipitation, 293T cells were transiently transfected with Flag-HA-OspG (wild type or indicated mutants). After 24 hours, cells were washed with PBS and lysed for 15 min in a buffer containing 50 mM HEPES (pH 7.4), 150 mM NaCl, and 1% Triton X-100.The lysates were cleared by centrifugation and proteins were immunoprecipitated with anti-Flag M2 beads (Sigma). The immunoprecipitates were washed four times with the lysis buffer and subjected to immunoblotting analysis.

Pulldown and Analytical gel-filtration Binding Assays

For the pulldown assay, ~ 2 μg of proteins were immobilized on Ni-NTA or glutathione-Sepharose resins and the resins were then incubated with 20 μg of prey proteins in 1 mL of binding buffer (25 mM HEPES, pH7.4, 150 mM NaCl, 1% Triton X-100) at 4°C for one hour. The resins were then centrifuged and extensively washed with the binding buffer. Proteins retained on the resins were eluted with an SDS loading buffer (50 mM Tris-HCl, pH6.8, 2% SDS, 10% glycerol, and 100 mM DTT).

To analyze complex formation on the gel filtration column, 200 μg of His6-OspG (23.6 kDa) and 100 μg of Flag-His6-ubiquitin (12.1 kDa) proteins were loaded onto the 24-ml Superdex 75 10/300 column (GE Healthcare) individually or after they were pre-mixed. The column buffer for chromatography contains 25 mM HEPES, pH 7.4, 150 mM NaCl and 1 mM DTT. Fractions of 300 μl each were collected. Aliquots of every other fraction were subjected to SDS-PAGE and Coomassie blue staining analysis.

Kinase and ATP Hydrolysis Assays

2 μg of OspG or GST-OspG were incubated with 2 μCi of [γ-P^{32}] ATP in the kinase assay buffer containing 10 mM HEPES, pH 7.4,10 mM $MgCl_2$ and 10 mM cold ATP at 30°C for 30 minutes.1 μg of ubiquitin and myelin basic protein (MBP) were added into the reaction as indicated. The reactions were quenched with the SDS loading buffer, loaded onto a 15% SDS-PAGE gel and transferred to a PVDF membrane (Millipore). Radioactivity was analyzed by autoradiography.

The ATPase activity of His6-OspG was determined by measuring the release of the inorganic phosphate. The reaction was carried out at 30°C for 30 minutes in a buffer containing 25 mM HEPES (pH 7.4), 150 mM NaCl, 10 mM $MgCl_2$, and 0.5 mM ATP. The reaction was initiated by addition of purified OspG, and quenched by adding 50 μl of molybdate dye/additive mixture (Promega). Following color development, the released inorganic phosphates were measured at the absorbance of 600 nm.

Genetic Manipulation of *Shigella* and Infection Assays

In-frame deletion of *ospG* from *Shigella flexneri* 2a 2457T was performed as previously described [11]. For infection, cultures of indicated *Shigella* strains were added to HeLa cells at MOI of 100 followed by centrifugation at 800 g for 10 min at RT to facilitate bacterial attachment. Infection was performed at 37°C for one hour, and the cells were then washed with PBS and incubated for additional four hours in fresh culture medium supplemented 100 ug/ml gentamicin to kill the extracellular bacteria. To examine ubiquitin recruitment to the bacteria, infected cells were fixed and subjected to immunofluorescence analysis. Bacteria were stained with anti-*Shigella* antibody (Abcam) and the polyubiquitinated proteins were stained with FK1 antibody (Millipore). To assay IκBα degradation, infected cells were treated with 10 ng/mL TNFα for indicated time periods. The cells were then lysed in 2X Laemmli buffer, and the protein samples were loaded onto an SDS-PAGE gel for immunoblotting analysis. For complementation in Δ*ospG* strain, 1 mM IPTG was added to the culture medium to induce OspG expression. To test OspG-ubiquitin interaction, HEK 293T cells were infected with indicated *Shigella* strains harboring Flag-OspG expression plasmid (the Flag tag was inserted into OspG after Asn-17) at MOI of 100 for five hours. Cells were lysed in a buffer containing 25 mM HEPES (pH 7.4), 150 mM NaCl and 0.1% Triton X-100. Cell lysates were cleared by centrifugation and then subjected to anti-Flag immunoprecipitation.

Supporting Information

Figure S1 Autophosphorylation site in GST-OspG and kinase assay of OspG. (**A**) Shown is the amino acid sequence of recombinant GST-OspG protein used in the kinase assay and subjected to mass spectrometry analysis. Residues in red correspond to the tryptic peptide sequence identified by mass spectrometry analysis. The sequence of OspG is underlined. The serine residue identified as the phosphorylation site is shown on a blue background. (**B**) OspG kinase assay using commercial histones as the artificial substrates. The assay was performed in the absence or presence of ubiquitin.

Figure S2 Ubiquitin does not stimulate the kinase activity of OspG-like effector NleH1/2. (**A**) Sequence alignment of *Shigella flexneri* OspG with NleH1/2 from enteropathogenic *Escherichia coli* O55:H7 (strain CB9615). The protein names are listed on the left of the alignment. Conserved residues are marked in pink, and similar residues are shown in green. (**B**) The kinase assay of GST-NleH1 (WT and K159A mutant) and GST-NleH2 (WT and K169A mutant) in the absence or presence of ubiquitin.

Acknowledgments

We thank members of the Shao lab for stimulating discussions and technical assistance.

Author Contributions

Conceived and designed the experiments: YZ FS. Performed the experiments: YZ. Analyzed the data: YZ FS. Contributed reagents/materials/analysis tools: ND LH. Wrote the paper: YZ FS.

References

1. Sansonetti PJ (1998) Pathogenesis of shigellosis: from molecular and cellular biology of epithelial cell invasion to tissue inflammation and vaccine development. Jpn J Med Sci Biol 51 Suppl: S69–80.
2. Sasakawa C, Buysse JM, Watanabe H (1992) The large virulence plasmid of Shigella. Curr Top Microbiol Immunol 180: 21–44.
3. Phalipon A, Sansonetti PJ (2007) Shigella's ways of manipulating the host intestinal innate and adaptive immune system: a tool box for survival? Immunol Cell Biol 85: 119–129.
4. Ogawa M, Handa Y, Ashida H, Suzuki M, Sasakawa C (2008) The versatility of Shigella effectors. Nat Rev Microbiol 6: 11–16.
5. Li H, Xu H, Zhou Y, Zhang J, Long C, et al. (2007) The phosphothreonine lyase activity of a bacterial type III effector family. Science 315: 1000–1003.
6. Arbibe L, Kim DW, Batsche E, Pedron T, Mateescu B, et al. (2007) An injected bacterial effector targets chromatin access for transcription factor NF-kappaB to alter transcription of host genes involved in immune responses. Nat Immunol 8: 47–56.
7. Kramer RW, Slagowski NL, Eze NA, Giddings KS, Morrison MF, et al. (2007) Yeast functional genomic screens lead to identification of a role for a bacterial effector in innate immunity regulation. PLoS Pathog 3: e21.
8. Huang Z, Sutton SE, Wallenfang AJ, Orchard RC, Wu X, et al. (2009) Structural insights into host GTPase isoform selection by a family of bacterial GEF mimics. Nat Struct Mol Biol 16: 853–860.
9. Ohya K, Handa Y, Ogawa M, Suzuki M, Sasakawa C (2005) IpgB1 is a novel Shigella effector protein involved in bacterial invasion of host cells. Its activity to promote membrane ruffling via Rac1 and Cdc42 activation. J Biol Chem 280: 24022–24034.
10. Handa Y, Suzuki M, Ohya K, Iwai H, Ishijima N, et al. (2007) Shigella IpgB1 promotes bacterial entry through the ELMO-Dock180 machinery. Nat Cell Biol 9: 121–128.
11. Dong N, Zhu Y, Lu Q, Hu L, Zheng Y, et al. (2012) Structurally Distinct Bacterial TBC-like GAPs Link Arf GTPase to Rab1 Inactivation to Counteract Host Defenses. Cell 150: 1029–1041.
12. Schwartz AL, Ciechanover A (1999) The ubiquitin-proteasome pathway and pathogenesis of human diseases. Annu Rev Med 50: 57–74.
13. Komander D, Rape M (2012) The ubiquitin code. Annu Rev Biochem 81: 203–229.
14. Rytkonen A, Holden DW (2007) Bacterial interference of ubiquitination and deubiquitination. Cell Host Microbe 1: 13–22.
15. Jiang X, Chen ZJ (2012) The role of ubiquitylation in immune defence and pathogen evasion. Nat Rev Immunol 12: 35–48.
16. Cui J, Yao Q, Li S, Ding X, Lu Q, et al. (2010) Glutamine deamidation and dysfunction of ubiquitin/NEDD8 induced by a bacterial effector family. Science 329: 1215–1218.
17. Sanada T, Kim M, Mimuro H, Suzuki M, Ogawa M, et al. (2012) The Shigella flexneri effector OspI deamidates UBC13 to dampen the inflammatory response. Nature 483: 623–626.
18. Rohde JR, Breitkreutz A, Chenal A, Sansonetti PJ, Parsot C (2007) Type III secretion effectors of the IpaH family are E3 ubiquitin ligases. Cell Host Microbe 1: 77–83.
19. Singer AU, Rohde JR, Lam R, Skarina T, Kagan O, et al. (2008) Structure of the Shigella T3SS effector IpaH defines a new class of E3 ubiquitin ligases. Nat Struct Mol Biol 15: 1293–1301.
20. Zhu Y, Li H, Hu L, Wang J, Zhou Y, et al. (2008) Structure of a Shigella effector reveals a new class of ubiquitin ligases. Nat Struct Mol Biol 15: 1302–1308.
21. Ashida H, Kim M, Schmidt-Supprian M, Ma A, Ogawa M, et al. (2010) A bacterial E3 ubiquitin ligase IpaH9.8 targets NEMO/IKKgamma to dampen the host NF-kappaB-mediated inflammatory response. Nat Cell Biol 12: 66–73; sup 61–69.
22. Buchrieser C, Glaser P, Rusniok C, Nedjari H, D'Hauteville H, et al. (2000) The virulence plasmid pWR100 and the repertoire of proteins secreted by the type III secretion apparatus of Shigella flexneri. Mol Microbiol 38: 760–771.
23. Le Gall T, Mavris M, Martino MC, Bernardini ML, Denamur E, et al. (2005) Analysis of virulence plasmid gene expression defines three classes of effectors in the type III secretion system of Shigella flexneri. Microbiology 151: 951–962.
24. Kim DW (2005) The Shigella flexneri effector OspG interferes with innate immune responses by targeting ubiquitin-conjugating enzymes. Proceedings of the National Academy of Sciences 102: 14046–14051.
25. Hurley JH, Lee S, Prag G (2006) Ubiquitin-binding domains. Biochem J 399: 361–372.
26. Husnjak K, Dikic I (2012) Ubiquitin-binding proteins: decoders of ubiquitin-mediated cellular functions. Annu Rev Biochem 81: 291–322.
27. Hochstrasser M (2009) Origin and function of ubiquitin-like proteins. Nature 458: 422–429.
28. van der Veen AG, Ploegh HL (2012) Ubiquitin-like proteins. Annu Rev Biochem 81: 323–357.
29. Cheek S, Zhang H, Grishin NV (2002) Sequence and structure classification of kinases. J Mol Biol 320: 855–881.
30. Taylor SS, Radzio-Andzelm E (1994) Three protein kinase structures define a common motif. Structure 2: 345–355.
31. Hemrajani C, Berger CN, Robinson KS, Marches O, Mousnier A, et al. (2010) NleH effectors interact with Bax inhibitor-1 to block apoptosis during enteropathogenic Escherichia coli infection. Proc Natl Acad Sci U S A 107: 3129–3134.
32. Chen G, Porter MD, Bristol JR, Fitzgibbon MJ, Pazhanisamy S (2000) Kinetic mechanism of the p38-alpha MAP kinase: phosphoryl transfer to synthetic peptides. Biochemistry 39: 2079–2087.
33. Mendelow M, Prorok M, Salerno A, Lawrence DS (1993) ATPase-promoting dead end inhibitors of the cAMP-dependent protein kinase. J Biol Chem 268: 12289–12296.
34. Young PR, McLaughlin MM, Kumar S, Kassis S, Doyle ML, et al. (1997) Pyridinyl imidazole inhibitors of p38 mitogen-activated protein kinase bind in the ATP site. J Biol Chem 272: 12116–12121.
35. Ward NE, O'Brian CA (1992) The intrinsic ATPase activity of protein kinase C is catalyzed at the active site of the enzyme. Biochemistry 31: 5905–5911.
36. Juris SJ, Rudolph AE, Huddler D, Orth K, Dixon JE (2000) A distinctive role for the Yersinia protein kinase: actin binding, kinase activation, and cytoskeleton disruption. Proc Natl Acad Sci U S A 97: 9431–9436.
37. Coaker G, Falick A, Staskawicz B (2005) Activation of a phytopathogenic bacterial effector protein by a eukaryotic cyclophilin. Science 308: 548–550.
38. Mittal R, Peak-Chew SY, Sade RS, Vallis Y, McMahon HT (2010) The acetyltransferase activity of the bacterial toxin YopJ of Yersinia is activated by eukaryotic host cell inositol hexakisphosphate. J Biol Chem 285: 19927–19934.

5

Characteristics of Diarrheal Illnesses in Non-Breast Fed Infants Attending a Large Urban Diarrheal Disease Hospital in Bangladesh

Sanjoy Kumer Dey[1], Mohammod Jobayer Chisti[2], Sumon Kumar Das[2], Chandan Kumar Shaha[1], Farzana Ferdous[2], Fahmida Dil Farzana[2], Shahnawaz Ahmed[2], Mohammad Abdul Malek[2], Abu Syed Golam Faruque[2]*, Tahmeed Ahmed[2], Mohammed Abdus Salam[3]

1 Department of Neonatology, Bangabandhu Sheikh Mujib Medical University (BSMMU), Dhaka, Bangladesh, **2** Centre for Nutrition and Food Security (CNFS), International Centre for Diarrhoeal Disease Research, Bangladesh (icddr,b), Dhaka, Bangladesh, **3** Research Administration Services (RAS), icddr,b, Dhaka, Bangladesh

Abstract

Background: Lack of breast feeding is associated with higher morbidity and case-fatality from both bacterial and viral etiologic diarrheas. However, there is very limited data on the characteristics of non-breastfed infants attending hospital with diarrheal illnesses caused by common bacterial and viral pathogens. Our objective was to assess the impact of lack of breast feeding on diarrheal illnesses in infants living in urban Bangladesh.

Methods: We extracted data of infants (0–11 months) for analyses from the data archive of Diarrheal Disease Surveillance System (DDSS) of the Dhaka Hospital of icddr,b for the period 2008–2011.

Results: The prevalence of breastfeeding in infants attending the hospital with diarrhea reduced from 31% in 2008 to 17% in 2011, with corresponding increase in the prevalence of non-breastfed (chi square for trend <0.001). Among breastfed infants, the incidence of rotavirus infections was higher (43%) among the 0–5 months age group than infants aged 9–11 months (18%). On the other hand, among non-breastfed infants, the incidence of rotavirus infections was much higher (82%) among 9–11 months old infants compared to those in 0–5 months age group (57%) (chi square for trend <0.001). Very similar trends were also observed in the incidence of cholera and ETEC diarrheas among different age groups of breastfed and non-breastfed infants (chi square for trend 0.020 and 0.001 respectively). However, for shigellosis, the statistical difference remained unchanged among both the groups (chi square for trend 0.240).

Conclusion and Significance: We observed protective role of breastfeeding in infantile diarrhea caused by the major viral and common bacterial agents. These findings underscore the importance of promotion and expansion of breastfeeding campaigns in Bangladesh and elsewhere.

Editor: Li-Min Huang, National Taiwan University Hospital, Taiwan

Funding: The Diarrhoeal Disease Surveillance System at the Dhaka Hospital of icddr,b was funded by icddr,b and the Government of the People's Republic of Bangladesh through its IHP under HNPSP. icddr,b acknowledges with gratitude the commitment of the Government of the People's Republic of Bangladesh to its research efforts. icddr,b also gratefully acknowledges the following donors which provide unrestricted support to the Centre's research efforts: Australian Agency for International Development (AusAID), Government of the People's Republic of Bangladesh, Canadian International Development Agency (CIDA), Embassy of the Kingdom of the Netherlands (EKN), Swedish International Development Cooperation Agency (Sida), Swiss Agency for Development and Cooperation (SDC), and Department for International Development, UK (DFID). The funders had no role in study design, data collection and analysis, decision to publish, or preparation of the manuscript.

Competing Interests: The authors have declared that no competing interests exist.

* E-mail: gfaruque@icddrb.org

Introduction

In developing countries, diarrheal diseases, as a group, remains the leading cause of illness and the second leading cause of death among young children, particularly during the first two years of their lives. Diarrheal diseases accounted for 11% of the estimated 7.6 million under-five deaths, globally, in 2010 [1]. In Bangladesh, 11% of all under-five deaths (n = 182,936) was due to diarrhea [2]. Guidelines for the management of diarrheal illnesses have been refined, and new strategies for prevention and control of this major health problem have also been developed [3]. In developing countries, children are exposed to a wide range of enteric bacterial pathogens even at a very early age and suffer from frequent episodes of diarrheal illnesses. The distribution of predominant bacterial pathogens varies with the age of the children, which also vary by geographic locations as well as demonstrates seasonal and secular trends. The diarrheagenic *Escherichia coli*, *Shigella* spp., *Campylobacter* spp., and *Vibrio* are the common bacterial pathogens causing diarrhea in young children in developing countries, including Bangladesh [3]. Globally, rotavirus is one of the most common causes of dehydrating gastroenteritis among children younger than two years, which accounts for one-third of all hospitalizations for diarrhea and an estimated 500,000 deaths each year [4]. Compared to industrialized countries, children in the developing countries experience their first severe infection with rotavirus at a younger age, which follows distinct seasonal pattern, with winter peak, and they often are infected with multiple or un-typable strains of rotavirus [5]. The relationship between lack of breast feeding and diarrhea is well established [6,7,8,9,10,11]. Non- breastfeeding is also associated with malnutrition, and diarrhea among this population caused by common enteric pathogens with higher risks for deaths [12,13].

The human-milk glycans, which include oligosaccharides in their free and conjugated forms, constitute a major and an innate immunologic mechanism by which human milk protects breast-fed infants against infections [10]. Although there is increased overall literacy rate as well as emphasis has been given on early initiation and continued breastfeeding, sustained, high level of continued breastfeeding has not been achieved. There is limited recent information on the etiology of infantile diarrhea and distribution of pathogens by breastfeeding status of the infants. We, therefore, used a large database to analyze distribution of breastfeeding status among infants attending a large diarrheal disease treatment facility in Bangladesh, and examined distribution of diarrhoeal pathogen among breastfed and non-breastfed infants as well as by their age groups.

Materials and Methods

Ethical Statement

The Diarrhoeal Disease Surveillance System of icddr,b is a routine activity of the Dhaka Hospital, which has been approved by the Research Review Committee (RRC) and Ethical Review Committee (ERC) of icddr,b and this study has been approved by the RRC and ERC of icddr,b. Verbal consent was taken from the caregivers, or guardians on the behalf of the patients, for their information to be stored in the hospital database and used for research. Although the Diarrhoeal Disease Surveillance System of icddr,b is a routine activity for hospital patients, and used to be done only with verbal consent from the parents or guardians of the patients following the hospital policy, parents or guardians were assured about the non-disclosure of information collected from them, and were also informed about the use of data for analysis and using the results for improving patient care activities as well as publication without disclosing the name or identity of their children. ERC was quite satisfied with voluntary participation, the maintenance of the rights of the participants and confidential handling of personal information by the hospital physicians and approved this consent procedure.

Study Population and Site

The study was conducted at the Dhaka Hospital of icddr,b. Located in the Dhaka, the capital city of Bangladesh, the hospital provides care and treatment to around 140,000 patients each year, vast majority of whom are under five children. Diarrhea is the common feature among the patients, whether or not they are associated with diarrhea-related complications or other health problems, while malnutrition is a common health problem in under-five children. The hospital also conducts research on enteric infections caused by common pathogens including rotavirus, ETEC, *V. cholerae*, and *Shigella*; acute respiratory infections; and malnutrition; and provides training to health care providers on case management and research methodology. Infants (0–11 months old), constitute about 28% of all attending patients. The majority of the patients come from poor socio-economic backgrounds, who live in urban and peri urban Dhaka.

Study Design

For this descriptive study, we stratified infants by their etiologic agents then compared them by their breastfeeding status. Infants receiving any amount of breast milk at their current episode of diarrhea were defined as breast-fed and those not receiving any amount of breast milk constituted non-breast-fed infants in our analyses. Age stratification was done taking into consideration that exclusive breastfeeding should be continued till the end of age as 0–5 months (recommended age of exclusive breastfeeding), 6–8 months are the time when most of the infants receive their

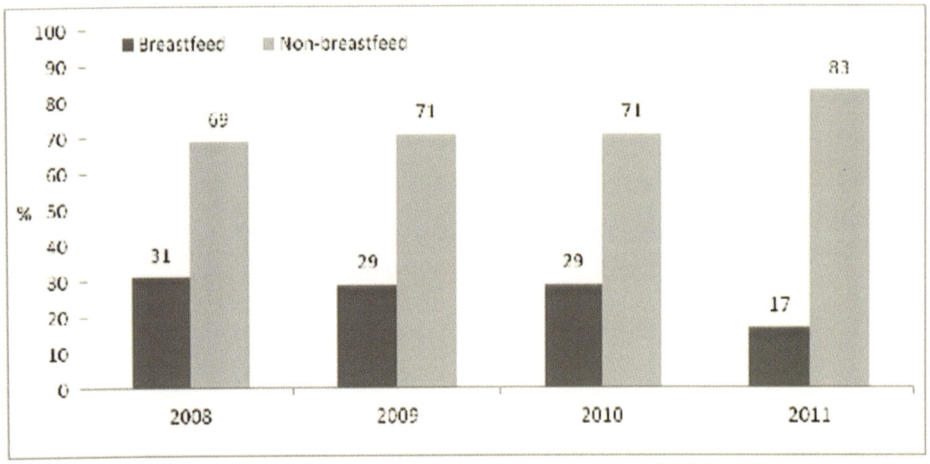

	Breastfeed	Non-breastfeed	OR (95% CI) p value
2008; n=690 (%)	214 (31)	476 (69)	1.36 (1.12, 1.65) 0.001
2009; n=658 (%)	190 (29)	468 (71)	1.18 (0.97, 1.44) 0.104
2010; n=754 (%)	221 (29)	533 (71)	1.12 (1.01, 1.48) 0.035
2011; n=767 (%)	131 (17)	636 (83)	0.49 (0.39, 0.60) <0.001

Figure 1. Yearly distribution of proportion of breastfeeding status of infants attending the hospital with diarrhea during 2008–11.

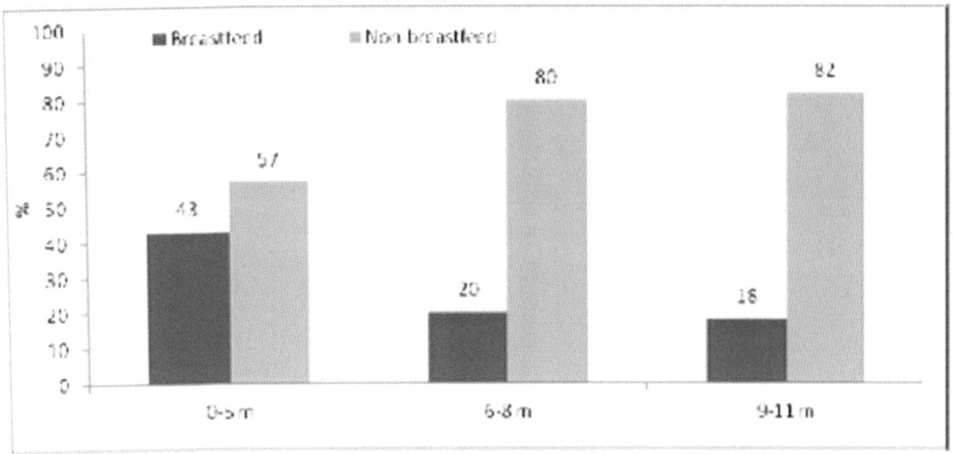

	Breastfeed	Non-breastfeed	OR (95% CI) p value
0-5 months; n=349 (%)	150 (43)	199 (57)	3.25 (2.48, 4.26) <0.001
6-8 months; n=575 (%)	112 (20)	463 (80)	0.70 (0.54, 0.90) 0.005
9-11 months; n=498 (%)	90 (18)	408 (82)	0.56 (0.42, 0.74) < 0.001

Figure 2. Age stratified proportion of rotavirus among breastfed and non-breastfed infants presented in the Dhaka Hospital, 2008–11.

complementary feeding (beginning of the weaning food), and 9–11 months (post supplementary feeding when infants gradually switch to their family food).

Source of Data and Hospital Surveillance System

icddr,b maintains a Diarrheal Disease Surveillance System (DDSS) at its Dhaka Hospital since 1979 [14]. The system currently enrolls a systematic 2% sample of all patients (every 50th patient, regardless of age, sex and diarrhea severity) and records their socio-demographic and environmental history; nutritional and clinical characteristics; immunization status and feeding practices (this data is collected for only those younger than 3 years); hygienic practices in the family; and determines the etiology of diarrhea along with antimicrobial susceptibility of common bacterial pathogens. Trained research assistants interview patients (patients or a female caregiver in the event of minors) using a standardized questionnaire, performs anthropometry using standard techniques, and records findings in pre-tested case report forms (CRFs). A physician obtains medical history, performs thorough physical examination, and records findings in the CRFs.

Specimen Collection and Laboratory Procedure

A fresh stool specimen is routinely collected from the surveillance patients for screening of common enteric pathogens

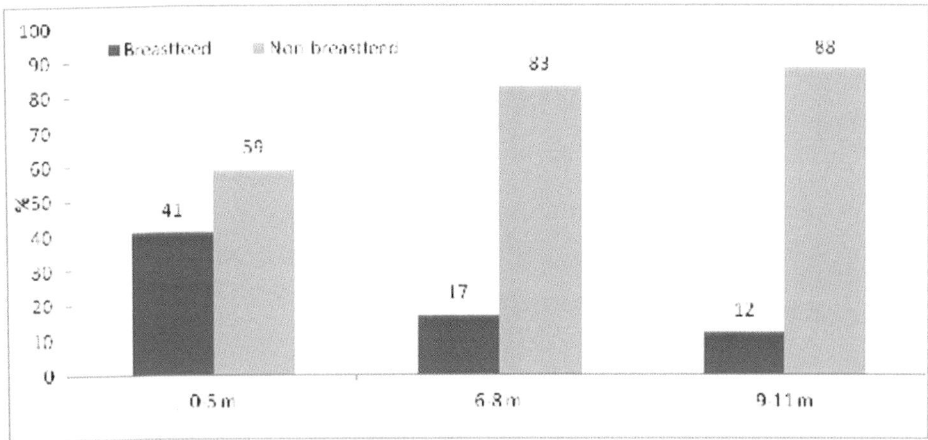

	Breastfeed	Non-breastfeed	OR (95% CI) p value
0-5 months; n=22 (%)	9 (41)	13 (59)	4.05 (1.10, 15.40) 0.033
6-8 months; n=23 (%)	4 (17)	19 (83)	0.61 (0.14, 2.47) 0.646
9-11 months; n=25 (%)	3 (12)	22 (88)	6.34 (0.07, 1.49) 0.188

Figure 3. Age stratified proportion of *Vibrio cholerae* O1 among breastfed and non-breastfed infants presented in the Dhaka Hospital, 2008–11.

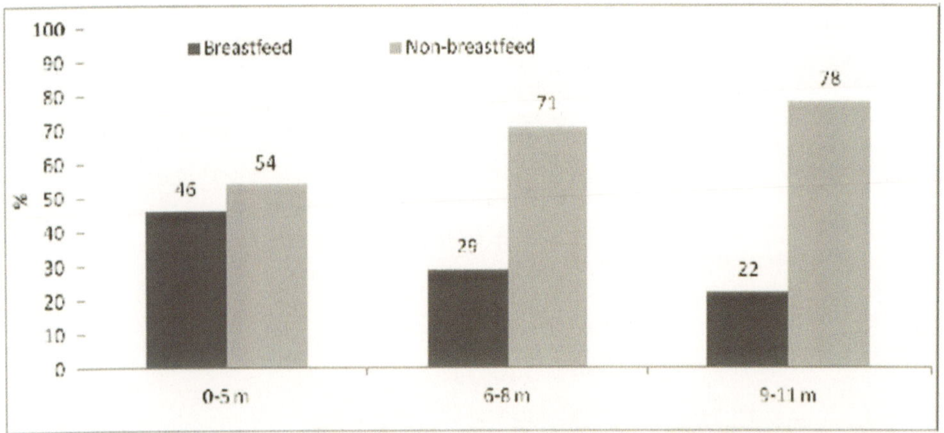

	Breastfeed	Non-breastfeed	OR (95% CI) p value
0-5 months; n=67 (%)	31 (46)	36 (54)	2.57 (1.38, 4.78) 0.002
6-8 months; n=90 (%)	26 (29)	64 (71)	0.88 (0.48, 1.60) 0.764
9-11 months; n=101 (%)	22 (22)	79 (78)	0.49 (0.26, 0.90) 0.019

Figure 4. Age stratified proportion of ETEC among breastfed and non-breastfed infants presented in the Dhaka Hospital, 2008–11.

such as rotavirus [15]; ETEC ([16]), *Vibrio cholerae* [17], and *Shigella* spp. [17] by standard methods.

Data Analysis

We extracted relevant information from the electronic database of the Diarrheal Disease Surveillance System for our analyses for the period 2008–2011. In total, 2,869 infants (aged 0–11 months) of both sex, attended the hospital during this study period.

We used Statistical Package for Social Sciences (SPSS) Windows (Version 15.2; Chicago, IL) for data entry and analysis. We calculated the proportion of both breastfed and non-breastfed infants infected with enteropathogens (rotavirus, ETEC, *V. cholerae*, and *Shigella*) causing diarrhea with a view to describe their hospital visit patterns due to diarrheal illnesses in a large urban diarrheal disease hospital in Bangladesh. We have also calculated age stratified proportion of diarrhea pathogens among the breastfed and non-breastfed infants and yearly distribution of different diarrhea pathogens among the breastfed infants. We used Chi-square for trend to test statistical significance of the changing trend by year and age [18] and the assumptions were; the sample was random, each observation was classified into one cell only, and sample size was sufficiently large with adequate cell counts, 5 or more in all cells [19]. A probability of less than 0.05 was considered statistically significant. Strength of association was determined by calculating odds ratio (OR) and their 95% confidence intervals (CIs).

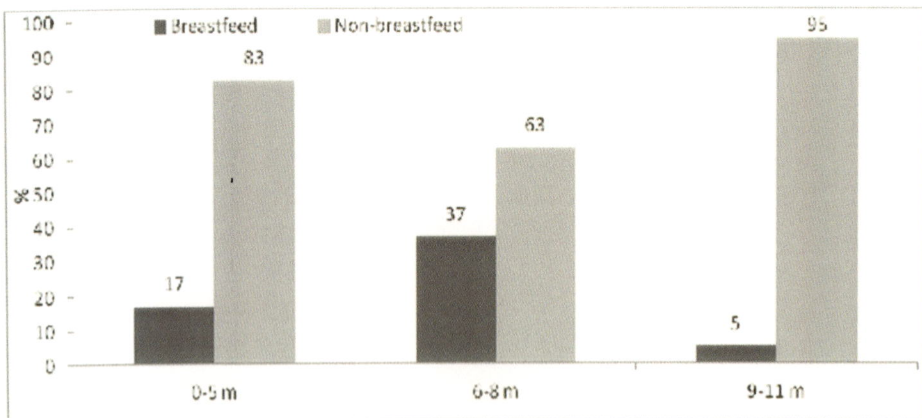

	Breastfeed	Non-breastfeed	OR (95% CI) p value
0-5 months; n=12 (%)	2 (17)	10 (83)	0.77 (0.10, 5.10) 1.000
6-8 months; n=19 (%)	7 (37)	12 (63)	5.64 (1.04, 33.90) 0.027
9-11 months; n=20 (%)	1 (5)	19 (95)	0.13 (0.01, 1.18) 0.067

Figure 5. Age stratified proportion of *Shigella* among breastfed and non-breastfed infants presented in the Dhaka Hospital, 2008–11.

Table 1. Age stratified proportion of diarrhea pathogens among the breastfed and non-breastfed infants.

	Breastfeed n = 756 (%)	Non-breastfeed n = 2113 (%)	OR (95% CI); p value
0–5 months	192 (25)	258 (12)	2.45 (1.97, 3.03); <0.001
6–8 months	149 (20)	558 (26)	0.68 (0.56, 0.84); <0.001
9–11 months	116 (15)	528 (25)	0.54 (0.43, 0.63); <0.001

Figures represent n (%) unless indicated otherwise.

Table 2. Yearly distribution of diarrhea pathogens among breastfed infants.

Name of the pathogens	2008 n = 214 (%)	2009 n = 190 (%)	2010 n = 221 (%)	2011 n = 131 (%)
Rotavirus	110 (52)	96 (51)	93 (43)	53 (41)
Vibrio cholerae O1	6 (3)	4 (2)	6 (3)	0
ETEC	35 (16)	15 (8)	15 (7)	14 (11)
Shigella	5 (2)	2 (1)	1 (0.5)	2 (2)

Figures represent n (%) unless indicated otherwise.

Results

The proportion of breast-fed infants gradually fell from 31% in 2008 to 17% in 2011, with gradual increase in the proportion of non-breast-fed infants from 69% to 83% during the same time period (chi square for trend <0.001) (Figure 1). Rotavirus was identified from 43% of breastfed infants aged 0–5 months which gradually reduced to 18% in 9–11 months old; while among the non-breast-fed the proportion infected with this pathogen was 57% in the 0–5 months age groups which increased to to 82% among 9–11 months (chi square for trend <0.001) (Figure 2). Similar observations were made for cholera and ETEC diarrheas among infants (Figure 3 and 4). Although the proportion of breast-fed infants with shigellosis increased to 37% at 6–8 months which was 17% at 0–5 months old, an insignificant rising trend with increasing age was observed among non-breastfed infants (chi square for trend 0.241) (Figure 5). Age stratified proportion of diarrhea pathogens among the breastfed and non-breastfed infants and yearly distribution of different diarrhea pathogens among the breastfed infants have also been shown in table 1 and 2 respectively as the summary results.

Discussion

We noted lesser proportion of hospital visits by breastfed infants infected with all the enteric pathogens we analyzed than non-breastfed infants. Breast milk contains non-inflammatogenic secretory immunoglobulin A (sIgA) antibodies that protects intestinal mucosa against the attack from *Vibrio cholerae*, ETEC, *Campylobacter*, and *Shigella* [11,20,21,22], which explains our findings. Literature suggests protective role of breastfeeding against shigellosis and cholera among infants older than 6 months. [8]. However, the breastfed compared to non-breastfed 0–5 months age groups infected with *Shigella* failed to gain statistical significance might be due to small sample size. Our observation of higher proportion of non-breastfed infants with rotavirus is also consistent with earlier observation [23]. The proportions were similar at the beginning but that changed later because of attrition of breastfeeding rate. A Bangladeshi study among infants reported high levels of neutralizing activity among only 20% of the breast milks and low protective efficacy of breast milks against rotavirus strains [24], another well designed case-control study from the same country reported significant protective role of breast milk during the infancy [25]. In another well designed epidemiologic study among Egyptian infants with rotavirus diarrhea, breastfeeding has been observed to be associated with a lower incidence of rotavirus diarrhea and recommended the promotion of breastfeeding along with improvements in water and sanitation for reducing rotavirus diarrhea [26]. We also noted protective role of breastfeeding in infants older than 5 months. However, the protective role in case of shigellosis at 6–8 months was less pronounced among breastfed and this could be due to more virulence of the organism, low infective dose, and lack of immune-competency among infants of that age group. As *Shigella* is the most virulent organism among the all organisms that have been studied here and consequently acquiring immunity against *Shigella* even during continuation of breast milk sometimes may take longer period and our observation of statistical insignificant difference of proportion of *Shigella* isolates in infants between 6–8 months of age among the breast-fed and non-breast-fed groups might also be due to the same reason [22,27,28].

The overall results from the study tell us that the proportion of breast-fed infants with diarrhea is reducing, while the national data gathered from the general population without diarrhoea suggests an increase in prevalence of exclusive breastfeeding among infants. Thus the data indicates lack of protection from breast milk against diarrhoeal disease among the non-breastfed infants. However, the population who reported to the facility was the special population with disease condition resulting from the lack of adherence to the breast feeding which had a potential role for this observation.

The main limitation of the study is that study observations are based on infants who attended the hospital and thus our data may not represent the general population because infants with less severe disease less often seek care from hospital facilities. However, systematic sampling of patients including infants and large data set are among strengths of our analyses. Moreover, despite variations, some differences were not statistically significant possibly due to lack of power with small sample size.

In summary, the present study documented the proportion of breastfed infants significantly decreased over the period.The study finding transparently produces evidence of the protective role of breastfeeding against the most common enteropathogens that cause diarrhea compared to those who were non-breastfed. So, there is a large scale need to give more emphasis on breastfeeding promotion campaigning as well as strengthen the current resources and infrastructures for breastfeeding counseling programs. At the same time, a cohort study in different facilities may be conducted to examine if the results of our study are similar in cases of children presenting with other non-diarrheal but infectious diseases.

Acknowledgments

We would like to express our sincere thanks to all physicians, clinical fellows, nurses, members of breast-feeding counselors, feeding team and cleaners of the hospital for their invaluable support and contribution during patient enrollment and data collection.

Author Contributions

Coordinated the writing within the authors: S. K. Dey. Patient care and management: MJC S. K. Das ASGF TA MAS. Conceived and designed the experiments: S. K. Dey MJC S. K. Das CKS FF FDF SA MAM ASGF TA MAS. Performed the experiments: S. K. Dey MJC S. K. Das CKS ASGF TA MAS. Analyzed the data: S. K. Dey MJC S. K. Das CKSS FF FDF SA MAM ASGF. Contributed reagents/materials/analysis tools: S. K. Dey MJC S. K. Das CKS FF FDF SA MAM ASGF TA MAS. Wrote the paper: S. K. Dey MJC S. K. Das CKS FF FDF SA MAM ASGF TA MAS.

References

1. Liu L, Johnson HL, Cousens S, Perin J, Scott S, et al. (2012) Global, regional, and national causes of child mortality: an updated systematic analysis for 2010 with time trends since 2000. Lancet.
2. Black RE, Cousens S, Johnson HL, Lawn JE, Rudan I, et al. (2010) Global, regional, and national causes of child mortality in 2008: a systematic analysis. Lancet 375: 1969–1987.
3. Podewils LJ, Mintz ED, Nataro JP, Parashar UD (2004) Acute, infectious diarrhea among children in developing countries. Semin Pediatr Infect Dis 15: 155–168.
4. Glass RI, Bresee J, Parashar UD (2003) The global burden of dehydrating disease In: Farthing MJ, Mahalanabis D, editors. The Control of Food and Fluid Intake in Health and Disease. Philadelphia: Vevey Nestec Ltd. and Lippincott Williams & Wilkins. 17–30.
5. Bresee JS, Glass RI, Ivanoff B, Gentsch JR (1999) Current status and future priorities for rotavirus vaccine development, evaluation and implementation in developing countries. Vaccine 17: 2207–2222.
6. Morrow AL, Rangel JM (2004) Human milk protection against infectious diarrhea: implications for prevention and clinical care. Semin Pediatr Infect Dis 15: 221–228.
7. Torres O, Cruz JR (1993) Protection against Campylobacter diarrhea: role of milk IgA antibodies against bacterial surface antigens. Acta Paediatr 82: 835–838.
8. Glass RI, Stoll BJ (1989) The protective effect of human milk against diarrhea. A review of studies from Bangladesh. Acta Paediatr Scand Suppl 351: 131–136.
9. Morrow AL, Ruiz-Palacios GM, Altaye M, Jiang X, Guerrero ML, et al. (2004) Human milk oligosaccharides are associated with protection against diarrhea in breast-fed infants. J Pediatr 145: 297–303.
10. Morrow AL, Ruiz-Palacios GM, Jiang X, Newburg DS (2005) Human-milk glycans that inhibit pathogen binding protect breast-feeding infants against infectious diarrhea. J Nutr 135: 1304–1307.
11. Ruiz-Palacios GM, Calva JJ, Pickering LK, Lopez-Vidal Y, Volkow P, et al. (1990) Protection of breast-fed infants against Campylobacter diarrhea by antibodies in human milk. J Pediatr 116: 707–713.
12. Rice AL, Sacco L, Hyder A, Black RE (2000) Malnutrition as an underlying cause of childhood deaths associated with infectious diseases in developing countries. Bull World Health Organ 78: 1207–1221.
13. Chisti MJ, Pietroni MA, Smith JH, Bardhan PK, Salam MA (2011) Predictors of death in under-five children with diarrhoea admitted to a critical care ward in an urban hospital in Bangladesh. Acta Paediatr 100: e275–279.
14. Faruque AS, Malek MA, Khan AI, Huq S, Salam MA, et al. (2004) Diarrhoea in elderly people: aetiology, and clinical characteristics. Scand J Infect Dis 36: 204–208.
15. Rahman M, De Leener K, Goegebuer T, Wollants E, Van der Donck I, et al. (2003) Genetic characterization of a novel, naturally occurring recombinant human G6P [6] rotavirus. J Clin Microbiol 41: 2088–2095.
16. Qadri F, Khan AI, Faruque AS, Begum YA, Chowdhury F, et al. (2005) Enterotoxigenic Escherichia coli and Vibrio cholerae diarrhea, Bangladesh, 2004. Emerg Infect Dis 11: 1104–1107.
17. (1987) Programme for control of diarrheal disease. In Manual for laboratory investigation of acute enteric infections. Geneva, Switzerland: World Health Organization. 9–20 p.
18. Armitage P (1955) Tests for Linear Trends in Proportions and Frequencies. Biometrics 11: 375–386.
19. Macaulay D, Blackhall MI (1961) Hypernatraemic dehydration in infantile gastro-enteritis. Arch Dis Child 36: 543–550.
20. Glass RI, Svennerholm AM, Stoll BJ, Khan MR, Hossain KM, et al. (1983) Protection against cholera in breast-fed children by antibodies in breast milk. N Engl J Med 308: 1389–1392.
21. Cruz JR, Gil L, Cano F, Caceres P, Pareja G (1988) Breast milk anti-Escherichia coli heat-labile toxin IgA antibodies protect against toxin-induced infantile diarrhea. Acta Paediatr Scand 77: 658–662.
22. Hayani KC, Guerrero ML, Morrow AL, Gomez HF, Winsor DK, et al. (1992) Concentration of milk secretory immunoglobulin A against Shigella virulence plasmid-associated antigens as a predictor of symptom status in Shigella-infected breast-fed infants. J Pediatr 121: 852–856.
23. Strina A, Rodrigues LC, Cairncross S, Ferrer SR, Fialho AM, et al. (2012) Factors associated with rotavirus diarrhoea in children living in a socially diverse urban centre in Brazil. Trans R Soc Trop Med Hyg 106: 445–451.
24. Glass RI, Stoll BJ, Wyatt RG, Hoshino Y, Banu H, et al. (1986) Observations questioning a protective role for breast-feeding in severe rotavirus diarrhea. Acta Paediatr Scand 75: 713–718.
25. Clemens J, Rao M, Ahmed F, Ward R, Huda S, et al. (1993) Breast-feeding and the risk of life-threatening rotavirus diarrhea: prevention or postponement? Pediatrics 92: 680–685.
26. Naficy AB, Abu-Elyazeed R, Holmes JL, Rao MR, Savarino SJ, et al. (1999) Epidemiology of rotavirus diarrhea in Egyptian children and implications for disease control. Am J Epidemiol 150: 770–777.
27. Hayani KC, Guerrero ML, Ruiz-Palacios GM, Gomez HF, Cleary TG (1991) Evidence for long-term memory of the mucosal immune system: milk secretory immunoglobulin A against Shigella lipopolysaccharides. J Clin Microbiol 29: 2599–2603.
28. Hanson LA, Hahn-Zoric M, Berndes M, Ashraf R, Herias V, et al. (1994) Breast feeding: overview and breast milk immunology. Acta Paediatr Jpn 36: 557–561.

6

Serotype Diversity of Astroviruses in Rawalpindi, Pakistan during 2009–2010

Muhammad Masroor Alam[1], Adnan Khurshid[2], Muhammad Suleman Rana[2], Shahzad Shaukat[2], Salmaan Sharif[2], Mehar Angez[2], Muhammad Naeem[1], Syed Sohail Zahoor Zaidi[2]*

1 Department of Biotechnology, Quaid-i-Azam University, Islamabad, Pakistan, **2** Department of Virology, National Institute of Health, Islamabad, Pakistan

Abstract

Astroviruses are globally known enteropathogens causing gastroenteritis and diarrhea, with eight well defined serotypes. Epidemiological studies have recognized serotype-1 as the most common subtype but no such data is available in Pakistan. During 2009–2010, we found astroviruses in 41 out of 535 (7%) samples collected from hospitalized children. Thirty one strains belonged to serotype-1 and clustered into two distinct lineages. Serotype-3, -4 and -6 were detected with 97–98% genetic homology to Indian and Chinese strains.

Editor: Li-Min Huang, National Taiwan University Hospital, Taiwan

Funding: The authors have no support or funding to report.

Competing Interests: The authors have declared that no competing interests exist.

* E-mail: zaidis@pak.emro.who.int

Introduction

Astroviruses have been known as the causative agents of gastroenteritis since 1975 [1]. The virion particles are non-enveloped, containing positive sense single stranded RNA of 6.8 to 7.2 kb in length enclosed in a nucleocapsid coat [2]. Three open reading frames have been identified; ORF1a and 1b encoding protease and polymerase proteins respectively while ORF2 encodes the capsid protein precursor [3,4]. ORF1b is expressed as a fusion protein generated through a ribosomal frameshift mechanism using a highly conserved heptameric slippery sequence between ORF1a and 1b [5,6]. These viruses comprise 2 genera, *Mamastroviruses* and *Avastroviruses* within the family *Astroviridae* infecting mammalian and avian species respectively [7]. The astrovirus taxonomy is mainly based on the species of origin and the serotypes within each species are defined on the basis of twenty-fold or greater cross-neutralization titers. The poor adaptation of astroviruses to laboratory growth systems led to the formation of genome based classification, based on the percentage similarity of nucleotide and amino acid sequence of ORF2 capsid protein [8]. In humans, eight classic serotypes of astroviruses are known (HAstV1-8) while five new species have been identified recently named as AstV-MLB-1 & -2 (Finkbeiner SR. Virol J. 2008 and Finkbeiner SR. Virol J. 2009), AstV-VA1 (Finkbeiner J Virol 2009), AstV-HMO-A (Kapoor A. JGV 2009) and AstV-HMO-B (Kapoor A. JGV 2009).

Human astroviruses mainly infect children (<2 years of age) along with adults as well as immunocompromised persons and are found to cause 20% of the sporadic non-bacterial diarrhea cases [9]. The prevalence rate varies from 10–30% depending upon the geographical region with 33–65% of mixed infections with rotavirus and norovirus [10,11].

Materials and Methods

This study was approved from the National Institute of Health internal review board committee. To investigate the role of astroviruses in childhood diarrhea and its contributing serotypes, we analyzed stool samples of children under 5 years of age who were admitted to a local hospital in Rawalpindi district of Pakistan. Samples from hospitalized children suspected of gastroenteritis were collected as per World Health Organization's standard case definitions that describe a suspected case if a child is reported with three or more loose stools or any vomiting during 24 hours. 535 samples were collected over a period of two years (2009–2010) with their epidemiological details as given in Figure 1. The samples were spun to get clarified fecal supernatant and frozen at −20°C until further analysis. RNA was purified using QIAamp viral RNA minikit (Qiagen Inc., USA) and kept at −80°C. Reverse-transcription PCR to detect astrovirus nucleic acid was performed using the ORF2 targeted primers, Mon-269/Mon-270, as described previously [12]. The amplified product was purified and bidirectionally sequenced using BigDye terminator v3.1 cycle sequencing kit (Applied Biosystems, USA). The raw sequence reads generated by automated Genetic Analyzer 3130xl were edited and refined to get a single consensus read using the program Sequencher version 5.0 (Gene Codes Corporation, Ann Arbor, MI USA). Nucleotide alignments and phylogenetic analysis were conducted using MEGA 4.0.

Results

Out of total 535 (368, 2009; 167, 2010) samples analyzed for astrovirus, 7.6% (n = 41) were found positive for astrovirus RNA with 7% (n = 26) and 9% (n = 15) during 2009 and 2010 respectively. Higher proportion of astrovirus infections was found in children between 3–12 months of age as compared to older children (85% and 15% respectively), while no significant

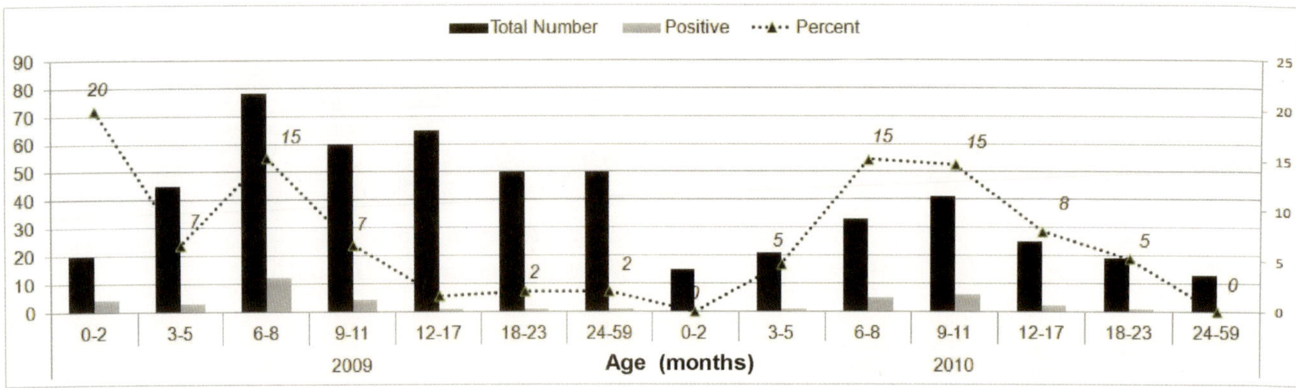

1a.

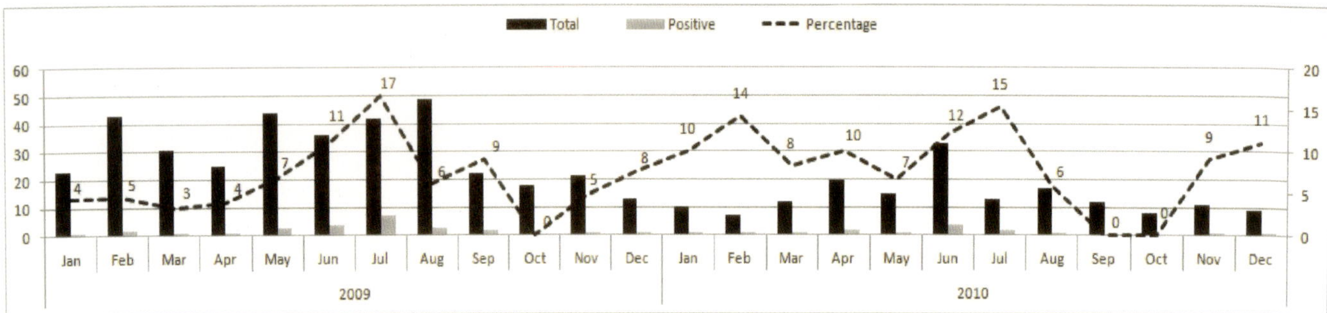

1b.

Figure 1. Astrovirus detection rates in various age groups of children hospitalized during 2009–2010. The data labels indicate the percentage of positive samples among each age group (1a). Month wise distribution of astrovirus positive samples between January, 2009 to December, 2010 (1b).

difference was found between males and females (Figure 1a and 1b). Co-infection with rotavirus and norovirus was found in 3% (16 out of 535) and 1% (5 out of 535) subjects respectively.

Molecular analysis revealed that the astroviruses found in Rawalpindi district belong to four different types HAstV-1, -3, -4 and -6 with 78%, 5%, 12% and 5% isolates respectively. Type-1, -3, -4 were detected in both years while serotype-6 was detected in two samples during 2010 only. Thirty two serotype-1 strains identified in this study had an inter-strain nucleotide similarity of 98–100% within the 348 bases of ORF2 region sequenced. Online BLAST search (www.ncbi.nlm.nih.gov/blast) revealed the closest nucleotide identity of all Pakistani astrovirus strains with those from the neighboring countries i.e. China and India. These closest matched type-1 viruses when compared and phylogeneticaly analyzed, presented ~4–5% nucleotide differences with Indian and Chinese strains and were grouped into two distinct lineages in the ORF2 based tree (Figure 2). In contrast, all of the viruses from serotypes-3, -4 and -6 were found clustered among the strains from India. The closest match for serotype-3 strains was Indian strain reported from Velore district in 2003 and 2004 (GenBank accession number JN871255 and JN871262). Similarly, the serotype-4 viruses were phylogeneticaly positioned among Indian strains found during 2004 (GenBank accession number JN871263). The serotype-6 strains from Pakistan presented two separate lineages, PAKNIH-2890 grouped with prototype strain (GenBank accession number L38507, isolated in UK) while the second lineage contained closely matched viruses from Beijing, China (GenBank accession number FJ755390) and Velore, India (GenBank accession number JN871267).

In addition, the Pakistani viruses detected in this study were also compared to sequences of prototype strains available in GenBank. For serotype-1 astroviruses, the nucleotide sequence of 348 bases from ORF2 region was aligned and compared to the four prototype strains reported from USA, United Kingdom, Japan and Germany. The closest identity of Pakistani strains was found with Japanese prototype strain showing 96–98% nucleotide similarity while the other prototype strains showed a greater degree of variance e.g. 91–93%, 88–89% and 88–91% divergence against USA, UK and Germany type 1 strains respectively. Significant nucleotide variance of 7% was found among serotype-3 viruses and its prototype (GenBank Accession No. L38505, Oxford strain). For serotype-4 and -6, the nucleotide variation was 5% and 1–2% with the prototype strains respectively (GenBank Accession No. L38506 and L38507).

Discussion

Unlike developed countries, epidemiological studies have never been conducted in Pakistan to investigate the burden of viruses in gastroenteritis and diarrhea related infections. Although a national program of laboratory based rotavirus surveillance was initiated in 2006, this program is based on the antigenic detection of rotavirus in stool samples. Similarly, no further investigation is routinely made at public health facilities for viral etiologies of diarrhea or gastroenteritis. Pakistan has been known to be among the top five

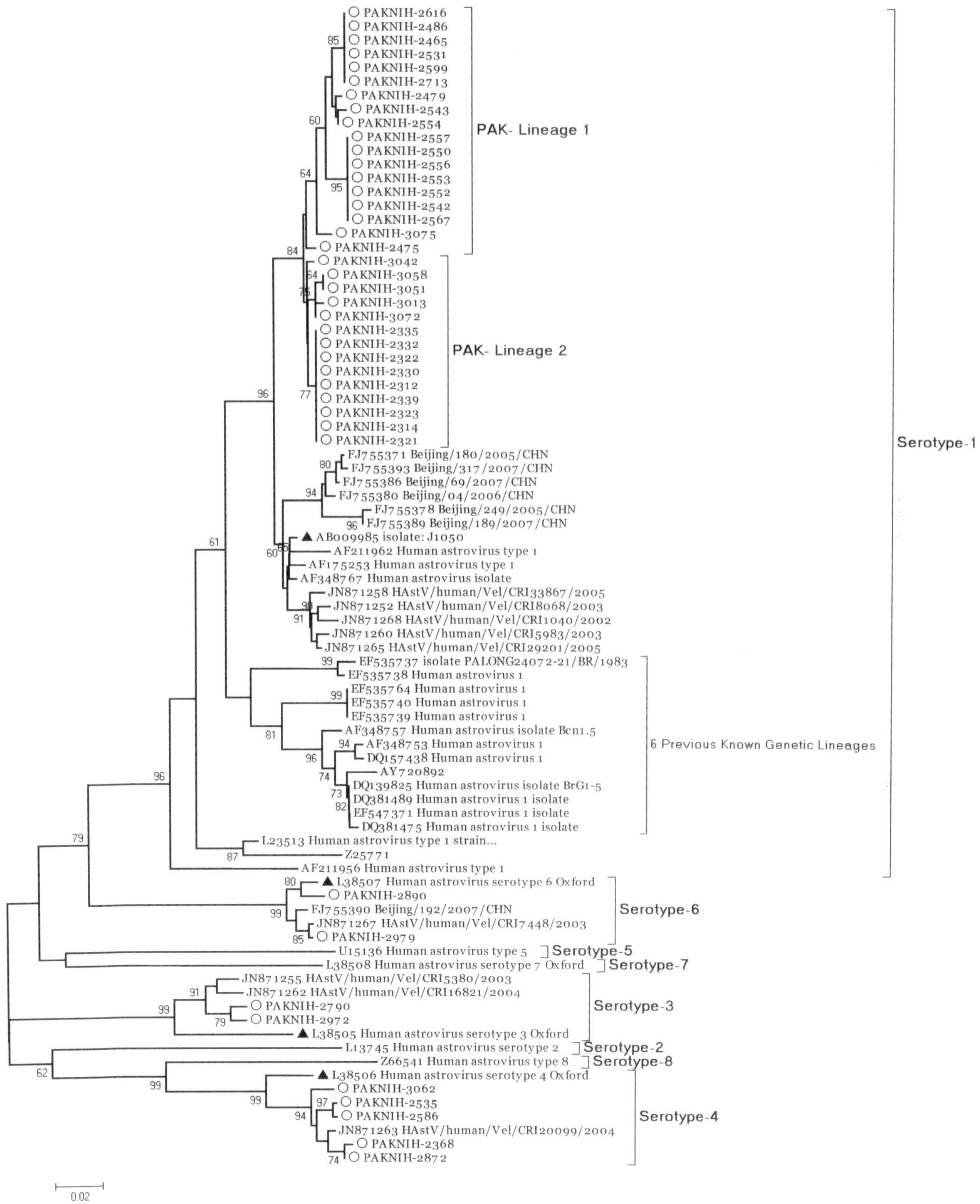

Figure 2. Phylogenetic analysis of Human Astrovirus strains identified in this study based on the partial ORF2 region (348 bases) encoding outer capsid precursor protein. The reference strains and closest match isolates detected through BLAST are given for genetic comparison. The phylogenetic tree with 500 bootstrap replicates was reconstructed using neighbor joining method and the K-2P model through MEGA 4.0. Serotype-1 strains were compared to four prototype strains (USA-GenBank accession number L23513, isolated in 1994), United Kingdom (GenBank accession number Z25771, isolated in 1990), Japan (GenBank accession number AB009985, isolated in 1997) and Germany (GenBank accession number AY720892). Taxa with arrow head indicates prototype strains within each serotype.

countries with highest number of reported childhood deaths due to diarrhea. To the best of our knowledge, we are, hereby, first to report the molecular epidemiology and genetic characterization of astroviruses in children admitted to a local tertiary care hospital in Pakistan. The only previous study in the country was conducted approximately two decades ago on samples collected during 1990–1994 in Karachi district and reported 11% samples positive for astrovirus type 1 [13]. Recently, novel astroviruses designated as AstV-HMO-A and AstV-HMO-B have been identified in Pakistan and Nigeria through metagenomic analysis of pediatric stool samples [14] but none of these new variants have been found in the present study which can be attributed to our use of highly specific primers targeting only the classical astrovirus serotypes. Upon nucleotide comparison of Mon-269/Mon-270 primers used in this study with the target region of ORF-2 (4526–4974 nucleotides based on astrovirus type 1; Genbank accession No. Z25771), several variations were found among the recently discovered astrovirus species necessitating the use of broad-range primers that can also detect the new astrovius species like AstV-MLB-1 and -2, AstV-HMO-A (highly similar to AstV-VA2), AstV-HMO-B (highly similar to AstV-VA3), and AstV-VA1 (highly similar to AstV-HMO-C) (Finkbeiner SR. Virol J. 2008 and Finkbeiner SR. Virol J. 2009, Finkbeiner J Virol 2009, Kapoor A. JGV 2009).

Our findings substantiate the data of epidemiological surveys in different countries that serotype-1 prevails as the most common subtypes while serotype-2, 3, 4 and 5 are less commonly detected, in addition to 6, 7 and 8 which are rarely found [15–17]. The current data represents the cases that were severely infected and required hospitalization but there may be the possibility of other serotypes prevailing in our population causing less severe or asymptomatic disease as reported previously from Australia [18]. The astrovirus strains identified in Rawalpindi during the two consecutive years period (2009–2010) does not represent any change in deduced amino acid sequence as compared to the prototype strains representing a stringent stability of the ORF2 region of virus genome. Similar findings have been observed by Mustafa et al.; Palombo et al., and Schnagl et al., where strains collected over 17 years period from Australia did not show any amino acid change in the same region of ORF2 encoded capsid protein [17–19]. Although the same genomic region has been utilized to identify the genotypic information [15,17,19,20] but this part of ORF2 does not provide sufficient information for evolutionary studies due to its high level of conservation and needs inclusion of other genomic regions. The serotype-1 astroviruses detected in our samples constitute a separate cluster and might reflect a different ancestral origin compared to those from neighboring countries. Recently, six lineages (1a–1f) have been proposed for astrovirus serotype-1 strains based on the 348 nucleotide region of ORF2 [21] but our viruses do not cluster with any of these lineages and thus support the circulation of type-1 strains with sufficient genetic variability as compared to the earlier known strains. Similar findings of geographical-specific clustering has been reported by Noel at al. [12] for type 1 viruses collected from different regions like Australia, New York and Colorado. Such findings also emphasize the role of continuous monitoring through large scale surveys to better understand the genetic diversity and astrovirus epidemiology in a particular population.

Conclusion

In Conclusion, Rawalpindi, one of the most populated city of Punjab province, is the only district for which more recent epidemiological information has been generated for astrovirus and its contributing serotypes. Further, Pakistani human population harbors a wide variety of astrovirus strains that require evaluation through large-scale incessant epidemiological surveys. As highlighted by Liu et al., such studies are helpful for formulating a more universal vaccine especially against serotype-1 which is found at significantly higher rates across the globe [20].

Acknowledgments

We are highly thankful to the staff of Virology department, National Institute of Health, Islamabad for their technical support in sample processing, handling and proper storage.

Author Contributions

Conceived and designed the experiments: SSZZ MN. Performed the experiments: MMA AK. Analyzed the data: S. Shaukat MA. Contributed reagents/materials/analysis tools: S. Sharif MSR. Wrote the paper: MMA SSZZ.

References

1. Madeley CR, Cosgrove BP (1975) Letter: 28 nm particles in faeces in infantile gastroenteritis. Lancet 2: 451–452.
2. Matsui SM, Greenberg HB (1996) Astroviruses. In: Fields BN, Knipe DM, Howley PM, Chanock RM, Melnick JL et al., editors. Fields Virology. 2nd ed: Lippincott-Raven, Philadelphia, Pa. pp. 811–824.
3. Jiang B, Monroe SS, Koonin EV, Stine SE, Glass RI (1993) RNA sequence of astrovirus: distinctive genomic organization and a putative retrovirus-like ribosomal frameshifting signal that directs the viral replicase synthesis. Proc Natl Acad Sci U S A 90: 10539–10543.
4. Willcocks MM, Brown TD, Madeley CR, Carter MJ (1994) The complete sequence of a human astrovirus. J Gen Virol 75 (Pt 7): 1785–1788.
5. Lewis TL, Matsui SM (1995) An astrovirus frameshift signal induces ribosomal frameshifting in vitro. Arch Virol 140: 1127–1135.
6. Marczinke B, Bloys AJ, Brown TD, Willcocks MM, Carter MJ, et al. (1994) The human astrovirus RNA-dependent RNA polymerase coding region is expressed by ribosomal frameshifting. J Virol 68: 5588–5595.
7. Mendez E, Arias CF (2007) Astroviruses. In: Knipe DM, Howley PM, editors. Fields Virology. 5th ed: Lippincott Williams and Wilkins, Philadelphia. pp. 981–1000.
8. De Benedictis P, Schultz-Cherry S, Burnham A, Cattoli G (2011) Astrovirus infections in humans and animals - molecular biology, genetic diversity, and interspecies transmissions. Infect Genet Evol 11: 1529–1544.
9. Kirkwood CD, Clark R, Bogdanovic-Sakran N, Bishop RF (2005) A 5-year study of the prevalence and genetic diversity of human caliciviruses associated with sporadic cases of acute gastroenteritis in young children admitted to hospital in Melbourne, Australia (1998–2002). J Med Virol 77: 96–101.
10. Colomba C, De Grazia S, Giammanco GM, Saporito L, Scarlata F, et al. (2006) Viral gastroenteritis in children hospitalised in Sicily, Italy. Eur J Clin Microbiol Infect Dis 25: 570–575.
11. Roman E, Wilhelmi I, Colomina J, Villar J, Cilleruelo ML, et al. (2003) Acute viral gastroenteritis: proportion and clinical relevance of multiple infections in Spanish children. J Med Microbiol 52: 435–440.
12. Noel JS, Lee TW, Kurtz JB, Glass RI, Monroe SS (1995) Typing of human astroviruses from clinical isolates by enzyme immunoassay and nucleotide sequencing. J Clin Microbiol 33: 797–801.
13. Phan TG, Okame M, Nguyen TA, Maneekarn N, Nishio O, et al. (2004) Human astrovirus, norovirus (GI, GII), and sapovirus infections in Pakistani children with diarrhea. J Med Virol 73: 256–261.
14. Kapoor A, Li L, Victoria J, Oderinde B, Mason C, et al. (2009) Multiple novel astrovirus species in human stool. J Gen Virol 90: 2965–2972.
15. Guix S, Caballero S, Villena C, Bartolome R, Latorre C, et al. (2002) Molecular epidemiology of astrovirus infection in Barcelona, Spain. J Clin Microbiol 40: 133–139.
16. Mendez-Toss M, Griffin DD, Calva J, Contreras JF, Puerto FI, et al. (2004) Prevalence and genetic diversity of human astroviruses in Mexican children with symptomatic and asymptomatic infections. J Clin Microbiol 42: 151–157.
17. Mustafa H, Palombo EA, Bishop RF (2000) Epidemiology of astrovirus infection in young children hospitalized with acute gastroenteritis in Melbourne, Australia, over a period of four consecutive years, 1995 to 1998. J Clin Microbiol 38: 1058–1062.
18. Schnagl RD, Belfrage K, Farrington R, Hutchinson K, Lewis V, et al. (2002) Incidence of human astrovirus in central Australia (1995 to 1998) and

comparison of deduced serotypes detected from 1981 to 1998. J Clin Microbiol 40: 4114–4120.

19. Palombo EA, Bishop RF (1996) Annual incidence, serotype distribution, and genetic diversity of human astrovirus isolates from hospitalized children in Melbourne, Australia. J Clin Microbiol 34: 1750–1753.

20. Liu MQ, Yang BF, Peng JS, Zhou DJ, Tang L, et al. (2007) Molecular epidemiology of astrovirus infection in infants in Wuhan, China. J Clin Microbiol 45: 1308–1309.

21. Gabbay YB, Leite JP, Oliveira DS, Nakamura LS, Nunes MR, et al. (2007) Molecular epidemiology of astrovirus type 1 in Belem, Brazil, as an agent of infantile gastroenteritis, over a period of 18 years (1982–2000): identification of two possible new lineages. Virus Res 129: 166–174.

7

Effect of Wild-Type *Shigella* Species and Attenuated *Shigella* Vaccine Candidates on Small Intestinal Barrier Function, Antigen Trafficking, and Cytokine Release

Maria Fiorentino[1], Myron M. Levine[2], Marcelo B. Sztein[2]❡, Alessio Fasano[1]*❡

1 Mucosal Immunology and Biology Research Center, Massachusetts General Hospital, Charlestown, Massachusetts, United States of America, 2 Center for Vaccine Development and the Departments of Pediatrics and Medicine, University of Maryland School of Medicine, Baltimore, Maryland, United States of America

Abstract

Bacterial dysentery due to *Shigella* species is a major cause of morbidity and mortality worldwide. The pathogenesis of *Shigella* is based on the bacteria's ability to invade and replicate within the colonic epithelium, resulting in severe intestinal inflammatory response and epithelial destruction. Although the mechanisms of pathogenesis of *Shigella* in the colon have been extensively studied, little is known on the effect of wild-type *Shigella* on the small intestine and the role of the host response in the development of the disease. Moreover, to the best of our knowledge no studies have described the effects of apically administered *Shigella flexneri* 2a and *S. dysenteriae* 1 vaccine strains on human small intestinal enterocytes. The aim of this study was to assess the coordinated functional and immunological human epithelial responses evoked by strains of *Shigella* and candidate vaccines on small intestinal enterocytes. To model the interactions of *Shigella* with the intestinal mucosa, we apically exposed monolayers of human intestinal Caco2 cells to increasing bacterial inocula. We monitored changes in paracellular permeability, examined the organization of tight-junctions and the pro-inflammatory response of epithelial cells. *Shigella* infection of Caco2 monolayers caused severe mucosal damage, apparent as a drastic increase in paracellular permeability and disruption of tight junctions at the cell-cell boundary. Secretion of pro-inflammatory IL-8 was independent of epithelial barrier dysfunction. *Shigella* vaccine strains elicited a pro-inflammatory response without affecting the intestinal barrier integrity. Our data show that wild-type *Shigella* infection causes a severe alteration of the barrier function of a small intestinal cell monolayer (a proxy for mucosa) and might contribute (along with enterotoxins) to the induction of watery diarrhea. Diarrhea may be a mechanism by which the host attempts to eliminate harmful bacteria and transport them from the small to the large intestine where they invade colonocytes inducing a strong inflammatory response.

Editor: Christopher R. Weber, University of Chicago, United States of America

Funding: These studies were funded by NIAID, NIH, DHHS grant U19 AI082655 (Cooperative Center for Translational Research in Human Immunology and Biodefense; CCHI) to M.B.S and A.F. The content is solely the responsibility of the authors and does not necessarily represent the official views of the National Institute of Allergy and Infectious Diseases or the National Institutes of Health. The funders had no role in study design, data collection and analysis, decision to publish, or preparation of the manuscript.

Competing Interests: Dr. M. M. Levine is co-inventor in patents for attenuated *Shigella* vaccines (gua mutants of *Shigella* spp. and vaccines containing the same. Patent US 5,783,196; Isolated DNA molecule encoding SHET1 of *Shigella flexneri* 2a and mutant *Shigella flexneri* 2a. Patent US 5,589,380). However, heretofore no company has licensed this technology and therefore there is no commercial "product" in development. The patent exists on paper only. Dr. A. F. is co-Founder and stock holder of Alba Therapeutics, a company working on treatments for celiac disease. No relation with the content of this manuscript. The remaining authors declare no conflicting financial interests.

* E-mail: afasano@mgh.harvard.edu

❡ These authors contributed equally to this work.

Introduction

Shigellosis is a leading cause of diarrheal disease, particularly in developing countries, estimated to have caused up to 1 million deaths per year between 1966–1997 [1]. Travelers and military personnel are at high risk of infection in the endemic countries. In the United States, there are approximately 14,000 laboratory-confirmed cases of shigellosis and an estimated 448,240 total cases that occur each year, according to the Center for Disease Control [2]. The peak incidence of shigellosis is among children 1 to 4 years of age, although no age groups are spared. Shigellosis can induce serious growth retardation [3]. Development of an efficacious vaccine against *Shigella* is a high priority for the protection of populations in developing countries, where the burden of *Shigella* causes much morbidity and claims many young lives. The same vaccines would also represent a potential tool to protect industrialized country travelers against the risk of travel shigellosis.

S. flexneri serotypes along with *S. sonnei* are responsible for most endemic disease in developing and transitional countries. *S. dysenteriae* type 1 is unique among *Shigella* in that it elaborates Shiga toxin (which exhibits potent neurotoxic, cytotoxic and enterotoxic activities), causes unusually severe clinical disease (including, rarely, hemolytic uremic syndrome) and is capable of large explosive outbreaks and true pandemic spread [4]. Two other enterotoxins are produced by *Shigella* strains and considerable evidence indicates that they are associated with the secretory diarrhea observed early in the clinical picture of shigellosis before the onset of dysentery (diarrheal stools with gross blood). These include *Shigella* enterotoxin 1 (ShET 1), restricted almost exclusively to the *S. flexneri* 2a serotype [5–8] and *Shigella* enterotoxin 2 (ShET2) which is found in all *Shigella* serotypes as it is encoded by genes located on the invasiveness plasmid [9,10].

Because the ingestion of as few as 10 organisms is sufficient to cause clinical shigellosis [11], this is a highly contagious infectious disease that is readily transmitted by fecal-oral contact.

There's a wealth of literature available describing the mechanisms by which *Shigella* cause dysentery. Most of these studies have focused on *S. flexneri* and *S. dysenteriae* 1 in animal models, including macaques, to assess the host response to infection with wild-type strains and immunogenicity and protection elicited by orally administered live attenuated vaccine candidates [12–20]. A few studies have also been performed in humans immunized and/or challenged with wild-type *Shigella* [21–26], using a model of human colonic explants [27,28] or mainly focusing on undifferentiated crypt-like cells [29,30]. While the mechanisms of pathogenesis of *Shigella* in the colon have been extensively studied, very limited and scattered information is available on the effect of wild-type *Shigella* on the small intestine and the role of the host response to infection of the small intestine itself in the development of the disease [28,31,32]. Similarly, most of the studies available on the effects of *Shigella* auxotrophic mutants on epithelial cells have been performed on basolaterally infected Caco2 cells, T84 or Hela cells and/or animal model colonic explants [30,33–35].

The aim of this study was therefore to assess the coordinated human epithelial responses, at both the functional and immunological levels evoked by apically administered strains of wild-type *Shigella* and candidate vaccines, by studying changes in Caco2 cell monolayer barrier integrity, tight junction function and secretion of pro-inflammatory cytokines.

Materials and Methods

Cell culture

Human Caco-2 intestinal epithelial cells [HTB-37, American Type Culture Collection (ATCC), Rockville, MD] were routinely grown in Dulbecco's Minimum Essential Medium (DMEM) supplemented with 20% fetal bovine serum. Monolayers (passages 22-35) were grown on 1.12 cm^2 permeable polyester filters with 0.4 um pore size (Corning, Lowell, MA) and utilized after 14–21 days until having reached a confluent, polarized and differentiated state.

Bacteria strains and growth conditions

S. flexneri 2a strain 2457T and *S. dysenteriae* 1 1617 are wild-type strains [36,37]. Bacteria were routinely grown at 37°C in Luria Bertani (LB) overnight. Two hundred microliters of a stationary phase culture were used to inoculate 5 ml of DMEM, and the bacteria were grown in a shaking incubator for approximately 2 h at 37°C to mid-exponential phase ($OD_{600nm}=0.3$). CVD 1208S and CVD 1256 are live, attenuated, oral vaccine candidates *de novo* constructed from their parental strains *Shigella flexneri* 2a strain 2457T and *Shigella dysenteriae* 1 1617, respectively. These attenuated strains harbor deletions in the guanine nucleotide synthesis pathway and in the genes encoding *Shigella* enterotoxins [30,38]. Vaccine strains were routinely grown on LB agar plates and in DMEM media supplemented with guanine [30]. The CVD 1208S strain used in this study has been reconstructed by using animal-free media [39].

Generation of conditioned media and heat-killed cultures

Aliquots of overnight precultured bacteria were grown in DMEM for 3 hours to a final OD_{600} of 0.3. Cells were pelleted, and supernatants filter sterilized by passing through a 0.22-um pore size filter. Supernatants, hereafter referred to as 'conditioned media', were immediately used. Bacteria grown in DMEM for 3 hours as described above were heat-killed by boiling at 100°C for 30 minutes.

In both cases, the effectiveness of filtration and killing by heat was confirmed by lack of bacterial growth from 100 μl of this media plated onto agar plates and then incubated overnight at 37°C.

Measurement of TEER

Transepithelial electric cell resistance (TEER) was used to monitor the integrity of the epithelial monolayer using a Millicel ERS Volt-ohm meter (World Precision Instruments, New Haven, CT). Monolayers with TEER values within ~800–1200 $\Omega.cm^2$ were considered to have an appropriate barrier function and were used in the study.

Caco2 cells were infected apically with the bacteria suspension, heat-killed bacteria or bacterial supernatants at an inoculation ratio (MOI) of 500, 50 and 5 bacteria/epithelial cell (corresponding to 10^7, 10^6 and 10^5 CFU) and incubated at 37°C. After 6 hours of incubation, cells were washed with PBS to remove non-adherent bacteria and treated with gentamicin. Monolayers were then incubated at 37°C overnight. TEER was measured at the time points indicated. Gentamicin-resistant intracellular bacteria counts were enumerated from representative infected monolayers after cell lysis for 30 min at 37°C with 1 ml 0.1% Triton X-100 in H_2O, by serial 10-fold dilution in PBS and plating on LB or LB agar (data not shown).

Cell viability

Caco2 cell monolayer viability after bacterial infection was assessed using a lactate dehydrogenase (LDH) secretion assay. The LDH secretion was measured from the cellular supernatant by a commercially available LDH assay kit (Cytotox 96, Promega, WI) and carried as described by the manufacturer's instructions. Lysis of the cells with 1% Triton X-100 served as positive control.

Assessment of Caco2 Cell Monolayer Permeability

The permeability of the Caco2 cell monolayer was evaluated by measuring the flux of Fluorescein isothiocyanate (FITC)-Bovine Serum Albumin (BSA) with a molecular weight of 66 kDa (Sigma).

FITC-BSA was dissolved in P buffer (10 mM HEPES, pH 7.4, 1 mM sodium pyruvate, 10 mM glucose, 3 mM $CaCl_2$, 145 mM NaCl) or P/EGTA buffer [(10 mM HEPES, pH 7.4, 1 mM sodium pyruvate, 10 mM glucose, 145 mM NaCl, 2 mM ethylene glycol-bis(ß-aminoethyl ether)-*N,N,N',N'* -tetraacetil acid (EGTA)].

Briefly, the apical surface of Caco2 cell monolayers was infected with either wild-type *S. flexneri* 2a or *S. dysenteriae* 1, CVD 1208S or CVD 1256 for 6 h, washed, treated with gentamicin and incubated at 37°C overnight. In order to measure the paracellular flux, the apical and basolateral cell culture media were replaced with P buffer containing FITC-BSA (10 mg/ml) and P buffer alone, respectively. P/EGTA buffer containing FITC-BSA (10 mg/ml) and P/EGTA buffer were used as positive controls. After incubation for 4 h, the amounts of FITC-BSA in the basolateral media were measured with a fluorometer (excitation at 492 nm and emission at 520 nm).

Western blot (Triton X-100 soluble and insoluble fractions)

Bacteria were added to the apical surface of Caco2 cell monolayers at a MOI of 50:1 for 4 hours at 37°C. Then cells were washed with PBS and incubated with DMEM supplemented with gentamicin overnight at 37°C. Cells were harvested at 6 and 24 hours post-infection and Triton X-100-soluble and -insoluble protein fractions were prepared. Monolayers were harvested on ice in lysis buffer [1% Triton X-100, 100 mM NaCl, 10 mM HEPES, 2 mM EDTA, 4 mM Na3VO4, 40 mM NaF 200 mM PMSF, and a protease inhibitor cocktail (Complete Mini, Roche Molecular Biochemicals, Mannheim, Germany) and phosphatase inhibitors (Sigma, St. Louis, MO)]. Lysates were rotated at 4°C, 30 min, centrifuged (14000 g for 30 min at 4°C) and the supernatant suspension, representing the Triton X-soluble fraction, was collected. The remaining pellet was re-suspended in lysis buffer supplemented with 1% SDS and sonicated (5 W, 5 s) two-three times on ice. The resulting suspension was centrifuged (14000 g for 5 min at 4°C) and the supernatant, representing the Triton X-insoluble fraction, was collected. Samples were used immediately or stored at −80°C. Protein concentration was quantified by the Bradford method (Bio-Rad, Hercules, CA). Samples were electrophoresed through a 10–20% gradient SDS polyacrylamide gel and transferred onto polyvinylidene difluoride membranes (Millipore, Bedford, MA). Membranes were blocked in blocking buffer (Tris-buffered saline, 0.1% Tween 20, 5% BSA), for 1 hour at room temperature. The blots were incubated overnight at 4°C with mouse anti-occludin diluted in blocking buffer. After washing, membranes were incubated for 1 hour at room temperature with the appropriate secondary antibody diluted in blocking buffer. The hybridized band was detected by chemiluminescence using an ECL kit (Amersham) according to the manufacturer's instructions. Membranes were stripped and reprobed (Blot restore solution, Millipore) for the detection of phosphothreonine followed by actin that served as the loading control. Band intensity was normalized to actin and quantitated by densitometry using Image J software (National Institutes of Health). Data represent the average of two separate experiments.

Cytokine assay

Media from both upper and lower transwell compartments were collected at 24 h postinfection. Samples were centrifuged at 2,000 rpm for 10 minutes to remove any residual cells or debris. Supernatants were stored at −80° until evaluated for cytokine secretion by Meso Scale Discovery (Rockville) technology, using a Human pro-inflammatory 7Plex Ultrasensitive Plate. Kits were run according to the manufacturer's instructions, with the exception of sample collection and processing as described above. Samples were run in duplicate.

Immunostaining

Cell monolayers on chamber slides were washed three times with PBS and fixed in PFA 4%/PBS or methanol for 20 min at room temperature or −20°C, respectively.

Cells were then blocked with 2% PBS diluted normal goat serum/1% BSA (blocking solution) for 30 min and incubated with blocking solution-diluted primary antibodies overnight at 4°C (anti-ZO-1, 1:100; anti-claudin 1, 1:1000).

After 3 washes with PBS, monolayers were incubated with 488 nm or 555 nm Alexa Fluor-conjugated secondary antibodies (1:800 in blocking solution) at room temperature for 1 h in the dark. Monolayers were washed with PBS and nuclei stained with DAPI (1:1000 in PBS) solution for 2 min at room temperature. Monolayers were analyzed with a Nikon Eclipse TE2000-E fluorescent microscope.

Antibodies

Rabbit anti-claudin-1(JAY-8, cat # 51-9000), mouse anti-occludin (OC-3F10, cat # 33-1500), mouse anti-ZO-1 (1A12, cat # 339100) and rabbit anti-phosphothreonine (ZPT1cat # 718200) antibodies were purchased from Invitrogen (Camarillo, CA). Mouse anti-actin protein antibody (5C, cat # 82353) was purchased by Thermo Fisher Scientific (IL).

Statistics

Data were analyzed by using GraphPad (San Diego, CA) software. Comparisons among time points within the same treatment group were made by two-way ANOVA. Comparisons among groups were made by one-way ANOVA. Differences were considered statistically significant if "p" values were <0.05.

Results

Shigella spp. adversely affect epithelial monolayer Trans-Epithelial Electric Resistance (TEER)

Shigella spp. are highly invasive bacteria affecting the mucosal layer of the intestine. To evaluate the effects of the interaction between the pathogens and the host on the mucosal barrier integrity and function, we apically infected Caco2 monolayers with bacteria at different inocula and monitored Transepithelial Electric Resistance (TEER) as a measure of tight junction function.

Caco2 cell monolayers were challenged with increasing amounts of wild-type *Shigella flexneri* 2a or *S. dysenteriae* 1. As shown in Fig. 1 (A, C) we found that wild-type *Shigella* species induced a marked drop in TEER in the epithelial cell monolayer at all inocula evaluated (10^5, 10^6 and 10^7 CFU/well, corresponding to MOIs of 5, 50 and 500:1 bacteria:epithelial cell, respectively). At 22 hours post infection with *S. flexneri* 2a we recorded the almost total disruption of the monolayer electric resistance, being TEER values comparable to those of initial cell seeding when no tight-junctions are still formed between cells (242 ± 22.6 Ω.cm^2, 203 ± 3.9 Ω.cm^2 and 171 ± 2.6 Ω.cm^2 for 10^5, 10^6 and 10^7 CFU/monolayer, respectively). *S. dysenteriae*-1 TEER values at 22 hour were similarly low (274 ± 15.4 Ω.cm^2, 231 ± 4.6 Ω.cm^2 and 193 ± 6.7 Ω.cm^2) suggesting that both wild-type *Shigella* species greatly affected monolayer barrier function integrity independent of the bacteria load.

Interestingly, and unlike our observations with *Salmonella* Typhi [40], we detected an increase in TEER in the initial few hours of infection (6 hours), when the monolayers were treated with bacteria at 10^5 and 10^6 CFU/monolayer. The greatest increase for both *Shigella* strains was observed when a 10^5 bacterial load was applied, for which we recorded TEER values of 1121 ± 59.9 Ω.cm^2 for *S. flexneri* 2a and 1094 ± 38.0 Ω.cm^2 for *S. dysenteriae* 1, compared to the uninfected monolayer (936 ± 49.1 Ω.cm^2 and 1004 ± 38.7 Ω.cm^2, respectively). Conversely, at the highest bacteria load, TEER decreased at 6 hours of about 50% and 25% of the initial value for *S. flexneri* 2a and *S. dysenteriae* 1, respectively (Fig. 1A, C).

At the end of the experiments, aliquots of lysates from the monolayers were plated on LB-agar to monitor for intracellular bacteria. Over 250 CFUs/monolayer were isolated following infection with *S. flexneri* 2a at 10^5, showing the ability of this pathogen to efficiently invade cells at their apical pole. Surprisingly, we observed much less bacteria/monolayer after infection with *S. dysenteriae* 1 ($\leq$50). As a further control, we plated on agar

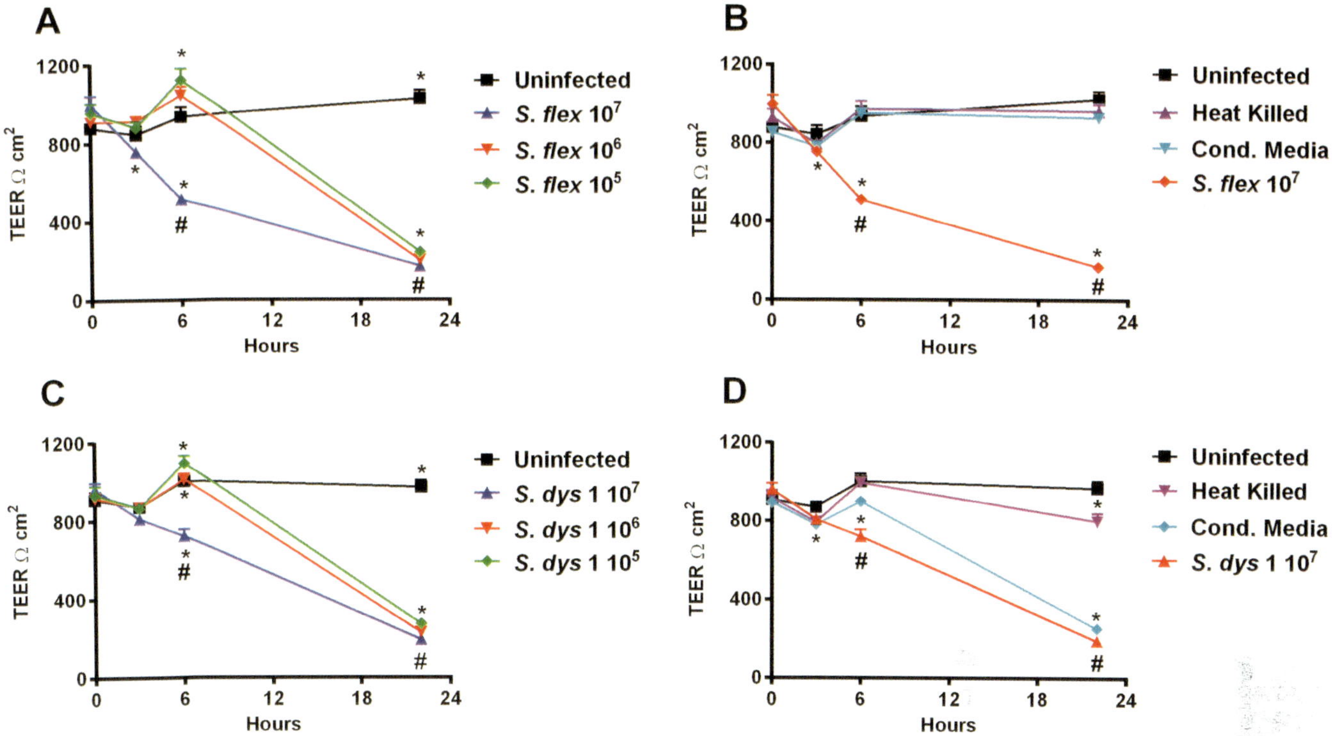

Figure 1. Wild type *Shigella* induce TEER decrease in Caco2 cell monolayers independent of MOIs. A. TEER responses to wild-type *S. flexneri* 2a applied at three different inocula. **B**. TEER responses to *S. flexneri* 2a heat-killed bacteria and culture supernatants (Cond. Media). **C**. TEER responses to wild-type *S. dysenteriae* 1 applied at three different inocula. **D**. TEER responses to *S. dysenteriae* 1 heat-killed bacteria and culture supernatants. Data are expressed as means ± SEM for triplicate samples for all conditions tested. * and # indicate statistically significant differences vs. t = 0 and vs. the uninfected control at the same time point, respectively; $p<0.05$ (ANOVA). These results are representative of 3 experiments with similar results.

an aliquot of media from the upper compartment supernatant, containing bacteria and did not observe any difference between the two strains at 6 hours, confirming that the monolayer had been infected with a comparable bacterial load. Both attenuated strains CVD 1208S and CVD 1256 showed a very small number of bacteria/monolayer (<5).

Further, we tested wild-type heat-killed bacteria and bacteria culture supernatant to determine whether viable organisms are required to affect the integrity of the epithelial barrier. As shown in Fig. 1 B and D, both heat-killed *S. flexneri* 2a and *S. dysenteriae* 1, applied at the same titer as viable wild-type bacteria, failed to significantly decrease the TEER of Caco2 cell monolayers. Unlike *S. flexneri* 2a, conditioned media from *S. dysenteriae* 1 had a decreasing effect on TEER at 22 hours, comparable to that of live cultures (Fig. 1D).

CVD 1208S and CVD 1256 strains designed for vaccine development, have an attenuated effect on epithelial barrier function

To evaluate their potential use as candidate vaccines, the effect of *S. flexneri* 2a and *S. dysenteriae* 1 attenuated strains was assessed on Caco2 monolayers. Caco2 cells were infected with CVD 1208S (Fig. 2A, C, E) or CVD 1256 (Fig. 2B, D, F) attenuated vaccine strains, in parallel with wild-type *S. flexneri* 2a and *S. dysenteriae* 1 strains, respectively. Vaccine strains were applied to Caco2 monolayers at the same titer as the wild-type bacteria. Both CVD 1208S and CVD 1256 attenuated strains induced a significant decline in TEER only when applied at the highest load (Fig. 2E, F). However, as the bacterial load was diminished, the milder effect on barrier function of the vaccine candidates compared to the wild-type became more apparent (Fig. 2C, D) with nearly no effect when applied at 10^5 (Fig. 2A, B).

Wild-type *Shigella* but not vaccine strains infection has a mild effect on Caco2 monolayer viability

To evaluate whether the disruption of the epithelial barrier function induced by *S. flexneri* 2a and *S. dysenteriae* 1 is mediated by enhanced apoptosis, the viability of the monolayer was assessed by measuring the levels of lactate dehydrogenase (LDH), released in the medium by cells undergoing the cell death pathway. As shown in Fig. 3, LDH levels at 24 hours post-infection showed small, albeit significant, increases after stimulation with wild-type bacteria at all inocula, compared to buffer alone. Similarly, wild-type *S. dysenteriae* 1 filtered supernatant and heat-killed bacteria also slightly affected cellular viability. Of note, the overall percentage of cell death observed after infection was never higher than 8% of positive control. Neither vaccine strains affected cell viability.

Shigella infection affects epithelial paracellular permeability to macromolecules

We assessed alterations in barrier function following infection with wild-type *S. flexneri* 2a and *S. dysenteriae* 1 and their isogenic attenuated strains CVD 1208S and CVD 1256, respectively, by measuring the transepithelial flux of fluorescently labeled Dextran (FITC-Dextran, 4 kDa) or Bovine Serum Albumin (FITC-BSA, 66 kDa). As shown in Fig. 4, Caco2 cells exposed to wild-type *S. flexneri* 2a (Fig. 4A) or *S. dysenteriae* 1 (Fig. 4B) showed a significantly

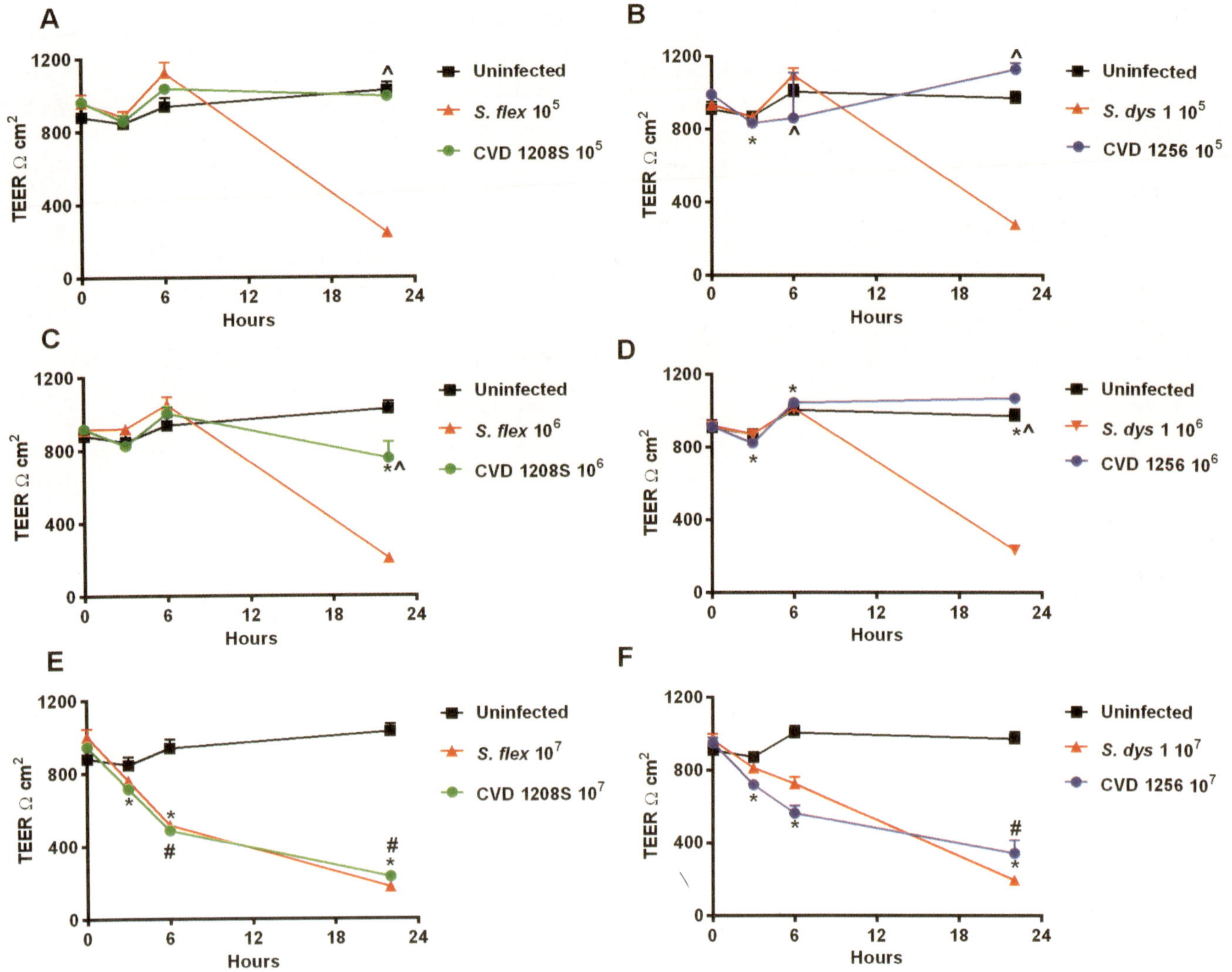

Figure 2. *Shigella* vaccine strains have attenuated effects on Caco2 monolayer barrier function, except at the highest inoculum. A, C, E. TEER of Caco2 cells infected with wild-type *S. flexneri* 2a and vaccine candidate *S. flexneri* 2a CVD 1208S applied apically at inocula of 10^5, 10^6 and 10^7 CFU. **B, D, F.** TEER of Caco2 cells infected with wild-type *S. dysenteriae* 1 and attenuated strain *S. dysenteriae* 1 CVD 1256 applied apically at inocula of 10^5, 10^6 and 10^7 CFU. Data are expressed as means ± SEM for triplicate samples for all conditions tested. * and ^ indicate statistically significant differences vs. t = 0 and vs. wild-type *Shigella* at the same inoculum and time point, respectively. # denotes statistically significant differences vs. the uninfected control at the same time point; $p<0.05$ (ANOVA). Statistical analysis results are shown only for the attenuated strains. Please, refer to Figure 1 for wild-type strains. These results are representative of 3 experiments with similar results.

increased transport of FITC-BSA from the apical to the basolateral chamber compared to uninfected controls at all inocula evaluated. Consistent with the TEER data, the vaccine candidates CVD 1208S and CVD 1256 elicited a slightly increased permeability to BSA only when applied at the highest MOI. Permeability to FITC-dextran was increased as well when wild-type *Shigella* was applied to Caco2 monolayers and interestingly only conditioned media from wild-type *S. dysenteriae* 1 induced a response entirely comparable to live bacteria (Fig. 4C). EGTA was used as a maximum permeability control for its ability to completely open tight-junctions.

Tight-junction disassembly in *Shigella* infected Caco2 monolayers

The data described above indicated that *S. flexneri* 2a and *S. dysenteriae* 1 affect epithelial barrier integrity by increasing Caco2 monolayer paracellular permeability, with some loss of cell viability. In a steady state status, the polarized epithelium maintains its relative impermeability to macromolecules through the correct functioning and integrity of intercellular tight junctions. We examined the effect of *Shigella* infection on Caco2 monolayer tight junction barrier by analyzing the tight junction-associated protein ZO-1 and the transmembrane proteins claudin-1 and occludin by immunofluorescence microscopy.

As shown in Fig. 5A, D, and G in uninfected monolayers ZO-1, claudin-1 and occludin are localized at the cell-cell boundary in a typical chicken wire-like pattern, indicating intact tight-junction complexes. In contrast, following infection with wild-type *S. flexneri* 2a at 10^6 (Fig. 5B) we observed the complete loss of the ZO-1 chicken-wire patterning. ZO-1 appeared unevenly distributed throughout the monolayer without a proper organization, indicating the total loss of cell-cell attachment. In contrast, CVD 1208S applied at the same inoculum had no effect on ZO-1

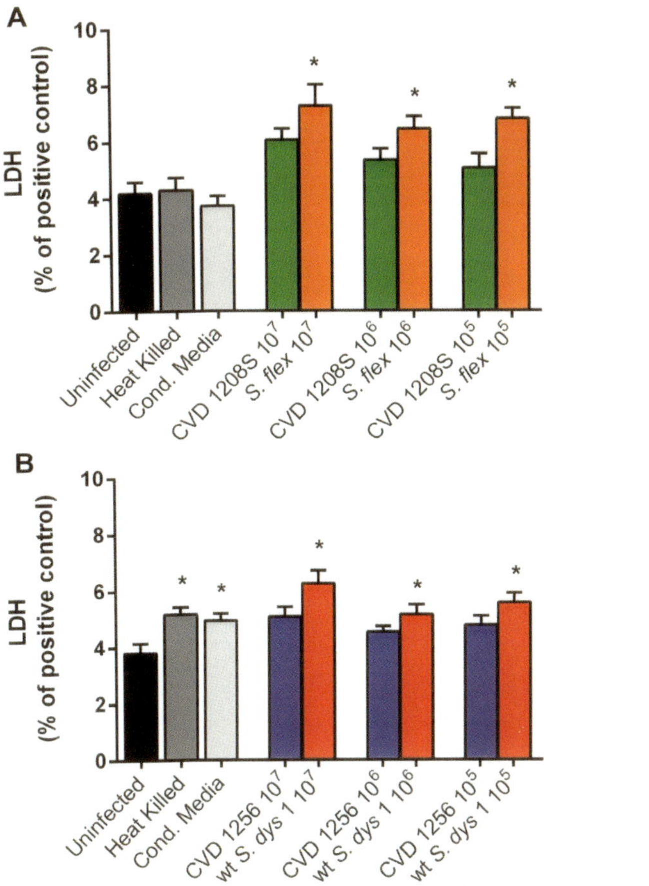

Figure 3. Wild type *Shigella*, but not vaccine strains, moderately affect Caco2 monolayer viability. A. LDH release after infection with wild-type *S. flexneri* 2a or its vaccine strain CVD 1208S at different inocula. **B**. LDH release after infection with wild-type *S. dysenteriae* 1 or its vaccine strain CVD 1256 applied at different inocula. Caco2 cells were infected with bacteria for 6 hours, washed and incubated overnight at 37°C. Apical supernatants were collected at 24 hours post-infection for LDH release measurement. Values represent LDH release from cells into the medium as a percentage of total LDH (Control). Data are expressed as means ± SEM for triplicate samples for all conditions tested. These results are representative of 3 experiments with similar results. *$p<0.05$ compared to uninfected cells (ANOVA).

organization (Fig. 5C). In monolayers infected with wild-type *S. flexneri* 2a at 10^6, we observed a derangement of both claudin-1 and occludin distribution throughout the monolayer (Fig. 5E, H), compared to uninfected cells (Fig. 5 D, G) whereas no alteration in the localization of these tight-junction proteins has been observed in CVD 1208S infected cells (Fig. 5F, I). Similar results to those obtained for wild-type *S. flexneri* 2a and CVD 1208S were obtained for ZO-1 with wild-type *S. dysenteriae* 1 and the CVD 1256 isogenic attenuated strain applied at the same inoculum (data not shown). Figs. 5K and L show ZO-1 distribution following wild type S. *dysenteriae* 1 or CVD 1256 infection at the lowest bacterial load, respectively. Interestingly, *S. dysenteriae* 1 culture supernatant altered ZO-1 organization (Fig. 5J) although not as severely as viable bacteria (Fig 5K).

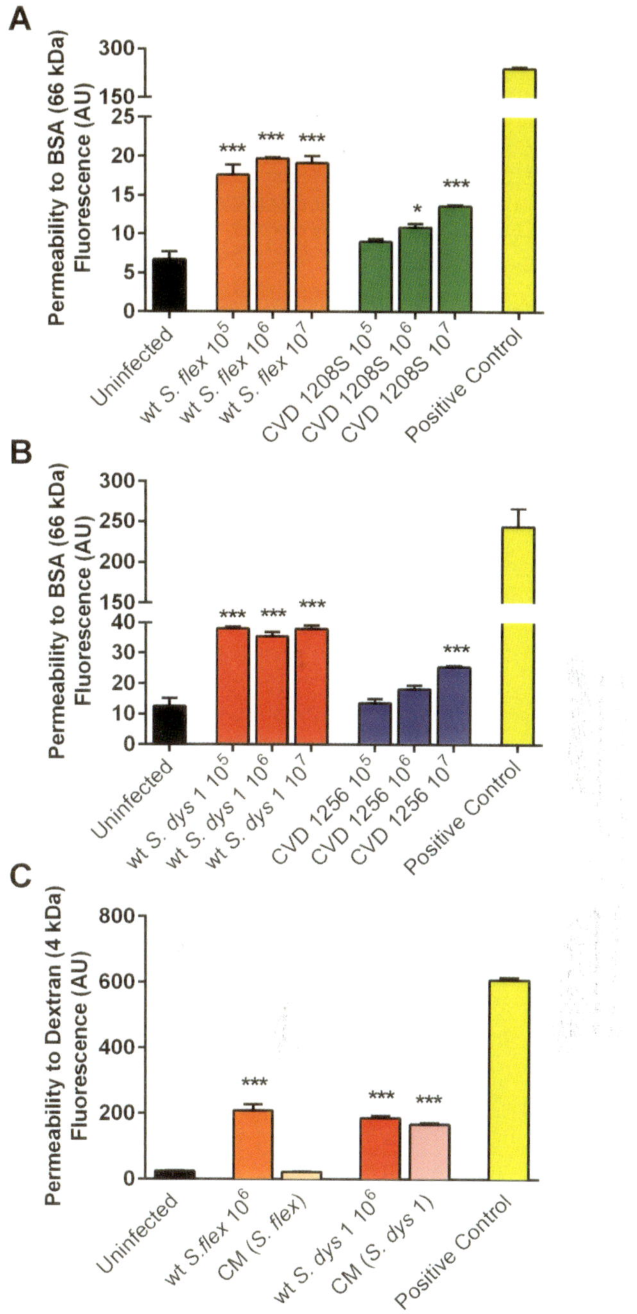

Figure 4. Wild type *Shigella* increase Caco2 monolayer paracellular permeability to macromolecules whilst vaccine candidates have no or markedly attenuated effect. A. FITC-BSA (66 kDa) net transport after infection with wild-type *S. flexneri* 2a or CVD 1208S applied at three different inocula. **B**. FITC-BSA (66 kDa) net transport after infection with wild-type *S. dysenteriae*-1 or CVD 1256 applied at three different inocula. C. FITC-Dextran (4 kDa) net transport after infection with wild-type filtered (Cond. Media: CM) or live *Shigella* applied at 10^6 CFU. Calcium-free medium supplemented with EGTA to disrupt TJs served as positive control. Results are expressed as mean ± SEM of triplicate samples for each condition and are representative of 3 experiments with similar results. ***$p<0.001$, *$p<0.05$ compared to uninfected control (ANOVA).

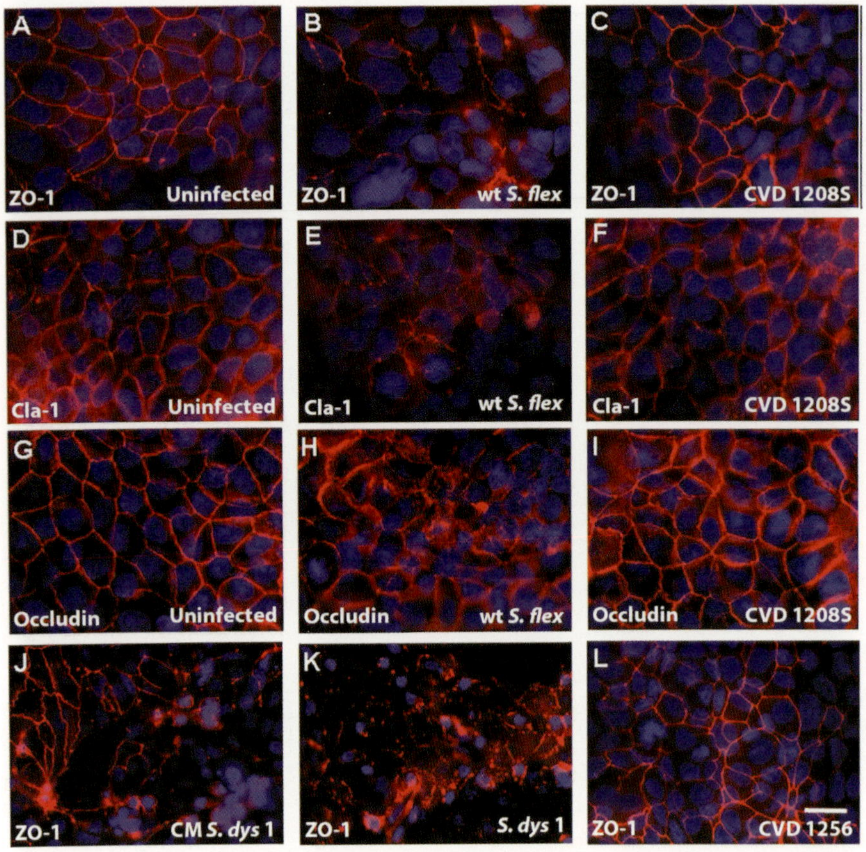

Figure 5. Tight-junction organization is disrupted following exposure to wild type *Shigella* but not to vaccine candidates. A, D, G. Uninfected monolayer immunostained for ZO-1, Claudin-1 or Occludin, respectively. **B, C.** Caco2 cells infected with wild-type *S. flexneri* 2a (B) or CVD 1208S (C) at 10^6 CFU, stained for ZO-1 (1:100). **E, F.** Caco-2 monolayers infected with wild-type *S. flexneri* 2a (E) or CVD 1208S (F) at 10^6 CFU and stained for Claudin-1 (1:1000). **H, I.** Monolayers infected with wild-type *S. flexneri* 2a (H) or CVD 1208S (I) at 10^6 CFU and stained for Occludin (1:100). **J, K, L.** Caco-2 cells treated with *S. dysenteriae* 1 filtered supernatant (J), live wild-type (K) or attenuated CVD 1256 (L) *S. dysenteriae* 1 strains applied at 10^5 CFU and stained for ZO-1 (1:100). Nuclei are stained with DAPI (blu). Bar 25 μm.

Shigella infection induces phosphorylation of occludin and its disengagement from the tight junction complex

Occludin plays an important role in the regulation of tight-junction integrity [41]. It has been shown that overexpression of occludin results in TEER elevation [42,43]. To understand the implication of occludin in the increased permeability caused by *Shigella* infection, we analyzed its solubility in the nonionic detergent Triton-X 100 in untreated controls and infected Caco2 monolayers (Fig. 6). In the untreated monolayer occludin was detected mostly in the insoluble fraction and was visible on western blots as a strong band of about 65 kDa [Low Molecular Weight (LMW) band; Fig. 6A, B upper panel]. Upon infection with wild-type *S. flexneri* 2a or *S. dysenteriae* 1 applied at 10^6 we detected an additional band of about 72–79 kD in the insoluble membrane fraction at 6 hours post-infection. This high molecular weight (HMW) band was observed in both CVD vaccine strain-treated cell lysates, as well and represents a hyperphosphorylated form of occludin, specifically associated with the functional sealing components of tight-junctions [44–46]. It has been shown that occludin undergoes dephosphorylation on Ser/Thr residues during the disruption of tight junctions by various insults. Analysis of the Thr phosphorylation status shows that occludin is phosphorylated in the resting epithelium. Following bacterial infection occludin undergoes hyperphosphorylation on Thr (Fig. 6A, B middle panel) interestingly coincident with the raise in TEER observed at 6 hours. At 24 hours, we observed the loss of the hyperphosphorylated form of occludin together with a decrease of occludin in the membrane fraction, in the infected cells (Fig. 6C, D upper and middle panels). Both attenuated strains had a similar although milder effect on occludin.

Shigella and attenuated strains induce a polarized secretion of IL-8

Cytokines analyzed in this study included IL-8, IL-6, IL-10, IL-12p70, IFNγ, IL1β and TNFα. With the exception of IL-8, all the other pro-inflammatory molecules were below detection level. IL-8 secretion was induced in Caco2 monolayers following infection with wild-type *S. flexneri* 2a and *S. dysenteriae* 1 and both vaccine candidate strains, at all inocula used in this study. Results from the analysis of media collected from the upper and lower chambers of transwells at 24 hours post infection are depicted in Fig. 7. As expected, we observed a polarized secretion of IL-8, predominantly in the basolateral side. Fig. 7A shows the levels of IL-8 measured in wild-type *S. flexneri* 2a and CVD 1208S infected monolayers. Overall, we observed a significantly higher level of IL-8 in cells infected with wild-type *Shigella* compared to the uninfected control, at all inocula evaluated. Likewise, IL-8 levels in wild type *Shigella* treated cells were significantly higher than CVD 1208S, except at the highest infection dose. Similarly, IL-8 basolateral levels in wild-type *S. dysenteriae* 1 treated cells were

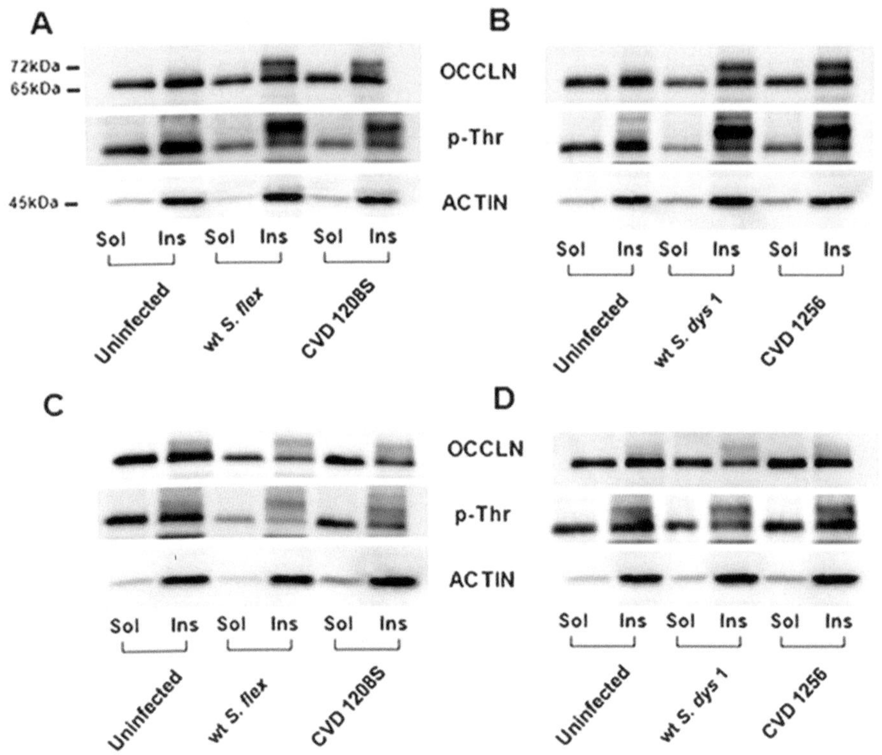

Figure 6. Occludin is hyperphosphorylated after infection with *Shigella* strains and disassembles from tight-junctions. A, B. Western blot of protein samples in the form of X-100 Triton soluble (Sol) and insoluble (Ins) fractions at 6 hours post-infection, blotted with anti-occludin (upper rows), anti-phosphothreonine (middle rows) and anti-actin (lower rows). **C, D**. Western blot of protein samples at 24 hours post-infection, blotted with anti-occludin (upper rows), anti-phosphothreonine (middle rows) and anti-actin (lower rows).

significantly higher than in uninfected controls at all inocula tested. CVD 1256 infected cells secreted a significant amount of IL-8 over uninfected control, only when applied at a MOI of 500 (10^7). Basolateral IL-8 levels in CVD 1256 treated monolayers were significantly lower than wild-type *S. dysenteriae* 1 at bacterial infections of 10^6 and 10^5. Interestingly, both heat-killed wild-type *Shigella* strains induced high levels of IL-8 and, only for *S. dysenteriae* 1, the conditioned media, as well.

Discussion

Shigellosis is typically characterized by two phases: an initial phase of watery diarrhea thought to arise in the jejunum, followed by a second phase characterized by stools containing blood, mucus and pus, as a result of bacterial invasion of the colonic epithelium. In milder cases, watery diarrhea may represent the only clinical presentation of the disease [47,48]. Unlike other enterobacteria, ingestion of as low as 10 microorganisms are sufficient to cause shigellosis implying that *Shigella* must have evolved an array of tools in order to resist the low pH of the stomach and safely and efficiently travel through the small intestine ultimately reaching their final colonizing/replicating niche in the colon. Although the pathophysiology of *Shigella* infection has been widely studied, little is known about the early stage interaction of the pathogens with the epithelium of the small intestine. By using Caco2 cell monolayers, morphologically and functionally mimicking the small intestinal mucosal barrier [49–51], we aimed at getting insights into the biological response of the small intestine to *Shigella* infection.

Our data show that exposure to *S. flexneri* 2a and *S. dysenteriae* 1 cause a permanent impairment of the mucosal barrier integrity independent of the bacterial inocula and associated to a minimal, although significant loss of cell viability. We further analyzed the effect of *Shigella* on barrier integrity and we were able to provide molecular evidence showing that intercellular tight-junctions were disassembled (Fig. 5) and that changes in the phosphorylation status of occludin (Fig. 6) contribute to the impairment of the epithelial fence. Interestingly, while in *S.* Typhi infected monolayers early occludin hyperphosphorylation was paralleled by a drop in TEER (40), in Caco2 cells exposed to low inocula *Shigella* the change in the phosphorylation status of occludin appears to be consistently paralleled by a slight TEER increase (Fig. 1A, C), suggesting a transient enhancement of barrier function. While several studies have demonstrated that depending on the kinases and the specific occludin residues phosphorylated, distinct effects on tight junctions' assembly and function can be observed [52–57], more in depth studies are needed to clarify the molecular mechanisms behind this discrepancy. Our results indicate that infection of enterocytes with wild-type *Shigella* induces molecular changes in occludin, leading to its disengagement from the tight junction complex that, together with the associated disruption of claudin-1 and ZO-1 organization, contribute to increase paracellular permeability to macromolecules. Our analysis of the vaccine candidates CVD 1208S and CVD 1256, demonstrates that both have a general attenuated effect on barrier integrity and function, except when applied at the highest inocula. Interestingly, the application of heat-killed bacteria had little or no consequence on mucosal barrier function whereas *S. dysenteriae* 1 conditioned media had a severe effect on Caco2 monolayer integrity and permeability comparable to live bacteria, suggesting that while direct interaction with epithelial cells by viable *S. flexneri* is required

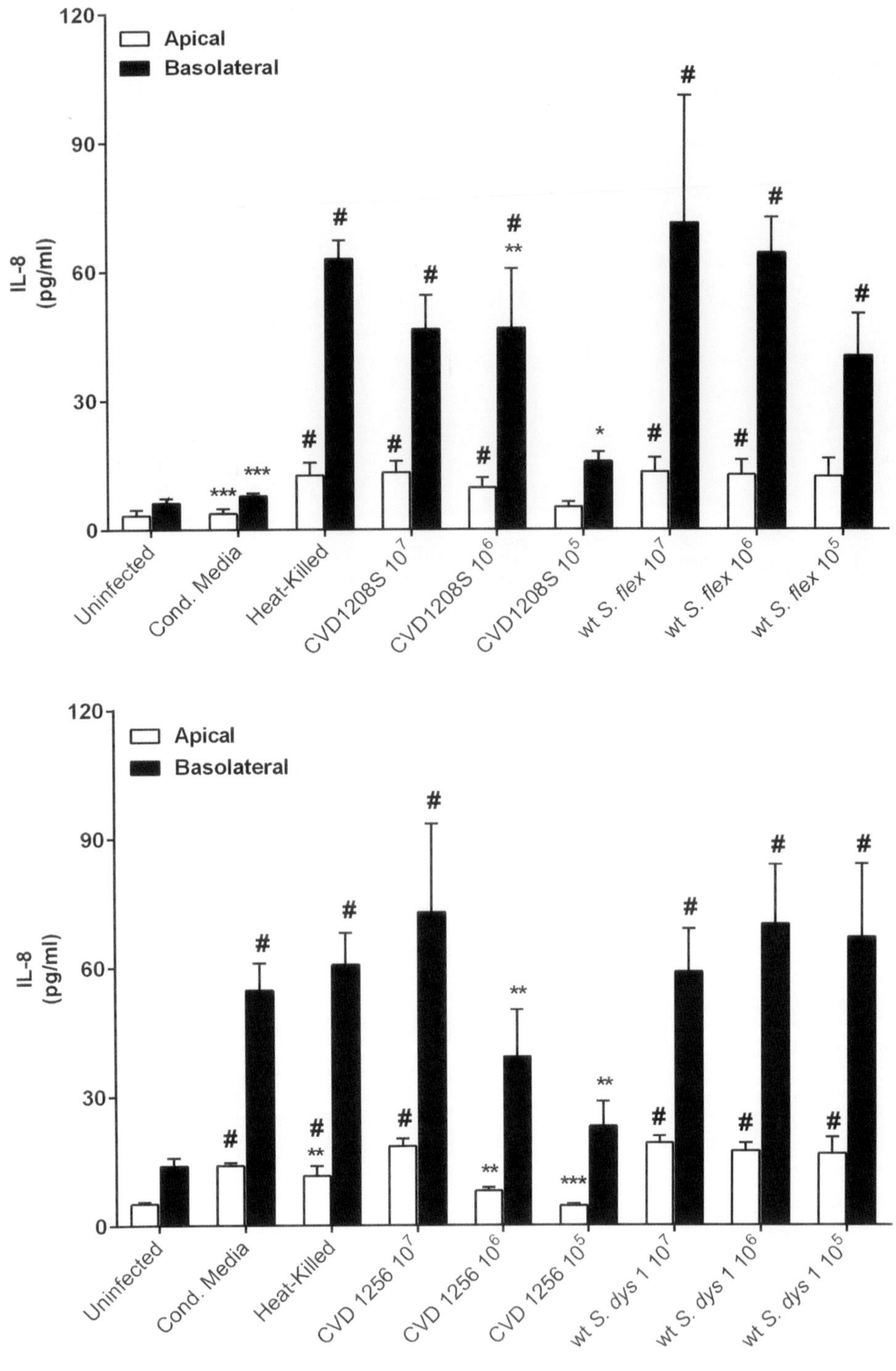

Figure 7. Wild type *Shigella* and attenuated strains induce Caco2 cells polarized secretion of IL-8. IL-8 secreted by Caco-2 cells infected with wild-type live, filtered and heat-killed *S. flexneri* 2a or vaccine candidate *S. flexneri* 2a CVD 1208S, applied at different inocula. **B**. IL-8 released by Caco2 cells infected with wild-type live, filtered and heat-killed *S. dysenteriae* 1 or *S. dysenteriae* 1 CVD 1256 applied at different inocula. Statistical comparisons are between infected and uninfected cells (#) or between the attenuated and the wild-type strains at the same inoculum (*). ***$p<0.001$, **$p<0.01$, * and #$p<0.05$ (ANOVA).

to affect barrier function, *S. dysenteriae* 1 releases into the surrounding environment mediators whose activity alone strongly impairs the monolayer integrity.

A challenge in developing effective and safe vaccines is the ability to elicit protection with minimal or no inflammatory reaction. Epithelial cells have the capability to release and array of pro-inflammatory molecules, including IL-8. *Shigella* spp. were reported to induce secretion of IL-8 in colonic T84, HT29 or Caco2 cell monolayers [58–61]. We have now extended these findings by showing the polarized secretion of IL-8 upon apical exposure of Caco2 cell monolayers to wild-type *S. flexneri* 2a or *S. dysenteriae* 1 and their vaccine candidates. Heat-killed bacteria from both wild-type *Shigella* strains cause a release of IL-8 comparable to live organisms, suggesting that viable bacteria/epithelial cell interaction is not required for the induction of IL-8 secretion. Moreover, while exposure of Caco2 cells to *S. flexneri* 2a conditioned media does not elicit the secretion of IL-8, conditioned media from wild-type *S. dysenteriae* 1 is able to induce the secretion of high levels of IL-8, indicating that the presence of bacteria-secreted mediators alone is sufficient to trigger an immune response. Although release of IL-8 following infection with CVD 1208S and CVD 1256 vaccine candidates was lower than that observed with the wild-type parental strains, especially at lower bacterial infection inocula, they still induce a remarkable pro-inflammatory response compared to uninfected cells. At higher bacterial inocula, no difference in IL-8 levels was observed between wild-type and vaccine strains.

These data, together with the initial results obtained from clinical trials with CVD 1208S [39] and the encouraging immunological Sereny test results on guinea pigs upon infection with CVD 1256 [30], make these vaccine candidates' future application as effective, safe and capable of eliciting protective immunity vaccines, very promising.

Overall, we have not observed differences between the two wild-type *Shigella* strains in their ability to disrupt mucosal barrier integrity and permeability. The two vaccine candidates showed a much smaller number of bacteria in the monolayer compared to their isogenic parents, in line with their attenuated properties [30].

With the present studies we have provided for the first time mechanistic insights on the early interaction of *Shigella* species with the small intestine leading to increased permeability (including the mechanisms leading to tight junction disassembly), antigen trafficking, and cytokine release. Our data demonstrate that wild-type *Shigella* spp. affect mucosal barrier function and immune response and that these two events are unrelated, suggesting a differential (biphasic?) pathogenic effect along the intestinal tract. However, *S. dysenteriae* 1 secretes active mediator(s) (e.g., Shiga toxin) capable by themselves of inducing the same barrier alteration and immune response as viable bacteria. The lack of effect following exposure to *S. flexneri* 2a conditioned media suggests that the enterotoxins ShET1 and/or ShET2 alone do not play a role in barrier function alteration and inflammation. We have previously shown that ShET1 and 2 alter electrolyte and water transport in rabbit small intestine both *in vitro* and *in vivo* [5,62], strongly suggesting their function as enterotoxins and a pivotal role in the onset of watery diarrhea in shigellosis. Recently, Faherty at al. [63] confirmed the enterotoxic activity of ShET 1 and 2 in an *ex-vivo* mouse model and identified a novel *S. flexneri* effector responsible for enterotoxic activity. All these studies have made use of highly concentrated supernatants from *Shigella* cultures. Since we have not tested either the amount or the activity of these toxins in our supernatants, we cannot exclude that they either have lost their activity during preparation or, more likely, are present in low concentrations, not sufficient to affect barrier function.

Nevertheless, data obtained following infection with the vaccine candidates, which are depleted of the major enterotoxins (ShET1/2 and stx), suggest that the increased paracellular permeability observed in Caco2 monolayers following exposure at the highest bacterial inoculum, might be attributed to a specific response of the host to infection rather than to bacterial toxins. The fact that attenuated *Shigella* strains induce a remarkable immune reaction, shows that the host immune response is not only independent of the functional impairment of the epithelial barrier but also of the bacteria main effector enterotoxic activities (ShET 1/2 and stx).

In summary, we speculate that wild-type *Shigella* infection causes a severe alteration of the small intestinal mucosa barrier function that might contribute to the induction of watery diarrhea as a mechanism for the host to eliminate harmful bacteria and for the pathogens to be efficiently transported to the large intestine where they invade the epithelium inducing a strong inflammatory response.

Acknowledgments

We thank Dr. Eileen M. Barry (University of Maryland) for critically reading the manuscript.

Author Contributions

Conceived and designed the experiments: MF AF. Performed the experiments: MF. Analyzed the data: MF AF MBS. Wrote the paper: MF AF MBS MML.

References

1. Kotloff KL, Winickoff JP, Ivanoff B, Clemens JD, Swerdlow DL, et al. (1999) Globalburden of Shigella infections: implications for vaccine development and implementation of control strategies. Bulletin of the World Health Organization 77: 651–666.
2. Gupta A, Polyak CS, Bishop RD, Sobel J, Mintz ED (2004) Laboratory-confirmed shigellosis in the United States, 1989-2002: epidemiologic trends and patterns. Clinical infectious diseases : an official publication of the Infectious Diseases Society of America 38: 1372–1377.
3. Black RE, Brown KH, Becker S (1984) Effects of diarrhea associated with specific enteropathogens on the growth of children in rural Bangladesh. Pediatrics 73: 799–805.
4. Levine MM, DuPont HL, Formal SB, Hornick RB, Takeuchi A, et al. (1973) Pathogenesis of Shigella dysenteriae 1 (Shiga) dysentery. The Journal of infectious diseases 127: 261–270.
5. Fasano A, Noriega FR, Maneval DR, Jr., Chanasongcram S, Russell R, et al. (1995) Shigella enterotoxin 1: an enterotoxin of Shigella flexneri 2a active in rabbit small intestine in vivo and in vitro. The Journal of clinical investigation 95: 2853–2861.
6. Yavzori M, Cohen D, Orr N (2002) Prevalence of the genes for shigella enterotoxins 1 and 2 among clinical isolates of shigella in Israel. Epidemiology and infection 128: 533–535.
7. Niyogi SK, Vargas M, Vila J (2004) Prevalence of the sat, set and sen genes among diverse serotypes of Shigella flexneri strains isolated from patients with acute diarrhoea. Clinical microbiology and infection : the official publication of the European Society of Clinical Microbiology and Infectious Diseases 10: 574–576.
8. Noriega FR, Liao FM, Formal SB, Fasano A, Levine MM (1995) Prevalence of Shigella enterotoxin 1 among Shigella clinical isolates of diverse serotypes. The Journal of infectious diseases 172: 1408–1410.
9. Nataro JP, Seriwatana J, Fasano A, Maneval DR, Guers LD, et al. (1995) Identification and cloning of a novel plasmid-encoded enterotoxin of enteroinvasive Escherichia coli and Shigella strains. Infection and immunity 63: 4721–4728.
10. Vargas M, Gascon J, Jimenez De Anta MT, Vila J (1999) Prevalence of Shigella enterotoxins 1 and 2 among Shigella strains isolated from patients with traveler's diarrhea. Journal of clinical microbiology 37: 3608–3611.
11. DuPont HL, Levine MM, Hornick RB, Formal SB (1989) Inoculum size in shigellosis and implications for expected mode of transmission. The Journal of infectious diseases 159: 1126–1128.
12. Shipley ST, Panda A, Khan AQ, Kriel EH, Maciel M, Jr., et al. (2010) A challenge model for Shigella dysenteriae 1 in cynomolgus monkeys (Macaca fascicularis). Comparative medicine 60: 54–61.
13. Shim DH, Suzuki T, Chang SY, Park SM, Sansonetti PJ, et al. (2007) New animal model of shigellosis in the Guinea pig: its usefulness for protective efficacy studies. Journal of immunology (Baltimore, Md: 1950) 178: 2476–2482.
14. Zhang Z, Jin L, Champion G, Seydel KB, Stanley SL, Jr. (2001) Shigella infection in a SCID mouse-human intestinal xenograft model: role for neutrophils in containing bacterial dissemination in human intestine. Infection and immunity 69: 3240–3247.
15. Perdomo OJ, Cavaillon JM, Huerre M, Ohayon H, Gounon P, et al. (1994) Acute inflammation causes epithelial invasion and mucosal destruction in experimental shigellosis. The Journal of experimental medicine 180: 1307–1319.

16. Rout WR, Formal SB, Giannella RA, Dammin GJ (1975) Pathophysiology of Shigella diarrhea in the rhesus monkey: intestinal transport, morphological, and bacteriological studies. Gastroenterology 68: 270–278.
17. Jeong KI, Zhang Q, Nunnari J, Tzipori S (2010) A piglet model of acute gastroenteritis induced by Shigella dysenteriae Type 1. The Journal of infectious diseases 201: 903–911.
18. Dinari G, Hale TL, Austin SW, Formal SB (1987) Local and systemic antibody responses to Shigella infection in rhesus monkeys. The Journal of infectious diseases 155: 1065–1069.
19. Katakura S, Reinholt FP, Karnell A, Huan PT, Trach DD, et al. (1990) The pathology of Shigella flexneri infection in rhesus monkeys: an endoscopic and histopathological study of colonic lesions. APMIS : Acta Pathologica, Microbiologica, et Immunologica Scandinavica 98: 313–319.
20. Oaks EV, Hale TL, Formal SB (1986) Serum immune response to Shigella protein antigens in rhesus monkeys and humans infected with Shigella spp. Infection and immunity 53: 57–63.
21. Porter CK, Thura N, Ranallo RT, Riddle MS (2012) The Shigella human challenge model. Epidemiology and infection: 1–10.
22. Levine MM, Kotloff KL, Barry EM, Pasetti MF, Sztein MB (2007) Clinical trials of Shigella vaccines: two steps forward and one step back on a long, hard road. Nature reviewsMicrobiology 5: 540–553.
23. Kotloff KL, Losonsky GA, Nataro JP, Wasserman SS, Hale TL, et al. (1995) Evaluation of the safety, immunogenicity, and efficacy in healthy adults of four doses of live oral hybrid Escherichia coli-Shigella flexneri 2a vaccine strain EcSf2a-2. Vaccine 13: 495–502.
24. Kotloff KL, Nataro JP, Losonsky GA, Wasserman SS, Hale TL, et al. (1995) A modified Shigella volunteer challenge model in which the inoculum is administered with bicarbonate buffer: clinical experience and implications for Shigella infectivity. Vaccine 13: 1488–1494.
25. Cohen D, Green MS, Block C, Slepon R, Ofek I (1991) Prospective study of the association between serum antibodies to lipopolysaccharide O antigen and the attack rate of shigellosis. Journal of clinical microbiology 29: 386–389.
26. DuPont HL, Hornick RB, Snyder MJ, Libonati JP, Formal SB, et al. (1972) Immunity in shigellosis. II. Protection induced by oral live vaccine or primary infection. The Journal of infectious diseases 125: 12–16.
27. Coron E, Flamant M, Aubert P, Wedel T, Pedron T, et al. (2009) Characterisation of early mucosal and neuronal lesions following Shigella flexneri infection in human colon. PloS one 4: e4713.
28. Flamant M, Aubert P, Rolli-Derkinderen M, Bourreille A, Neunlist MR, et al. (2011) Enteric glia protect against Shigella flexneri invasion in intestinal epithelial cells: a role for S-nitrosoglutathione. Gut 60: 473–484.
29. Sakaguchi T, Kohler H, Gu X, McCormick BA, Reinecker HC (2002) Shigella flexneri regulates tight junction-associated proteins in human intestinal epithelial cells. Cellular microbiology 4: 367–381.
30. Wu T, Grassel C, Levine MM, Barry EM (2011) Live attenuated Shigella dysenteriae type 1 vaccine strains overexpressing shiga toxin B subunit. Infection and immunity 79: 4912–4922.
31. Mounier J, Vasselon T, Hellio R, Lesourd M, Sansonetti PJ (1992) Shigella flexneri enters human colonic Caco-2 epithelial cells through the basolateral pole. Infection and immunity 60: 237–248.
32. Vasselon T, Mounier J, Hellio R, Sansonetti PJ (1992) Movement along actin filaments of the perijunctional area and de novo polymerization of cellular actin are required for Shigella flexneri colonization of epithelial Caco-2 cell monolayers. Infection and immunity 60: 1031–1040.
33. Lindberg AA, Karnell A, Stocker BA, Katakura S, Sweiha H, et al. (1988) Development of an auxotrophic oral live Shigella flexneri vaccine. Vaccine 6: 146–150.
34. Lindberg AA, Karnell A, Pal T, Sweiha H, Hultenby K, et al. (1990) Construction of an auxotrophic Shigella flexneri strain for use as a live vaccine. Microbial pathogenesis 8: 433–440.
35. Cersini A, Salvia AM, Bernardini ML (1998) Intracellular multiplication and virulence of Shigella flexneri auxotrophic mutants. Infection and immunity 66: 549–557.
36. Formal SB, Dammin GJ, Labrec EH, Schneider H (1958) Experimental Shigella infections: characteristics of a fatal infection produced in guinea pigs. Journal of Bacteriology 75: 604–610.
37. Venkatesan MM, Hartman AB, Newland JW, Ivanova VS, Hale TL, et al. (2002) Construction, characterization, and animal testing of WRSd1, a Shigella dysenteriae 1 vaccine. Infection and immunity 70: 2950–2958.
38. Kotloff KL, Pasetti MF, Barry EM, Nataro JP, Wasserman SS, et al. (2004) Deletion in the Shigella enterotoxin genes further attenuates Shigella flexneri 2a bearing guanine auxotrophy in a phase 1 trial of CVD 1204 and CVD 1208. The Journal of infectious diseases 190: 1745–1754.
39. Kotloff KL, Simon JK, Pasetti MF, Sztein MB, Wooden SL, et al. (2007) Safety and immunogenicity of CVD 1208S, a live, oral DeltaguaBA Deltasen Deltaset Shigella flexneri 2a vaccine grown on animal-free media. Human vaccines 3: 268–275.
40. Fiorentino M, Lammers KM, Levine MM, Sztein MB, Fasano A (2013) In vitro Intestinal Mucosal Epithelial Responses to Wild-Type Salmonella Typhi and Attenuated Typhoid Vaccines. Frontiers in immunology 4: 17.
41. Rao R (2009) Occludin phosphorylation in regulation of epithelial tight junctions. Annals of the New York Academy of Sciences 1165: 62–68.
42. Balda MS, Whitney JA, Flores C, Gonzalez S, Cereijido M, et al. (1996) Functional dissociation of paracellular permeability and transepithelial electrical resistance and disruption of the apical-basolateral intramembrane diffusion barrier by expression of a mutant tight junction membrane protein. The Journal of cell biology 134: 1031–1049.
43. McCarthy KM, Skare IB, Stankewich MC, Furuse M, Tsukita S, et al. (1996) Occludin is a functional component of the tight junction. Journal of cell science 109 (Pt 9): 2287–2298.
44. Seth A, Sheth P, Elias BC, Rao R (2007) Protein phosphatases 2A and 1 interact with occludin and negatively regulate the assembly of tight junctions in the CACO-2 cell monolayer. The Journal of biological chemistry 282: 11487–11498.
45. Sakakibara A, Furuse M, Saitou M, Ando-Akatsuka Y, Tsukita S (1997) Possible involvement of phosphorylation of occludin in tight junction formation. The Journal of cell biology 137: 1393–1401.
46. Wong V (1997) Phosphorylation of occludin correlates with occludin localization and function at the tight junction. The American Journal of Physiology 273: C1859–1867.
47. Taylor DN, Echeverria P (1986) Etiology and epidemiology of travelers' diarrhea in Asia. Reviews of infectious diseases 8 Suppl 2: S136–141.
48. Taylor DN, Houston R, Shlim DR, Bhaibulaya M, Ungar BL, et al. (1988) Etiology of diarrhea among travelers and foreign residents in Nepal. JAMA : the journal of the American Medical Association 260: 1245–1248.
49. Pignata S, Maggini L, Zarrilli R, Rea A, Acquaviva AM (1994) The enterocyte-like differentiation of the Caco-2 tumor cell line strongly correlates with responsiveness to cAMP and activation of kinase A pathway. Cell growth & differentiation : the molecular biology journal of the American Association for Cancer Research 5: 967–973.
50. Hidalgo IJ, Raub TJ, Borchardt RT (1989) Characterization of the human colon carcinoma cell line (Caco-2) as a model system for intestinal epithelial permeability. Gastroenterology 96: 736–749.
51. Artursson P (1990) Epithelial transport of drugs in cell culture. I: A model for studying the passive diffusion of drugs over intestinal absorptive (Caco-2) cells. Journal of pharmaceutical sciences 79: 476–482.
52. Dorfel MJ, Huber O (2012) Modulation of tight junction structure and function by kinases and phosphatases targeting occludin. Journal of biomedicine & biotechnology 2012: 807356.
53. Suzuki T, Elias BC, Seth A, Shen L, Turner JR, et al. (2009) PKC eta regulates occludin phosphorylation and epithelial tight junction integrity. Proceedings of the National Academy of Sciences of the United States of America 106: 61–66.
54. Sundstrom JM, Tash BR, Murakami T, Flanagan JM, Bewley MC, et al. (2009) Identification and analysis of occludin phosphosites: a combined mass spectrometry and bioinformatics approach. Journal of proteome research 8: 808–817.
55. Murakami T, Felinski EA, Antonetti DA (2009) Occludin phosphorylation and ubiquitination regulate tight junction trafficking and vascular endothelial growth factor-induced permeability. The Journal of biological chemistry 284: 21036–21046.
56. Dorfel MJ, Westphal JK, Bellmann C, Krug SM, Cording J, et al. (2013) CK2-dependent phosphorylation of occludin regulates the interaction with ZO-proteins and tight junction integrity. Cell communication and signaling : CCS 11: 40-811X-811-840.
57. Raleigh DR, Boe DM, Yu D, Weber CR, Marchiando AM, et al. (2011) Occludin S408 phosphorylation regulates tight junction protein interactions and barrier function. The Journal of cell biology 193: 565–582.
58. Farfan MJ, Toro CS, Barry EM, Nataro JP (2011) Shigella enterotoxin-2 is a type III effector that participates in Shigella-induced interleukin 8 secretion by epithelial cells. FEMS immunology and medical microbiology 61: 332–339.
59. Zurawski DV, Mumy KL, Faherty CS, McCormick BA, Maurelli AT (2009) Shigella flexneri type III secretion system effectors OspB and OspF target the nucleus to downregulate the host inflammatory response via interactions with retinoblastoma protein. Molecular microbiology 71: 350–368.
60. Nandakumar NS, Pugazhendhi S, Ramakrishna BS (2009) Effects of enteropathogenic bacteria & lactobacilli on chemokine secretion & Toll like receptor gene expression in two human colonic epithelial cell lines. The Indian journal of medical research 130: 170–178.
61. Jung HC, Eckmann L, Yang SK, Panja A, Fierer J, et al. (1995) A distinct array of proinflammatory cytokines is expressed in human colon epithelial cells in response to bacterial invasion. The Journal of clinical investigation 95: 55–65.
62. Fasano A, Noriega FR, Liao FM, Wang W, Levine MM (1997) Effect of shigella enterotoxin 1 (ShET1) on rabbit intestine in vitro and in vivo. Gut 40: 505–511.
63. Faherty CS, Harper JM, Shea-Donohue T, Barry EM, Kaper JB, et al. (2012) Chromosomal and plasmid-encoded factors of Shigella flexneri induce secretogenic activity ex vivo. PloS one 7: e49980.

8

Plasmid-Mediated Sulfamethoxazole Resistance Encoded by the sul2 Gene in the Multidrug-Resistant *Shigella flexneri* 2a Isolated from Patients with Acute Diarrhea in Dhaka, Bangladesh

Mohd S. Iqbal[1,2]*, Mostafizur Rahman[1], Rafiad Islam[1], Atanu Banik[1], M. Badrul Amin[1], Fatema Akter[1], Kaisar Ali Talukder[1]

1 Centre for Food and Waterborne Diseases (CFWD), icddr,b, Dhaka, Bangladesh,, **2** Centre for Control of Chronic Diseases (CCCD), icddr,b, Dhaka, Bangladesh

Abstract

In this study, mechanisms of plasmid-mediated sulfamethoxazole resistances in the clinical strains of multi-drug resistant (MDR) *Shigella flexneri* 2a were elucidated for the first time in Bangladesh. From 2006 to 2011, a total of 200 *S. flexneri* 2a strains were randomly selected from the stock of the Enteric and Food Microbiology Laboratory of icddr,b. Antimicrobial susceptibility of the strains showed 73%, 98%, 93%, 58%, 98%, 64% and 4% resistance to trimethoprim-sulfamethoxazole, nalidixic acid, ampicillin, erythromycin, tetracycline, ciprofloxacin and ceftriaxone respectively. Plasmid profiling revealed heterogeneous patterns and interestingly, all the trimethoprim-sulfamethoxazole resistant (SXT^R) strains yielded a distinct 4.3 MDa plasmid compared to that of the trimethoprim-sulfamethoxazole susceptible (SXT^S) strains. Curing of this 4.3 MDa plasmid resulted in the susceptibility to sulfamethoxazole alone suggesting the involvement of this plasmid in the resistance of sulfamethoxazole. Moreover, PCR analysis showed the presence of *sul2* gene in SXT^R strains which is absent in SXT^S strains as well as in the 4.3 MDa plasmid-cured derivatives, confirming the involvement of *sul2* in the resistance of sulfamethoxazole. Furthermore, pulsed-field gel electrophoresis (PFGE) analysis revealed that both the SXT^R and SXT^S strains were clonal. This study will significantly contributes to the knowledge on acquired drug resistance of the mostly prevalent *S. flexneri* 2a and further warrants continuous monitoring of the prevalence and correlation of this resistance determinants amongst the clinical isolates of *Shigella* and other enteric pathogens around the world to provide effective clinical management of the disease.

Editor: Oliver Schildgen, Kliniken der Stadt Köln gGmbH, Germany

Funding: This study was funded by icddr,b (www.icddrb.org) and its donors which provide unrestricted support to icddr,b for its operations and research. Current donors providing unrestricted support include: Government of the People's Republic of Bangladesh; Canadian International Development Agency (CIDA), Embassy of the Kingdom of the Netherlands (EKN), Swedish International Development Cooperation Agency (Sida), and the Department for International Development, UK (DFID). The authors gratefully acknowledge these donors for their support and commitment to icddr,b research efforts. The funders had no role in study design, data collection and analysis, decision to publish, or preparation of the manuscript.

Competing Interests: The authors have declared that no competing interests exist.

* E-mail: msiqbal@icddrb.org

Introduction

Shigellosis is becoming an increasing public health problem due to the emergence of multiple antimicrobial resistances, leading to high rate of global morbidity and mortality especially in the endemic areas like Bangladesh. Approximately 165 million cases of *Shigella* infection occur annually worldwide with 1.1 million deaths with most of the causality are children under 5 years of age [1]. It is well established that *S. flexneri* is the most commonly isolated species in the developing countries; in contrast, *S. sonnei* predominates in developed countries. In developing countries like Bangladesh, the predominant serotype of *S. flexneri* is 2a which is also the most common strain in industrialized countries [1]. Previously efficacious first-line antimicrobial drugs such as sulphonamides, tetracycline, ampicillin, and trimethoprim-sulfamethoxazole have become largely ineffective against prevalent *Shigella* strains in many parts of the world and the recently reported emergence of ciprofloxacin and third-generation cephalosporin resistance, further narrows the choice of effective antimicrobials [2]. The American Academy of Pediatrics and the Infectious Disease Society of America recommend azithromycin as an alternative drug for the treatment of Shigellosis [3]. However, resistance and reduced susceptibility to azithromycin has also been emerged [4,5]. Thus, the urge for new antibiotics is more pressing than ever. Sulfamethoxazole, a short acting derivative of sulfonamide, is an antibacterial drug widely used since 1930s in the clinical and veterinary medicine to treat bacterial and protozoal infections [6]. The sul2 is one of the three sulfonamide resistance genes and was first identified on a small nonconjugative plasmid of *Escherichia coli* [6]. Plasmid-mediated multidrug resistance is a grave concern for the treatment of infectious diseases. Multiple plasmid-mediated mechanisms of resistance against the fluoroquinolones and aminoglycosides have been described, and the combination of plasmid-mediated resistance with chromosomally encoded resistance mechanisms of multiple drug classes now results in strains that are resistant to all of the main classes of commonly used antimicrobial drugs [7].

In this study, we have characterized 200 clinical MDR *S. flexneri* 2a strains and shown for the first time that the sul2 gene encoded by a small 4.3 MDa plasmid is responsible for the sulfamethoxazole resistance, which eventually will lead to better understanding of effective clinical management of Shigellosis around the world.

Materials and Methods

Bacterial strains and serotyping

Two hundred *S. flexneri* 2a strains were randomly selected from patients attending the Dhaka treatment center operated by the International Centre for Diarrhoeal Diseases Research, Bangladesh (icddr,b) in between 2006 and 2011. These strains were isolated and identified in the clinical microbiology laboratory by standard microbiological and biochemical methods [8] and confirmed serologically by using commercially available antisera kit (Denka Saiken, Co. Ltd.,Japan) specific for all type- and group-factor antigens as described earlier [8]. A version of *S. flexneri* 2a without the 4.3 MDa plasmid was constructed by curing with acridine orange. *E. coli* strains PDK-9 and V-517 were used as plasmid molecular weight standard [8]. The *Salmonella enterica* serovar Braenderup H9812 was used as molecular size marker for PFGE [8].

Antimicrobial susceptibility

Bacterial susceptibility to antimicrobial agents was determined as described previously [3] with commercial antimicrobial discs (Oxoid, Basingstoke, UK). The antibiotic discs used in this study were ampicillin (AMP, 10 µg), azithromycin (AZM, 15 µg), ceftriaxone (CRO, 30 µg), chloramphenicol (CHL, 30 µg), ciprofloxacin (CIP, 5 µg), nalidixic acid (NA, 30 µg), sulfamethoxazole (SMX, 25 µg), trimethoprim (TMP, 5 µg), norfloxacin (NOR, 10 µg), trimithoprim/sulfamethoxazole (SXT, 1.25/23.75 µg), streptomycin (STR, 10 µg), tetracycline (TET, 30 µg), mecillinum (MEL, 30 µg), gentamycin (GEN, 10 µg), kanamycin (KAN, 30 µg) and amikacin (AK, 15 µg). *Escherichia coli* ATCC 25922 and *Staphylococcus aureus* ATCC 25923 were used as control strains for susceptibility studies.

Plasmid profiling

Plasmid DNA was prepared by the simplified alkaline lysis method of Kado and Liu with some modifications as described previously [8]. The molecular mass of the unknown plasmid DNA was assessed by comparison with the mobilities of plasmids with known molecular masses and plasmid DNA of reference *E. coli* strains PDK-9 and V517 were used as molecular mass standards [8].

Curing of plasmids

The minimum inhibitory concentration (MIC) and sub inhibitory concentration of acridine orange were determined by the agar dilution method [9]. *S. flexneri* 2a strain was grown in Muller-Hinton agar (Becton, Dickinson and Company, USA) plates in the presence of acridine orange (Sigma, St Louis, MO) at variable concentration for 24 h at 37°C. The MIC was defined as the lowest concentration of acridine orange that completely inhibited the visible growth of the test organism after incubation. Plasmid curing was performed as described previously [9]. *S. flexneri* 2a strain was inoculated with Tryptic Soy Broth (TSB) (Becton, Dickinson and Company, USA) containing 0.3% yeast extract in the presence of acridine orange of different concentrations (180, 200, 220, 240 and 260 µg/mL) and then incubated for 24hrs at 37°C. Overnight grown broth culture was then plated on MacConkey agar (Becton, Dickinson and Company, USA) plate and isolated colonies were then subjected to colony patch. Colonies that failed to grow in Tryptic Soy agar (Becton, Dickinson and Company, USA) containing trimethoprim-sulfamethoxazole were considered as putative cured derivatives. Physical loss of the plasmid in the cured derivative was confirmed by agarose gel electrophoresis following extraction of the plasmid DNA from the respective cultures. The percentages of curing efficiency were expressed as the number of colonies with cured phenotype per 100 colonies tested. Antibiotic resistance profiles of plasmid-harboring and plasmid-cured strains were reconfirmed by the disk diffusion method as described earlier [3].

PCR analysis

Total DNA of SXT^R, SXT^S and 4.3 MDa plasmid cured derivatives of *S.flexneri* 2a strains were prepared according to the procedures described earlier [10]. The *sul1, sul2, sul3, integron1 and integron2* genes were detected by PCR using the primers recommended earlier [11]. Amplifications were performed with a final volume of 30 µl on an thermal cycler (Biorad) with each reaction mixture contained 3.0 µl 5x Green GoTaq Flexi buffer (Promega, USA), 2.0 µl dNTPs (Invitrogen), 10 pmol of each primer, (Integrated DNA Technologies, Inc. USA), 1 µl of total DNA and 1 U of GoTaq Flexi DNA polymerase enzyme (Promega, USA). PCR conditions were adopted from elsewhere [11].

Pulsed-field gel electrophoresis (PFGE)

PFGE analysis was performed according to the PulseNet standardized protocol [12] using *Xba I* as the restriction enzyme (New England Biolabs, Ipswich, MA). The *Salmonella enterica* serovar Braenderup H9812 was used as molecular size marker [8]. Dendrogram analysis was performed using algorithms available within the Bionumerics software package v.4.5. The unweighted pair group method arithmetic means (UPGMA), with a 2.0% tolerance limit and 1.00% optimization was used to obtain the dendrogram. Strains with a coefficient of similarity ≥90% were considered as genetically closely related.

Results

Serotyping and antimicrobial susceptibility testing

All (n = 200) the strains were serologically subtyped and reconfirmed as *S. flexneri* 2a. In order to clarify the association of small plasmids in the drug resistance of *Shigella*, 200 *S. flexneri* 2a clinical strains were subjected to antimicrobial susceptibility testing and found that 73%, 98%, 93%, 58%, 98%, 64% and 4% resistance to SXT, NA, AMP, E, TET, CIP and CRO respectively (Data not shown).

Plasmid profiling

Plasmid profiling revealed heterogeneous patterns ranging in sizes from approximately 140 to 2.1 MDa among the MDR *S. flexneri* 2a strains. Three plasmids of approximately 140, 2.7 and 2.1 MDa in size were present in more than 90% of the strains and were considered to be the core plasmids of *S. flexneri* 2a (Table 1). Interestingly, all the SXT^R (n = 146) strains harbored 4.3 MDa plasmid which is absent in all the SXT^S strains (Table 1) and among the eight different plasmid patterns, pattern P1 (140, 4.3, 2.7 and 2.1 MDa) and P6 (140, 2.7, 2.1 MDa) were predominant in SXT^R (n = 146) (91.2%) and SXT^S (n = 54) (84%) strains

Table 1. Plasmid patterns of MDR *S. flexneri* 2a strains isolated in Dhaka, Bangladesh in between 2006 and 2011.

Serotypes	Plasmid patterns	Plasmid sizes (MDa)	Percentage
SXT resistant strains (n = 146)	P1	140, 4.3,2.7, 2.1	91.2%
	P2	4.3, 2.7, 2.1	4%
	P3	140, 52, 4.3, 2.7, 2.1	3.2%
	P4	105, 4.3, 2.7, 2.1	0.8%
	P5	140, 4.3, 2.7, 2.1, 1.4	0.8%
SXT susceptible strains (n = 54)	P6	140, 2.7, 2.1	84%
	P7	2.7, 2.1	12%
	P8	140, 3.2	4%

respectively (Table 1). The frequency of rest of the patterns was very low.

Plasmid curing

Typical in vitro plasmid curing experiments involve exposure of plasmid containing cells to a drug throughout the growth cycle and subsequent assay of the population for the loss of plasmid specific traits. The minimum inhibitory concentration (MIC) of acridine orange against two different clinical strains of MDR *S. flexneri* 2a was found to be 280 µg/ml (Table 2), indicating that acridine orange was not a potent antibacterial agent for the test strains. Acridine orange cured the 4.3 MDa plasmid in the clinical strains of MDR *S. flexneri* 2a (Figure 1a). Curing activity was investigated at different concentrations of acridine orange ranging from 180 µg/mL to 260 µg/mL. The curing efficiency was expressed as the number of colonies with cured phenotype per 100 colonies tested. The highest curing efficiency (3.2%) was observed below the MIC at subinhibitory concentration 260 µg/mL (Table 2).

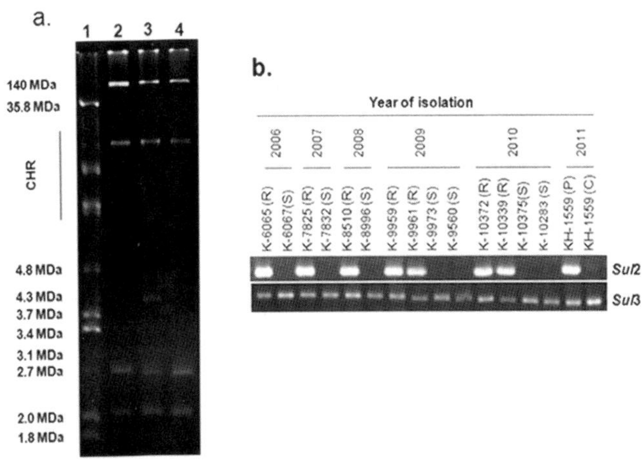

Figure 1. Involvement of 4.3 MDa plasmid and the sul2 gene in the resistance of sulfamethoxazole. a. Agarose gel electrophoresis pattern of plasmid DNA isolated from SXT^R *S. flexneri* 2a clinical strain KH-1559 and its plasmid cured derivative. Lanes 1 and 2, represents *Escherichia coli* V517 and PDK-9 respectively as size determination markers. Lanes 3 and 4 represent KH-1559(P) SXT^R strains and its 4.3 MDa plasmid cured derivative KH-1559 (C) respectively. **b.** *sul2 and sul*3 gene expressions in the representative SXT^R (R) and SXT^S (S) strains of *S. flexneri* 2a from 2006 to 2011.

Detection of *sul1, sul2, sul3, integron1* and *integron2* genes in the SXT-resistant and susceptible strains

To investigate the possible mechanisms of SXT resistance, we have checked the presence of *sul1*, *sul2*, *sul3*, *integron1* and *integron2* genes in all the MDR *S. flexneri* 2a strains and found that *sul2* was present in all the SXT^R strains (n = 146) and absent in all the SXT^S strains (n = 54) (Figure 1b). However, no change was observed in the expressions of *sul1*, *sul3*, *integron1 and integron2* genes among the SXT^R and SXT^S strains. Interestingly, curing of the 4.3 MDa plasmid resulted in the loss of *sul2* and sulfamethoxazole sensitivity in the cured strains confirming the involvement of 4.3 MDa plasmid and *sul2* in the resistance of sulfamethoxazole (Figure 1 and Table 3), as has also been supported by others. [6,13–15].

Pulsed-field gel electrophoresis (PFGE)

PFGE has been used for the identification of new strains within a community and determining the clonal diversity among the circulating pathogens [8]. PFGE analysis of the *Xba*I-digested chromosomal DNA of the MDR *S. flexneri* 2a strains and their plasmid cured derivatives yielded DNA fragments ranging in size approximately from 20 to 670 Kb. Dendrogram analysis exhibited the same PFGE patterns among the representative SXT^R and SXT^S strains indicating that they have originated from a common ancestor (Figure 2). Besides, both the parent and 4.3 MDa plasmid cure derivatives were very much close in their homology (95%)

Table 2. Effect of acridine orange concentration on curing efficiency of MDR *S. flexneri* 2a*.

Strain ID	Concentration (µg/ml)	Curing efficiency (%)
KH 1559	260	3.20
	240	1.82
	220	0.62
	200	0.13
KH 1972	260	2.76
	240	1.34
	220	0.27
	200	0.12

*Five hundred colonies (at each concentration) were tested for curing of the antibiotic resistant phenotype.

Table 3. Antibiogram of two MDR *S. flexneri* 2a strains and their 4.3 MDa plasmid-cured derivatives*.

Antimicrobial agents	Diameter of inhibition zone (mm)			
	Before curing		After curing	
	Resistance	Susceptibility	Resistance	Susceptibility
Ampicillin (AMP)	8	-	8	-
Azithromycin (AZM)	-	25	-	26
Ceftriaxone (CRO)	-	36	-	35
Chloramphenicol (C)	12	-	11	-
Ciprofloxacin (CIP)	-	30	-	30
SXT	8	-	-	27
Sulfamethoxazole(SMX)	8	-	-	25
Trimethoprim (TMP)	8	-	8	-
Amikacin (AK)	-	22	-	21
Nalidixicacid (NA)	8	-	8	-
Gentamicin (GEN)	-	25	-	24
Kanamycin (KAN)	-	25	-	26
Norfloxacin (NOR)	-	30	-	29
Streptomycin (STR)	8	-	8	-
Tetracycline(TET)	10	-	10	-
Mecillinam (MEL)	-	26	-	27

SXT, trimethoprim-sulfamethoxazole (Co-trimoxazole).
*Wild-type MDR *S. flexneri* 2a strains were resistant to eight antibiotics and susceptible to eight; the plasmid-cured derivatives showed that the antibiotic resistance loci of sulfamethoxazole were plasmid-encoded.

demonstrating no effect of acridine orange treatment on chromosomal DNA (Figure 2).

Discussion

The emergence and dissemination of multi-drug resistant strains of *Shigella* are particularly of greater importance in developing countries like Bangladesh due to the accessibility of multiple drugs which further augments the resistance rate resulting in frequent treatment failures. Our study demonstrates an increasing incidence of antimicrobial resistance of the mostly prevalent *S. flexneri* 2a serotype isolated in between 2006 to 2011 and also determines a 4.3 MDa plasmid-mediated sulfamethoxazole resistance encoded by the sul2 *gene*. Moreover, these MDR strains were concurrently resistant to ≥3 of the eight antimicrobial agents used and were detected in 95% of the *S. flexneri* 2a isolates. Resistance to ampicillin + nalidixic acid + trimethoprim-sulfamethoxazole was the most common pattern whereas resistances to at least four, five and six antimicrobial agents were found to be 92%, 77% and 33% respectively. None of the strains were found to be resistant to at least seven or eight antibiotics. Alarmingly, significant increase (32%) in the multi-drug resistance

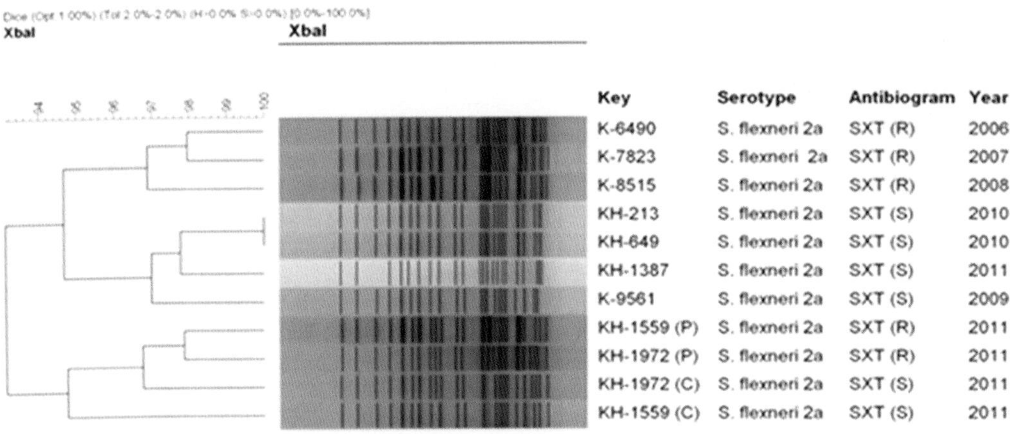

Figure 2. PFGE patterns of representative SXT^R (R) and SXT^S (S) *S. flexneri* 2a strains and their plasmid cured (C) derivatives. The dendrogram was constructed with Bionumerics v.4.5 software using the unweighted pair group method with arithmetic means (UPGMA). Dendrogram analysis showed that the plasmid cured strains and the parent strains are very close (95%) in their homology.

was observed among the *S. flexneri 2a* strains as compared to that of the 2001–2002 isolates reported by Rahman M et al. [5]. This increased resistance phenomena could be explicated by widespread and indiscriminate use of antibiotics over longer periods to treat Shigellosis, resulting in the positive selection pressure and maintenance of drug resistance [16]. Almost all the strains from 2010 were found to be resistant (95%) to ciprofloxacin as has also been found in neighboring Kolkata, India during 2007–2009, where the resistance was 91.6%. Moreover, similar trend has been reported in many South Asian countries [3]. Interestingly, almost all the tested strains from 2009 and 2010 were susceptible to mecillinam and thus currently used as an empirical drug for the treatment of Shigellosis in Bangladesh [5]. Plasmid profiling could be an attractive tool in epidemiological investigations of various enteric pathogens [17]. Our study revealed heterogeneous populations of plasmids in *S. flexneri* 2a strains ranging from two to five in numbers. Of these 200 strains, 12% lost the large, 140 MDa plasmid, mostly known for the invasiveness of the bacteria and possibly due to prolonged storage at −70°C and repeated sub-culturing as has also been described by Vargas et al. [18]. In addition to the large plasmid, about 98% of the strains contained two plasmids of approximately 2.7 MDa and 2.1 MDa in size and these two along with the 140 MDa plasmid are considered as the core plasmid (140, 2.7 and 2.1 MDa) of *S. flexneri* 2a as reported earlier [19]. Interestingly, all the SXT^R (n = 146) strains harbored a unique 4.3 MDa plasmid which is absent in all the SXT^S (n = 54) strains and paved us the way towards further investigation (Table 1). Curing of this 4.3 MDa plasmid from two of the recently isolated SXT^R strains showed resistance to six drugs (AMP, C, NA, TMP, STR, TET) and susceptibility to ten drugs (SXT, SMX, AZM, CRO, CIP, NOR, MEL, GEN, KAN, AK). In contrast, wild type strains were resistant to SXT, SMX, TMP AMP, C, NA, STR and TET (Table 3) and thus confirming the involvement of 4.3 MDa plasmid in the resistance to sulfamethoxazole alone as has also been reported elsewhere [9]. In gram-negative clinical isolates, spread of antibiotic resistance determinants by integrons underlies the rapid evolution of MDR phenotypes [20]. Both *sul1* and *sul3* genes are thought to be associated with class 1 integrons while the sul2 with the class 2 integrons [11,20]. In our study, sulfamethoxazole resistance observed in *S. flexneri* 2a strains was conferred by the sul2 gene encoded by a small non-conjugative plasmid as reported earlier [9,21]. However, apart from *sul2*, no significant difference was observed in *integron1*, *integron2*, *sul1* and *sul3* gene expressions among all the 200 strains irrespective of SXT resistance which might be attributable to possible promoter inactivation or other environmental factors. Similarly, Hu LF and colleagues showed the involvement of 7.3 kb plasmid encoded the sul2 gene conferring high SXT resistance in the clinical isolates of *Stenotrophomonas maltophilia* [13].

In conclusion, this study collectively demonstrates for the first time the association of *sul2* and 4.3 MDa plasmid in the sulfamethoxazole resistance of the MDR clinical strains of *S. flexneri* 2a in Bangladesh. Further analysis of the function of small plasmids as well as the comparative analysis of virulence plasmids from other *Shigella* serotypes will allow a more complete characterization of the evolution of these plasmids. Although, more severe approaches should be taken to clarify the precise molecular mechanism; this study will significantly contributes to the knowledge on acquired drug resistance of the mostly prevalent *S. flexneri* 2a and thereby warrants continuous monitoring of the prevalence and correlation of this resistance determinants amongst the clinical isolates of *Shigella* and other enteric pathogens around the world to provide effective clinical management of the disease.

Acknowledgments

We gratefully acknowledge Mr. Dilip K. Dutta and Abu I. M. S. Ud-Din for their technical assistances. The authors would like to thank the members of the Enteric and Food Microbiology Laboratory, CFWD, icddr,b for their sincere cooperation throughout the study.

Author Contributions

Conceived and designed the experiments: MSI. Performed the experiments: MSI MR RI AB MBA FA. Analyzed the data: MSI MR RI AB MBA FA. Contributed reagents/materials/analysis tools: MR RI AB MBA. Wrote the paper: MSI MR. Critical revision: MSI MR AB KAT. Final approval of manuscript: MSI MR RI AB MBA FA KAT.

References

1. Kotloff KL, Winickoff JP, Ivanoff B, Clemens JD, Swerdlow DL, et al. (1999) Global burden of *Shigella* infections: implications for vaccine development and implementation of control strategies. Bull World Health Organ 77(8): 651–666.
2. Niyogi SK (2007) Increasing antimicrobial resistance — an emerging problem in the treatment of shigellosis. Clin Microbiol Infect 13(12): 1141–1143.
3. Ghosh S, Pazhani GP, Chowdhury G, Guin S, Dutta S, et al. (2011) Genetic characteristics and changing antimicrobial resistance among *Shigella* spp. isolated from hospitalized diarrhoeal patients in Kolkata, India. J Med Microbiol 60: 1460–1466.
4. Howie RL, Folster JP, Bowen A, Barzilay EJ, Whichard JM (2010) Reduced azithromycin susceptibility in *Shigella sonnei*, United States. Microb Drug Resist 16(4): 245–8.
5. Rahman M, Shoma S, Rashid H, Arifeen SE, Baqui AH, et al. (2007) Increasing spectrum in antimicrobial resistance of *Shigella* strains in Bangladesh: Resistance to azithromycin and ceftriaxone and decreased susceptibility to ciprofloxacin. J Health Popul Nutr 25(2): 158–167.
6. Byrne-Bailey KG, Gaze WH, Kay P, Boxall AB, Hawkey PM, et al. (2009) Prevalence of sulfonamide resistance genes in bacterial isolates from manured agricultural soils and pig slurry in the United Kingdom. Antimicrob Agents Chemother 53(2): 696–702.
7. Schultsz C, Geerlings S (2012) Plasmid-mediated resistance in Enterobacteriaceae: changing landscape and implications for therapy. Drugs 72(1): 1–16.
8. Talukder KA, Islam MA, Dutta DK, Hassan F, Safa A, et al. (2002) Phenotypic and genotypic characterization of serologically atypical strains of *Shigella flexneri* type 4 isolated in Dhaka, Bangladesh. J Clin Microbiol 40: 2490–2497.
9. Barman S, Chatterjee S, Koley H (2010) Plasmid-mediated streptomycin and sulfamethoxazole resistance in *Shigella flexneri* 3a. Int J Antimicrob Agents 36: 348–351.
10. Talukder KA, Islam Z, Islam MA, Dutta DK, Safa A, et al. (2003) Phenotypic and genotypic characterization of provisional serotype *Shigella flexneri* 1c and clonal relationships with 1a and 1b strains isolated in Bangladesh. J Clin Microbiol 41(1): 110–117.
11. Vrints M, Mairiaux E, Meervenne EV, Collard JM, Bertrand S (2009) Surveillance of antibiotic susceptibility patterns among *Shigella sonnei* strains isolated in Belgium during the 18-year period 1990 to 2007. J Clin Microbiol 47(5): 1379–85.
12. Ribot EM, Fair MA, Gautom R, Cameron DN, Hunter SB, et al. (2006) Standardization of pulsed-field gel electrophoresis protocols for the subtyping of *Escherichia coli* O157:H7, *Salmonella*, and *Shigella* for PulseNet. Foodborne Pathog Dis 3: 59–67.
13. Hu LF, Chang X, Ye Y, Wang ZX, Shaoa YB, et al. (2011) *Stenotrophomonas maltophilia* resistance to trimethoprim/sulfamethoxazole mediated by acquisition of *sul* and *dfra* genes in a plasmid-mediated class 1 integron. Int J Antimicrob Agents 37(3): 230–4.
14. Nigro SJ, Hall RM (2011) GI*sul2*, a genomic island carrying the *sul2* sulphonamide resistance gene and the small mobile element CR2 found in the *Enterobacter cloacae* subspecies *cloacae* type strain ATCC 13047 from 1890, *Shigella flexneri* ATCC 700930 from 1954 and *Acinetobacter baumannii* ATCC 17978 from 1951. J Antimicrob Chemother 66(9): 2175–217.
15. Toleman MA, Bennett PM, Bennet DMC, Jones RN, Walsh TR (2007) Global emergence of trimethoprim/sulfamethoxazole resistance in *Stenotrophomonas maltophilia* mediated by acquisition of *sul* genes. Emerg Infect Dis 13(4): 559–565.
16. Faiz MA, Basher A (2011) Antimicrobial resistance: Bangladesh experience. Regional Health Forum – Vol 15 No 1: 1–18. Available: http://www.searo.who.int/publications/journals/regional_health_forum/issues/rhfv15n1/en/index.html. Accessed 2013 Nov 25.

17. Talukder KA, Islam Z, Dutta DK, Islam MA, Khajanchi BK, et al. (2006) Antibiotic resistance and genetic diversity of *Shigella sonnei* isolated from patients with diarrhoea between 1999 and 2003 in Bangladesh. J Med Microbiol 55: 1257–1263.
18. Vargas M, Gascon J, Anta M, Vila J (1999) Prevalence of Shigella enterotoxins 1 and 2 among Shigella strains isolated from patients with traveler's diarrhea. J Clin Microbiol 37: 3608–3611.
19. Haider k, Hijq ML, Talukder KA, Ahmad QS (1989) Electropherotyping of plasmid DNA of different serotypes of *Shigella flexneri* isolated in Bangladesh. Epidem Inf 102: 421–428.
20. Magnus A, Guerout MA, Maze D (2002) Bacterial resistance evolution by recruitment of super-integron gene cassettes. Mol Microbiol 43: 1657–1669.
21. Antunes P, Machado J, Sousa JC, Peix L (2005) Dissemination of sulfonamide resistance genes (*sul1, sul2, and sul3*) in Portuguese Salmonella enterica strains and relation with integrons. Antimicrob Agents Chemother 49: 836–839.

9

The Duration of Gastrointestinal and Joint Symptoms after a Large Waterborne Outbreak of Gastroenteritis in Finland in 2007 – A Questionnaire-Based 15-Month Follow-Up Study

Janne Laine [1,2]*¶, Jukka Lumio[3], Salla Toikkanen[2], Mikko J. Virtanen[2], Terhi Uotila[1], Markku Korpela[1,3], Eila Kujansuu[4¤], Markku Kuusi[2]

1 Tampere University Hospital, Department of Internal Medicine, Tampere, Finland, **2** National Institute of Health and Welfare, Epidemiologic Surveillance and Response Unit, Helsinki, Finland, **3** University of Tampere, School of Medicine, Tampere, Finland, **4** Nokia Health Centre, Nokia, Finland

Abstract

An extensive drinking water-associated gastroenteritis outbreak took place in the town of Nokia in Southern Finland in 2007. 53% of the exposed came down with gastroenteritis and 7% had arthritis-like symptoms (joint swelling, redness, warmth or pain in movement) according to a population-based questionnaire study at 8 weeks after the incident. *Campylobacter* and norovirus were the main pathogens. A follow-up questionnaire study was carried out 15 months after the outbreak to evaluate the duration of gastrointestinal and joint symptoms. 323 residents of the original contaminated area were included. The response rate was 53%. Participants were inquired about having gastroenteritis during the outbreak and the duration of symptoms. Of those with gastroenteritis, 43% reported loose stools and abdominal pain or distension after the acute disease. The prevalence of symptoms declined promptly during the first 3 months but at 15 months, 11% reported continuing symptoms. 32% of the respondents with gastroenteritis reported subsequent arthritis-like symptoms. The disappearance of arthritis-like symptoms was more gradual and they levelled off only after 5 months. 19% showed symptoms at 15 months. Prolonged gastrointestinal symptoms correlated to prolonged arthritis-like symptoms. High proportion of respondents continued to have arthritis-like symptoms at 15 months after the epidemic. The gastrointestinal symptoms, instead, had declined to a low level.

Editor: Oliver Schildgen, Kliniken der Stadt Köln gGmbH, Germany

Funding: This study was financially supported by the Competitive Research Funding of the Tampere University Hospital (Grants 9E129 and 9M124). The funders had no role in study design, data collection and analysis, decision to publish, or preparation of the manuscript.

Competing Interests: The authors have declared that no competing interests exist.

* E-mail: janne.laine@pshp.fi

¤ Current address: Department of Social Services and Health Care, Tampere, Finland

¶ The Pirkanmaa Waterborne Outbreak Study Group: Jaakko Antonen[1,3], Pekka Collin[1,3], Tina Katto[1], Anna-Leena Kuusela [1,3], Sami Mustajoki[1], Jukka Mustonen[1,3], Heikki Oksa[1,3], Petri Ruutu[2] and Sirpa Räsänen[1]

Introduction

Although acute gastroenteritis is a common disease, little is known about its consequences after passing the acute phase of the disease. As nearly everyone meets episodes of acute gastroenteritis occasionally, the possible connection with later health problems is easily missed. Food- and waterborne epidemics give special opportunity to study this connection prospectively as a cohort of people is infected in a relatively short period, often with identified pathogens. Epidemics large enough to conduct a study are, however, uncommon in developed countries with a good level of investigation capabilities.

Reactive arthritis (ReA) and milder forms of joint complaints are well known and fairly common acute complications of bacterial gastroenteritis [1]. There is also growing evidence of increased incidence of irritable bowel syndrome (IBS) after bacterial [2,3] and possibly viral [4] gastroenteritis. The most intensively studied waterborne outbreak is the Walkerton epidemic in Ontario, Canada. According to the Walkerton Health Study, increased risk of reactive arthritis, irritable bowel syndrome, pregnancy-related hypertension, hypertension, kidney disease, and even cardiovascular events has been observed after the epidemic [5,6,7,8,9,10].

A large drinking-waterborne epidemic occurred in a Finnish town Nokia in November–December 2007. Shortly after the incident, a comprehensive outbreak investigation of short- and long-term health effects was initiated. Details on the epidemiology, microbial findings, and early arthritic complaints have been published previously [11,12,13,14,15]. We performed a questionnaire study at 15 months after the exposure to contaminated water to observe the duration of symptoms and the remaining health complaints at 15 months after the incident. Here, we present data on the persistence of gastrointestinal and joint symptoms after the outbreak.

Methods

Setting

The town of Nokia is located in Southern Finland and has a population of 30 000. At the end of November 2007, maintenance work was carried out in the town's wastewater plant. During the work, a valve connecting the wastewater plant's effluent line and household water distribution line was opened and it was accidentally left open for two days. Approximately 450 m^3 of plant's effluent water contaminated the drinking water of 9 500 residents. This resulted in a large gastroenteritis outbreak in the contaminated area of the town. Some excess morbidity was also detected in the uncontaminated area [11]. The epidemic peaked four days after the incident, and most gastroenteritis cases occurred within two weeks.

Seven pathogens were found from the patients' stools. Six of those were also detected from tap water or water-distribution network samples. *Campylobacter* was the most common pathogen found in 27% (N = 148) of stool samples. In addition, norovirus was also considered as a major pathogen [16]. Non-typhoidal *Salmonellae* and *Giardiae* [13] were detected in less number of samples. In a study focusing on children with gastroenteritis, other viruses and infections with mixed pathogens were also observed [12].

According to a population-based questionnaire survey performed eight weeks after the incident 53% of the population in the contaminated area reported falling ill with gastroenteritis and 6.7% reported having arthritis-like joint symptoms [15]. In spite of active encouragement to refer new cases of probable arthritis to a rheumatologist at the local university hospital, only 21 confirmed cases of ReA were detected [14].

Questionnaire studies

Two consecutive questionnaires were mailed 13 months apart. The first was mailed eight weeks after the incident to detect the immediate morbidity [15]. The second, a follow-up study, was performed fifteen months after the outbreak in order to study the persistence of gastrointestinal and joint symptoms.

Details of the first questionnaire at 8 weeks were presented in previous articles [11,15]. In brief, two target populations were defined from Nokia; those residing in the part of town with contaminated water supply ("contaminated group") and those residing in the uncontaminated area ("uncontaminated group"). A third group ("control group") was chosen among the citizens of another municipality in the same district. Approximately, 1000 participants were randomly picked from the national population registry for each group (Table 1). All the ages were included and the groups were matched for age and gender. Only one participant per household was allowed.

The second questionnaire at 15 months ("follow-up") was mailed to persons who had participated in the first survey and given their consent for being contacted again. Therefore, the groups became smaller (Table 1.). No reminder was mailed to those who did not respond. Participants were asked whether they had gastroenteritis during the outbreak period (from November 28 to December 31 2007). They were also asked for how long (weeks or months) abdominal or joint symptoms persisted after the acute gastroenteritis.

Gastrointestinal symptoms, such as the presence of loose stools, constipation, nausea, abdominal pain, and abdominal distension were recorded. After analyzing these symptoms separately, a combination of gastrointestinal symptoms was created to observe IBS-like symptoms, such as loose stools and abdominal pain or distension. This combination is close to the Manning 3 and/or Rome I IBS-criteria [17].

Of joint symptoms, joint pain, pain in joint movement and the presence of swelling, redness, or warmth of the joint were recorded. The condition was classified as arthritis-like if pain in joint movement or any of the symptoms of joint swelling, redness, or warmth was present as defined in our previous study of early joint symptoms [15].

The persistence of gastrointestinal and arthritis-like symptoms was then analyzed as the remaining prevalence of a symptom in the course of time among those who had declared as having had gastroenteritis during the epidemic.

Use of microbiological data

Data of the stool specimens sent for microbiological analysis were obtained from the database of the Fimlab laboratories. This institution is a district-wide and public-run clinical laboratory serving the entire public health-care sector in the district. From year 2005 to 2009, the quantity, dates, and microbiological findings among the residents of Nokia and the control municipality were collected for comparison.

Statistical methods

Completed forms were stored in a database and analysed in the National Institute of Health and Welfare. Estimation of the effect of selection was done in two steps. First, the probability to be included in the study (i.e., those who gave permission to be contacted again) within all the initial study subjects was estimated by using univariate logistic regression. Secondly, the probability of returning the questionnaire within the included subjects was estimated in a similar manner. Confidence intervals for the proportion of subjects continuing to have symptoms at each time point were calculated by using ordinary bootstrap. All analyses were done with R version 2.15.2.

Ethical considerations

When answering the first questionnaire, participants were asked whether they would accept a follow-up contact. An informed consent was attached in the second questionnaire. The follow-up study was approved by the ethical committee of the Tampere University Hospital.

Results

Response rates and selection

Answer on the first questionnaire was received from 808 (79%) persons of the contaminated group, 717 (73%) of the uncontaminated group and 598 (60%) of the control group (Table 1). Taking all groups together, 667 (31.4%) of those responding declined the request for further contact. Response rates to the follow-up questionnaire were 53% (323/615), 46% (230/498), and 54% (186/343), respectively.

The odds ratios (ORs) for probability to be included in the follow-up questionnaire (i.e., giving permission to be contacted again) were 1.2 (95% CI 1.0–1.5) for the female gender, 1.7 (1.3–2.1) for those who had reported gastroenteritis and 1.7 (1.3–2.2) for those reporting joint symptoms in the first questionnaire. For these features the ORs for responding to the follow-up questionnaire were 1.1 (0.9–1.3), 1.0 (0.8–1.2) and 1.03 (0.8–1.3), respectively.

Of those participating in the follow-up study, 54% (174/323) in the contaminated group, 13% (31/230) in the uncontaminated group, and 3% (6/186) in the control group reported that they had gastroenteritis during the outbreak.

Table 1. Evolution of the study groups in the follow-up study.

	Nokia, contaminated	Nokia, uncontaminated	Control population
Population 2007	9 538	20 478	27 259
Size of the study groups in the first study	1 021	979	1 000
Responded to the first study	808	717	598
Sample size in the follow-up study (i.e., those who gave permission to be contacted again)	615	498	343
Responded to the follow-up study	323	230	186
Gastroenteritis during the epidemic, according to the follow-up study	174		

Study groups were based on the original population samples that were used in the first survey. The study groups became step-wise smaller because of lack of response to the first survey, denying further contact, and lack of response to the follow-up survey.

Gastrointestinal symptoms

Of the 174 persons in the contaminated group who had gastroenteritis, 53.6% (93) reported continuing loose stools, 47.9% (83) abdominal pain, and 32.7% (57) abdominal distension after the acute disease. 42.7% (74) experienced loose stools and abdominal pain or distension in the beginning of the follow-up (Figure 1). After a rapid decrease in the proportion of symptomatic persons in one month, the decline started to level off. At 15 months, 10.9% (19) of the respondents continued to have loose stools and abdominal pain or distension. This figure was 11.5% for adults 16 years of age or older and 8.9% for children.

Arthritis-like symptoms

Among the 174 participants in the contaminated group who had experienced gastroenteritis, 31.8% (55/174) reported arthritis-like symptoms after acute gastroenteritis. The proportion of persons with arthritis-like symptoms declined more slowly over time than the corresponding proportion with gastrointestinal symptoms (Figure 1). At 15 months, 19.0% (33/174) reported as continuing to have arthritis-like symptoms. The persistence of gastrointestinal symptoms (loose stools and abdominal pain or distension) predicted the presence of arthritis-like symptoms at 3 and 15 months (Table 2).

Use of microbiological tests

In Nokia, a sharp peak in the number of microbiological stool specimens was observed during the outbreak. Thereafter, the number of specimens diminished gradually and reached the pre-outbreak level in six months. In Nokia, the incidence of positive findings was high during the outbreak and for two months thereafter, but no difference was observed compared to the control municipality after one month (Figure 2).

Discussion

The faecal contamination of household water and the subsequent large epidemic of gastroenteritis was an exceptional accident [11]. The contamination was extensive as over half of the exposed population became ill. A remarkable proportion of the population suffered also from joint symptoms within the following eight weeks [15]. Two questionnaire surveys done thirteen months apart, based on representative population samples, focused on short- and long-term health effects of the epidemic. The 15-month follow-up questionnaire study reported here describes the duration of gastrointestinal and arthritis-like symptoms after the epidemic.

53.6% of those having had gastroenteritis during the epidemic reported loose stools and abdominal pain after the acute disease and 42.7% loose stools and abdominal pain or distension. Although the prevalence decreased rapidly within five months, 10.9% was still having symptoms resembling IBS (loose stools and abdominal pain or distension) at 15 months.

Irritable bowel syndrome (IBS) is a condition characterized by altered bowel function and abdominal pain or discomfort. The studies on the prevalence of symptoms compatible with IBS in the general population have given widely variable figures depending on the definition used. For example, in a population-based Finnish study, the prevalence of IBS ranged from 5.1% to 16.2%, depending on diagnostic criteria [17]. According to a recent systematic review of worldwide IBS-studies, the pooled prevalence of IBS was 11.2% among adult subjects [18].

IBS occurring after an episode of infective gastroenteritis has been referred as post-infectious irritable bowel syndrome (PI-IBS). Generally about 10% of IBS-patients regard that their symptoms began after an infective gastroenteritis [3]. According to a meta-analysis of eight studies published until December 2005, the median prevalence of IBS was 9.8% in the infective gastroenteritis groups and 1.2% in the control groups [19]. The observed frequency of PI-IBS is likely to depend on the pathogen(s) involved. In Walkerton, Canada, the prevalence of IBS was 27.5% among adult subjects who had had gastroenteritis during the epidemic while the prevalence among those without gastroenteritis was 10.1% at 2–3 years after the outbreak [9]. Diarrhoea was found to be a more prominent feature in gastroenteritis-associated IBS than in the case of sporadic IBS. The prognosis of PI-IBS is thought to be better than IBS without infectious onset [3]; however, the condition can still take more than 8 years to resolve as was observed by the Walkerton group [3,20]. If PI-IBS occurs after viral gastroenteritis, it is short lived and rarely lasts for 6 months or longer [4,21].

Commonly used diagnostic criteria for IBS were not utilized in this study. However, abdominal pain or discomfort or distension and loose stools are the principal parts of these criteria. Analyzing these symptoms in such a combination makes it reasonably close to Manning 3 and/or Rome I criteria for IBS. The high prevalence of gastrointestinal symptoms within the first five months after the epidemic in our study may therefore indicate PI-IBS. However, at the end of the follow-up, the prevalence of these symptoms was 11.5% among adults ≥16 years of age. In the population-based study among adults in Finland, the prevalence of IBS was 9.7% according to the Manning 3 criteria [17]. Therefore, the

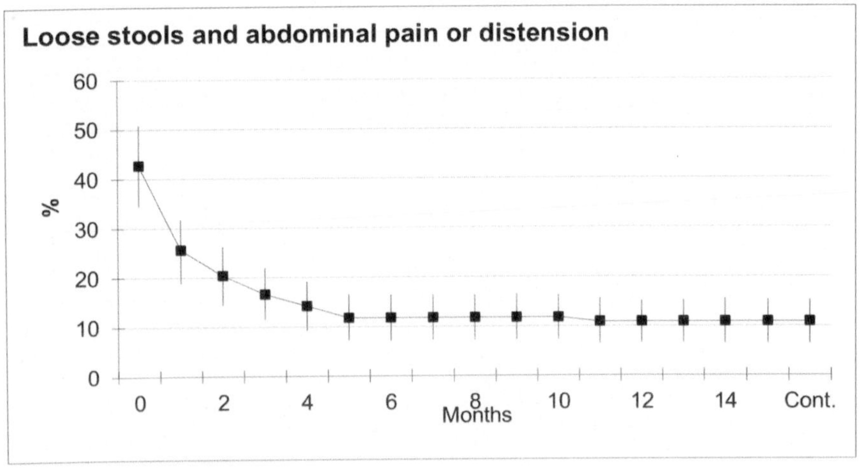

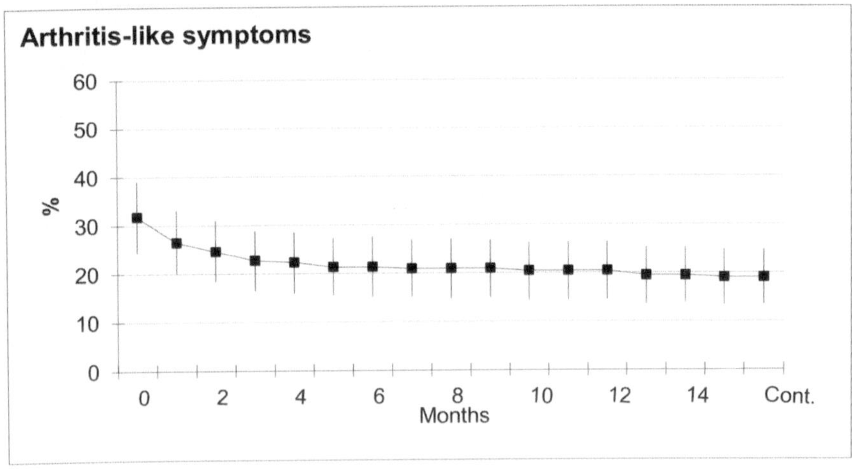

Figure 1. The prevalence of gastrointestinal and arthritis-like symptoms in the contaminated group within fifteen months from the outbreak. The proportions were counted as dividing the number of subjects with symptoms by the number of subjects having fallen ill with gastroenteritis at the time of the outbreak (N = 174). The curves represent the proportion of subjects with symptoms and the vertical lines are the 95% confident intervals.

remaining prevalence of gastrointestinal symptoms in the present study may be close to the natural occurrence of these symptoms.

Other reasons for long-lasting symptoms than PI-IBS must be considered in an epidemic where more than half of the exposed residents fell ill with gastroenteritis caused by mixed pathogens. There may have been prolonged circulation of the pathogens in the population leading to secondary infections. Bacterial stool cultures were extensively examined during the following months in the affected town. No excess frequency of positive findings could be noticed after the peak of the epidemic (Figure 2). This evidence does not support the prolonged circulation of bacterial pathogens in the population. Viral pathogens (especially, norovirus), are highly contagious and could well have started to spread horizontally after the outbreak. Such a possibility could not be excluded reliably because samples for viral diagnostics were not routinely taken during the study period. Giardiasis often causes long-lasting gastrointestinal symptoms. This epidemic was the first domestic *Giardia*-cluster in Finland [13]. The whole population was informed about the possibility of giardiasis and individuals were called for parasitological investigation if they suffered from prolonged symptoms. In spite of that, only 55 cases were found out of the 872 persons tested, a number that is probably too low to solely explain the magnitude of prolonged gastrointestinal symptoms.

As the data relies on self-reported symptoms, psychological factors like anger, anxiety or distress may have influenced the participants' expressions. The connection of psychological factors on the duration of IBS has been observed in epidemics caused by drinking water [20]. The public anger and anxiety in the town of Nokia was considerable for several months after the epidemic.

Table 2. The prevalence of arthritis-like symptoms among participants with and without gastrointestinal symptoms (loose stools and abdominal pain or distension) at 3 and 15 months after the water contamination.

	At 3 months	At 15 months
With gastrointestinal symptoms	54.3% (19/35)	52.2% (12/23)
Without gastrointestinal symptoms	10.9% (6/55)	10.4% (7/67)
p-value	<0.0001	<0.0001

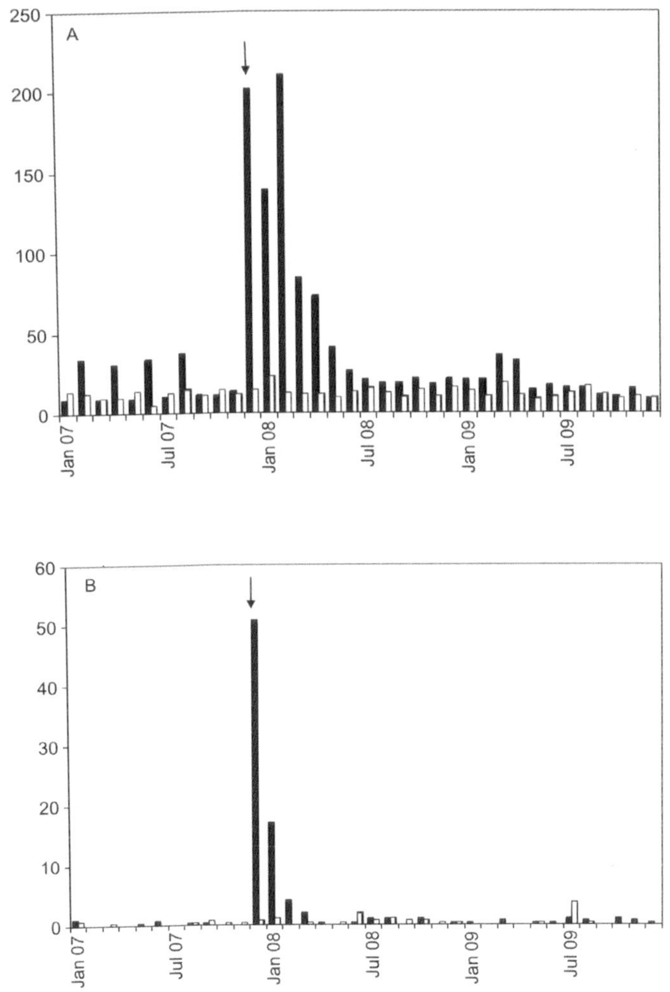

Figure 2. a–b. Monthly incidence (/10 000 inhabitants) of microbiological stool specimens (Fig. 2a) and positive findings (Fig. 2b). Black bars represent the town of Nokia and white bars the control municipality. The arrows indicate the outbreak month, December 2007. Only findings of *Campylobacter* and *Giardia* from January 2007 to December 2009 were counted.

Psychological influences of the incident on health experience will be investigated in another project and reported later.

Previously, we have reported a frequency of 6.7% of arthritis-like symptoms among the participants of the contaminated group within eight weeks from the incident [15]. According to the follow-up study, 31.8% of those who reported having had gastroenteritis during the epidemic announced subsequent arthritis-like symptoms. The explanation for the difference lies in the fact that joint symptoms in the follow-up study were asked for only from those with gastroenteritis and through a selection bias towards those with joint symptoms in the first study.

The arthritis-like symptoms were fairly longstanding. About a third of the symptoms were resolved within five months. Thereafter, the decline was slow and 19% of the respondents were still experiencing arthritis-like symptoms 15 months after the epidemic. In a previously published population-based study of verified ReA cases related to this outbreak, 21 cases of ReA were observed [14], mostly relatively mild cases. According to a follow-up study (one year) of this cohort, over a half of all the patients were still taking analgesics because of ReA symptoms and 33% was on antirheumatic medication [22]. This proportion of residual symptoms among verified ReA-cases is quite well in line with the findings of the present study.

ReA is a well-known complication of bacterial gastroenteritis [1]. *Giardia* has also been associated rarely with ReA [23]. To our knowledge, there are hardly any observations possibly linking rotavirus or norovirus to ReA. Considering this and the microbiological findings, we regard that campylobacter infections probably have been the major trigger of joint symptoms in this epidemic.

There are few population-based studies on the duration of self-reported joint symptoms following gastroenteritis epidemics. The previous literature deals with those fulfilling the criteria for ReA, either according to self-reporting or clinical judgement. In studies done in Finland, the average duration of ReA symptoms has been 3–5 months [1]. Symptoms persisting over six months have often been considered as a sign of chronic disorder. Development to the chronic condition has been reported in 12–16% of the cases [1]. The proportion of subjects with arthritis-like symptoms (19%), after 15 months in this study, is therefore, reasonably well in line with previous observations, especially, since this was a questionnaire study with no clinical verification of the symptoms.

The persistence of gastrointestinal symptoms correlated with the presence of arthritis-like symptoms (Table 2.). As PI-IBS and ReA are inflammatory disorders, pathogenesis of both gastrointestinal and arthritis-like symptoms may have common immunological mechanisms, although the genetic predisposition for these two conditions seems to be different [24].

There are some limitations of this study. First, although the initial sample for the first questionnaire was carefully randomized, there were three subsequent steps in which a selection bias could have taken place. They are responding to the first questionnaire, giving permission to be re-contacted, and finally responding to the follow-up survey (Table 1). The response rates of the first survey were good and the authors concluded that the survey was representative. For the follow-up survey, some selection in sample formation took place, but not any more in responding to the follow-up survey. Those with joint symptoms in the original cohort were more prone (OR 1.7, 95% CI 1.3–2.2) to participate in the 15-month follow-up. As the aim of the present study was to observe the duration of symptoms, selection towards participants who experienced symptoms during the outbreak does not seriously hamper the conclusions. Secondly, prolonged symptoms were asked only from those who fell ill with gastroenteritis during the outbreak. As one could assume, there were hardly any such cases in the control group and this made meaningful comparisons impossible. Thirdly, as the follow-up survey was done 15 months after the exposure, recalling the symptoms by those surveyed may have been difficult, thereby, creating a recall-bias of some degree. Fourthly, the outbreak and the faults causing it were widely discussed in the public media and several claims for compensation were made. Therefore, it is possible that some subjects with a disease that may have been potentially connected to the water contamination were prone to overweigh their symptoms.

The contamination of drinking water and the subsequent epidemic in the town of Nokia was a potentially dangerous situation. Large amounts of pathogens were distributed through household water and thousands of people fell ill. Given these circumstances, consequences could have been much more serious. In addition, more virulent bacterial strains, such as *Escherichia coli* O157:H7 were avoided. Despite the relatively favourable outcome of this epidemic, however, there were cases of people who suffered from consequences, especially, joint symptoms up to one year or more. In addition, individual patients have suffered from serious, prolonged, or permanent damages caused by joint destruction [22], IBS, or chronic fatigue syndrome.

In conclusion, prolonged gastrointestinal and joint symptoms were common among those who fell ill with gastroenteritis during the epidemic. The frequency of gastrointestinal symptoms declined during the follow-up period of 15 months. However, over half of the subjects with arthritis-like symptoms after the outbreak were still symptomatic at the end of the follow-up.

Acknowledgments

We thank Anneli Keinonen for providing the register data of microbiological specimens.

Author Contributions

Conceived and designed the experiments: JLaine JLumio MJV MKuusi. Performed the experiments: JLaine JLumio MJV MKuusi. Analyzed the data: JLaine JLumio ST MJV TU MKorpela EK MKuusi. Wrote the paper: JLaine JLumio ST MJV TU MKKorpela EK MKuusi.

References

1. Leirisalo-Repo M (2005) Reactive arthritis. Scand J Rheumatol 34: 251–259.
2. DuPont AW (2008) Postinfectious irritable bowel syndrome. Clin Infect Dis 46: 594–599.
3. Spiller R, Garsed K (2009) Postinfectious irritable bowel syndrome. Gastroenterology 136: 1979–1988.
4. Marshall JK, Thabane M, Borgaonkar MR, James C (2007) Postinfectious irritable bowel syndrome after a food-borne outbreak of acute gastroenteritis attributed to a viral pathogen. Clin Gastroenterol Hepatol 5: 457–460.
5. Clark WF, Sontrop JM, Macnab JJ, Salvadori M, Moist L, et al. (2010) Long term risk for hypertension, renal impairment, and cardiovascular disease after gastroenteritis from drinking water contaminated with Escherichia coli O157:H7: a prospective cohort study. Bmj 341: c6020.
6. Garg AX, Moist L, Matsell D, Thiessen-Philbrook HR, Haynes RB, et al. (2005) Risk of hypertension and reduced kidney function after acute gastroenteritis from bacteria-contaminated drinking water. Cmaj 173: 261–268.
7. Garg AX, Pope JE, Thiessen-Philbrook H, Clark WF, Ouimet J (2008) Arthritis risk after acute bacterial gastroenteritis. Rheumatology (Oxford) 47: 200–204.
8. Marshall JK (2009) Post-infectious irritable bowel syndrome following water contamination. Kidney Int Suppl: S42–43.
9. Marshall JK, Thabane M, Garg AX, Clark WF, Salvadori M, et al. (2006) Incidence and epidemiology of irritable bowel syndrome after a large waterborne outbreak of bacterial dysentery. Gastroenterology 131: 445–450; quiz 660.
10. Moist LM, Sontrop JM, Garg AX, Clark WF, Suri RS, et al. (2009) Risk of pregnancy-related hypertension within five years of exposure to bacteria-contaminated drinking water. Kidney Int Suppl: S47–49.
11. Laine J, Huovinen E, Virtanen MJ, Snellman M, Lumio J, et al. (2011) An extensive gastroenteritis outbreak after drinking-water contamination by sewage effluent, Finland. Epidemiol Infect: 1–9.
12. Rasanen S, Lappalainen S, Kaikkonen S, Hamalainen M, Salminen M, et al. (2010) Mixed viral infections causing acute gastroenteritis in children in a waterborne outbreak. Epidemiol Infect 138: 1227–1234.
13. Rimhanen-Finne R, Hanninen ML, Vuento R, Laine J, Jokiranta TS, et al. (2010) Contaminated water caused the first outbreak of giardiasis in Finland, 2007: a descriptive study. Scand J Infect Dis 42: 613–619.
14. Uotila T, Antonen J, Laine J, Kujansuu E, Haapala AM, et al. (2011) Reactive arthritis in a population exposed to an extensive waterborne gastroenteritis outbreak after sewage contamination in Pirkanmaa, Finland. Scand J Rheumatol 40: 358–362.
15. Laine J, Uotila T, Antonen J, Korpela M, Kujansuu E, et al. (2012) Joint symptoms after a large waterborne gastroenteritis outbreak–a controlled, population-based questionnaire study. Rheumatology (Oxford) 51: 513–518.
16. Maunula L, Kllemola P, Kauppinen A, Söderberg K, Nguyen T, et al. (2009) Enteritic viruses in a large waterborne outbreak of acute gastroenteritis in Finland. Food Environ Virol 1: 31–36.
17. Hillila MT, Farkkila MA (2004) Prevalence of irritable bowel syndrome according to different diagnostic criteria in a non-selected adult population. Aliment Pharmacol Ther 20: 339–345.
18. Lovell RM, Ford AC (2012) Global Prevalence of, and Risk Factors for, Irritable Bowel Syndrome: a Meta-analysis. Clin Gastroenterol Hepatol.
19. Halvorson HA, Schlett CD, Riddle MS (2006) Postinfectious irritable bowel syndrome–a meta-analysis. Am J Gastroenterol 101: 1894–1899; quiz 1942.
20. Marshall JK, Thabane M, Garg AX, Clark WF, Moayyedi P, et al. (2010) Eight year prognosis of postinfectious irritable bowel syndrome following waterborne bacterial dysentery. Gut 59: 605–611.
21. Porter CK, Faix DJ, Shiau D, Espiritu J, Espinosa BJ, et al. (2012) Postinfectious gastrointestinal disorders following norovirus outbreaks. Clin Infect Dis 55: 915–922.
22. Uotila TM, Antonen JA, Paakkala AS, Mustonen JT, Korpela MM (2013) Outcome of reactive arthritis after an extensive Finnish waterborne gastroenteritis outbreak: a 1-year prospective follow-up study. Clin Rheumatol.
23. Morris D, Inman RD (2012) Reactive arthritis: developments and challenges in diagnosis and treatment. Curr Rheumatol Rep 14: 390–394.
24. Nielsen H, Steffensen R, Ejlertsen T (2012) Risk and prognosis of campylobacteriosis in relation to polymorphisms of host inflammatory cytokine genes. Scand J Immunol 75: 449–454.

10

Host and Bacterial Proteins That Repress Recruitment of LC3 to *Shigella* Early during Infection

Leigh A. Baxt[1,2], Marcia B. Goldberg[1,2]*

1 Department of Medicine, Massachusetts General Hospital, Cambridge, Massachusetts, United States of America, **2** Department of Microbiology and Immunobiology, Harvard Medical School, Boston, Massachusetts, United States of America

Abstract

Shigella spp. are intracytosolic gram-negative pathogens that cause disease by invasion and spread through the colonic mucosa, utilizing host cytoskeletal components to form propulsive actin tails. We have previously identified the host factor Toca-1 as being recruited to intracellular *S. flexneri* and being required for efficient bacterial actin tail formation. We show that at early times during infection (40 min.), the type three-secreted effector protein IcsB recruits Toca-1 to intracellular bacteria and that recruitment of Toca-1 is associated with repression of recruitment of LC3, as well as with repression of recruitment of the autophagy marker NDP52, around these intracellular bacteria. LC3 is best characterized as a marker of autophagosomes, but also marks phagosomal membranes in the process LC3-associated phagocytosis. IcsB has previously been demonstrated to be required for *S. flexneri* evasion of autophagy at late times during infection (4–6 hr) by inhibiting binding of the autophagy protein Atg5 to the *Shigella* surface protein IcsA (VirG). Our results suggest that IcsB and Toca-1 modulation of LC3 recruitment restricts LC3-associated phagocytosis and/or LC3 recruitment to vacuolar membrane remnants. Together with published results, our findings suggest that IcsB inhibits innate immune responses in two distinct ways, first, by inhibiting LC3-associated phagocytosis and/or LC3 recruitment to vacuolar membrane remnants early during infection, and second, by inhibiting autophagy late during infection.

Editor: Dipshikha Chakravortty, Indian Institute of Science, India

Funding: This work has been supported by National Institutes of Health (NIH) R01 AI081724 (to MBG), NIH R21 AI083624 (to MBG) and NIH F32 AI092967 (to LAB). The funders had no role in study design, data collection and analysis, decision to publish, or preparation of the manuscript.

Competing Interests: The authors have declared that no competing interests exist.

* E-mail: marcia.goldberg@mgh.harvard.edu

Introduction

Shigella spp. are intracytoplasmic bacterial pathogens that cause diarrheal disease by invasion and spread through the colonic epithelium [1–3]. *Shigella* entry into cells is mediated by a type three secretion system, a needle-like apparatus that injects effector proteins directly into the host cell cytoplasm to modulate host cell functions. Contact with host cells triggers delivery of early effector proteins, which induce rearrangements of the actin cytoskeleton resulting in membrane ruffling and bacterial uptake, which is followed shortly thereafter by bacterial escape from the uptake vacuole [4,5]. Within the host cytoplasm, *Shigella* triggers the polymerization of a propulsive tail that consists of polymerized host actin and leads to dissemination of *Shigella* in the intestinal epithelium [6].

The *Shigella* outer membrane protein IcsA, the host actin nucleation-promoting factor N-WASP, and Toca-1 are required for efficient actin tail formation [7–11]. In resting cells, N-WASP is maintained in an auto-inhibited state [6,12,13]. In the context of *Shigella* actin tail formation, Toca-1 activates N-WASP by relieving N-WASP auto-inhibition [11]. Toca-1 is recruited to bacteria in a manner that depends on type three secretion [11], although the effector protein responsible for Toca-1 recruitment has been unknown.

We sought to characterize the mechanism and function of Toca-1 recruitment to intracellular *Shigella*. We identified IcsB as being required for recruitment of Toca-1. We found that early during infection, IcsB and Toca-1 repress recruitment of LC3 to the vicinity of intracellular *S. flexneri*. LC3 is best characterized as a marker of autophagy, a bulk degradation process used by cells to eliminate from the cytosol undesirable or invasive components, including protein aggregates, damaged organelles, and intracellular pathogens [14]. Of note, late during infection, IcsB has been shown to inhibit anti-*Shigella* autophagy [15]. However, LC3 is also central to LC3-associated phagocytosis, a process that occurs early upon uptake of pathogens and other cargo, involves several components of the classical autophagy pathway, and promotes phagosome maturation [16–18]. We demonstrate that the function of IcsB we characterize here is distinct from its previously described role in inhibition of autophagy [15] and is most consistent with LC3-associated phagocytosis and/or LC3 recruitment to vacuolar membrane remnants. Together, these findings indicate that IcsB and the host protein Toca-1 modulate LC3 recruitment around *S. flexneri* early during infection.

Materials and Methods

Bacterial strains, plasmids, and growth conditions

Strains and plasmids used in this study are listed in Table 1. All *S. flexneri* strains are isogenic to 2457T, and infectivity was similar for all strains. To generate the Δ*icsB* strain, the kanamycin cassette was removed from strain 2457T Δ*icsB*::FRT-km-FRT using FLP recombinase to generate a nonpolar, unmarked isogenic *icsB* mutant [19]. Cultures of *S. flexneri* strains were started from colonies that were Congo red positive. All strains were cultured in tryptic soy or Luria broth or agar with appropriate antibiotics and with or without addition of 0.2% glucose. Bacteria were grown at 37°C with shaking. Induction of transcription of genes under the control of IPTG-inducible promoters was performed at 37°C for 1 hr by addition IPTG to 100 μM.

Myc-Toca-1 truncation mutants used in this study were generated by PCR amplification of the DNA fragments encoding the relevant portions of Toca-1, using Myc-Toca-1 as template and subcloning of these fragments into pCS2+MT. Sequence analysis was performed to verify that each construct was correct. The sequences of the primers used in this study are available from the authors upon request.

Cell lines and culture conditions and transfection

Cells were cultured in high glucose DMEM (Gibco) supplemented with 10% fetal calf serum and pen/strep at 37°C with 5% CO_2. A431 human epidermoid carcinoma cells, originally derived from a solid tumor [20], stably containing either an empty lentiviral plasmid or plasmid encoding shRNA directed against Toca-1 (gift of Andrew Craig [21]) were maintained under selection with 1 μg/ml puromycin. HeLa cells (ATCC), 293T cells (ATCC), and mouse embryonic fibroblasts (MEFs) ([22]; gift of David Sacks) were maintained under the same conditions.

On the day prior to transfections, 3×10^5 cells were seeded onto glass coverslips. Monolayers of HeLa and A431 cells were transfected using 1.5 μg DNA and 4.5 μl Fugene 6 (Promega) transfection reagent in DMEM to a total volume of 100 μl, followed by 20 min incubation at room temperature before adding to the cells. Transfected cells were infected with bacteria 24 hr after transfection.

Immunoprecipitation, co-precipitation, and western blot analysis

293T cells were transfected with selected plasmids using the calcium phosphate method. Forty-eight hr after transfection, cells were lysed in chilled lysis buffer (150 mM NaCl, 1 mM EDTA, 50 mM Tris pH 7.4, 1% Triton X-100, protease inhibitor cocktail (Roche)) for 30 min and cleared by centrifugation in a microfuge at 15,000 rpm for 15 min at 4°C. Secreted bacterial proteins were bound to antibody-conjugated beads by incubation of the beads with bacterial culture supernatants 1 hr at 4°C, followed by 3 washes in lysis buffer. The prepared beads were then incubated with cleared cell lysates overnight at 4°C, followed by recovery by centrifugation. Beads were then washed 6 times with lysis buffer, resuspended in SDS-PAGE sample buffer, and analyzed by western blot. Primary antibodies used for western blot analysis were anti-Myc (Clontech), anti-Flag M2 (Sigma), anti-HA (Covance), each used at 1:1000. Secondary antibodies were HRP-conjugated True Blot antibodies (eBioscience), used at 1:5000.

For bacterial co-precipitation experiments, proteins were synthesized in *E. coli* BL21-DE3. Overnight cultures were back diluted and grown at 16°C for several hours before inducing

Table 1. Strains and plasmids used in this study.

Strain or Plasmid	Genotype or description	Reference
Bacterial strains		
Wild-type	Wild-type serotype 2a *S. flexneri* strain 2457T	[47]
Δ*icsB* (km)	2457T *icsB*::FRT-km-FRT	Gift of Cammie Lesser
Δ*icsB*	2457T *icsB*::FRT	This study
icsA	2457T pWR100 *icsA*::Ω	[48]
icsA Δ*icsB*	2457T pWR100 *icsA*::Ω *icsB*	This study
Δ*ipaB* Δ*ipaC*	2457T *ipaB ipaC*	Gift of Cammie Lesser
SL1344	*S.* Typhimurium	Lab stock
BL21 DE3	*E. coli* K-12	Lab stock
Plasmids		
Myc-Toca-1	pCS2+MT full length Toca-1,	[12]
Toca-1_{1-477}	pCS2+MT Toca-1 truncation mutant (amino acids 1-477)	[12]
Toca-1_{1-293}	pCS2+MT Toca-1 truncation mutant (amino acids 1–293)	[12]
Toca-$1_{105-547}$	pCS2+MT Toca-1 truncation mutant (amino acids 105–547)	[12]
Toca-$1_{245-547}$	pCS2+MT Toca-1 truncation mutant (amino acids 245–547)	[12]
Toca-$1_{372-547}$	pCS2+MT Toca-1 truncation mutant (amino acids 372–547)	[12]
Toca-$1_{483-547}$	pCS2+MT Toca-1 truncation mutant (amino acids 483–547)	[12]
Toca-$1_{105-477}$	pCS2+MT Toca-1 truncation mutant (amino acids 105–477)	This study
Toca-$1_{245-477}$	pCS2+MT Toca-1 truncation mutant (amino acids 245–477)	This study
Toca-$1_{105-373}$	pCS2+MT Toca-1 truncation mutant (amino acids 105–373)	This study
Toca-$1_{245-373}$	pCS2+MT Toca-1 truncation mutant (amino acids 245–373)	This study
LC3-GFP	pEGFP-C1-LC3	[49]
pDSW206-flag	IPTG inducible expression of 3xflag	Gift of Jon Beckwith
pDSW206-OspF-flag	IPTG inducible expression of OspF-3xflag	Gift of Cammie Lesser
pDSW206-IcsB-flag	IPTG inducible expression of IcsB-3xflag	Gift of Cammie Lesser

expression of the target proteins from IPTG-inducible and arabinose-inducible promoters with 100 µM IPTG and 0.2% arabinose overnight. The following day, bacteria were recovered by centrifugation and lysed with sonication in chilled lysis buffer (150 mM NaCl, 1 mM EDTA, 50 mM Tris pH 7.4, protease inhibitor cocktail). Lysates were centrifuged in a microfuge at 15,000 rpm for 5 min at 4°C. Soluble fractions were incubated with amylose or cobalt resin for 2 hr at 4°C. Resins with bound protein were then washed 4 times in lysis buffer, recovered by centrifugation, and resuspended in SDS-PAGE sample buffer.

Bacterial infections of mammalian cells

Bacteria were grown in liquid media at 37°C with aeration to an absorbance 600 of 0.2–0.5, recovered by centrifugation, resuspended in cell culture media, and added to cell monolayers at a multiplicity of infection of 100–200 for *S. flexneri* and 50–100 for *S.* Typhimurium (bacteria:cell). When appropriate, 100 µM IPTG was added to the bacterial culture for the last 1 hr of growth and throughout the cell infection. To bring bacteria into close contact with the cells, infected monolayers were centrifuged for 10 min at 2,000 rpm. Infected monolayers were then incubated at 37°C for 15 min, washed once with pre-warmed cell culture media, and incubated at 37°C for an additional 15 min for *S. flexneri* or 35 min for *S.* Typhimurium. Monolayers were then fixed in 3.7% paraformaldehyde in F-buffer for 20 min and permeabilized with 1% Triton-X-100. Immunofluorescence labeling was performed using as primary antibodies, Toca-1 (gift of G. Scita, used at a dilution of 1:20), P62 (BD Biosciences, used at a dilution of 1:100), NDP52 (Abcam, used at a dilution of 1:100), FK2 (Enzo Life Sciences, used at a dilution of 1:100), and Galectin-3 (used at a dilution of 1:100, BD) with as secondary antibodies, anti-mouse Alexa 488, anti-rabbit Alexa 488, anti-mouse Alexa 568, and anti-rabbit Alexa-568 (each used at a 1:100 dilution, and each from Invitrogen). Staining of actin, cholesterol and DNA was performed using Alexa 568 phalloidin (Invitrogen), filipin complex (Sigma) and 5 µM DAPI (Invitrogen).

For the quantification of bacterial survival in cells (gentamicin protection assay), MEFs were seeded at 3×10^5 cells per well in 12-well plates the day prior to infection, giving approximately 95% confluence on the day of infection. *S. flexneri* strains were grown as described above and added to cell monolayers at a multiplicity of infection of 0.0001 (bacteria:cell). The bacterial inoculum was plated for quantification. Infected monolayers were centrifuged for 10 min at 2,000 rpm and incubated at 37°C for 45 min. Cell monolayers were then washed once with pre-warmed DMEM and incubated for an additional 4 hrs at 37°C with fresh DMEM containing 25 µg/ml gentamicin, which kills extracellular but not intracellular bacteria. Infected monolayers were then washed twice with phosphate buffered saline and lysed in 1% Triton X-100 to release the intracellular bacteria. Lysates containing the bacteria were plated on Congo red agar and bacterial colonies were quantified 16 hrs later.

Microscopy analysis

Experimental samples were blinded, infected cells were identified using the DAPI channel, and a minimum of ten cells was analyzed for each condition. For the analysis of Toca-1 and LC3 recruitment, a bacterium was counted as positive if labeling was observed anywhere on the periphery of the bacterium. For quantification of actin tail formation, bacteria were counted as having a tail if the polymerized actin adjacent to the bacterium was ≥0.83 uM in length, as described [11]. For quantification of autophagosome formation in MEFs, cells were counted as positive if at least one intracellular bacterium was surrounded by LC3-GFP.

Data analysis

For all sets of experiments, three or more independent experiments were performed, data were collected in a blinded manner, and standard statistical tools were applied to assess for significant differences among experimental results.

Results

The type three-secreted effector IcsB is required for recruitment of Toca-1 around intracellular *Shigella*

Previous studies from our lab have shown that Toca-1 is recruited to intracellular *Shigella* in a manner that depends on type three secretion [11]. To determine which type three-secreted effector protein was required for recruitment of Toca-1 to bacteria, we screened for loss of Toca-1 recruitment in HeLa cells infected with each among a panel of 21 isogenic *S. flexneri* strains harboring single deletions of genes encoding type three effector proteins for 40 min., the time at which Toca-1 recruitment peaks (Fig. S1). A single mutant, Δ*icsB*, showed a dramatic decrease in recruitment of Myc-Toca-1 (wild-type, 62±14% versus Δ*icsB*, <1±2% of intracellular bacteria, p = 0.006, Fig. 1A and B). Expression of IcsB from a plasmid in the Δ*icsB* mutant restored Toca-1 recruitment to wild-type levels (Fig. 1B), confirming that the defect in Toca-1 recruitment observed for the deletion strain was due to the absence of IcsB. Immunolocalization revealed that like Toca-1, IcsB formed rings around intracellular bacteria (Fig. 1C) and that IcsB and Toca-1 co-localized around the same intracellular bacteria (Fig. 1C). Identical results were observed using an antibody to endogenous Toca-1 (Fig. 1D), indicating that the over-expression of transfected Myc-Toca-1 *per se* did not contribute to the recruitment phenotype. Toca-1 was detectable around bacteria within membrane ruffles (Fig. S2), suggesting that Toca-1 is recruited as extracellular bacteria are taken up into vacuoles. These data demonstrate that IcsB is required for recruitment of Toca-1 to *S. flexneri* and suggest that this occurs during bacterial entry.

IcsB interacts with Toca-1

The dependence of Toca-1 recruitment on IcsB and the co-localization of IcsB with Toca-1 (Fig. 1) suggested that IcsB might interact with Toca-1. To test this, IcsB-flag that had been recovered on beads from bacterial culture supernatants was used to precipitate proteins from lysates of 293T cells that had been transfected with Myc-Toca-1 (see Methods). IcsB-flag beads precipitated Myc-Toca-1 in a specific manner, since Myc-Toca-1 was not precipitated by beads that had been incubated with culture supernatant alone or with a flag-tagged derivative of the type three secreted protein OspF (Fig. 2A).

To define the region of Toca-1 that interacts with IcsB, we tested the ability of IcsB-flag to precipitate derivatives of Toca-1 in which specific domains had been deleted (Fig. 2B). The results of this analysis narrowed the interaction to a region of Toca-1 that includes the protein kinase C-related kinase homology region 1 (HR1) and a coiled coil domain that lies between the Fer/Cip4 homology (FCH) and HR1 domains (Fig. 2B–D). To determine whether the region required for *in vitro* interaction between the two proteins correlated with that required for recruitment of Toca-1 to *Shigella* in infected cells, we analyzed recruitment of each truncation mutant to intracellular *S. flexneri* in HeLa cells (Figs. 2B and S3). The recruitment of the Toca-1 truncation mutants to intracellular bacteria correlated with the precipitation

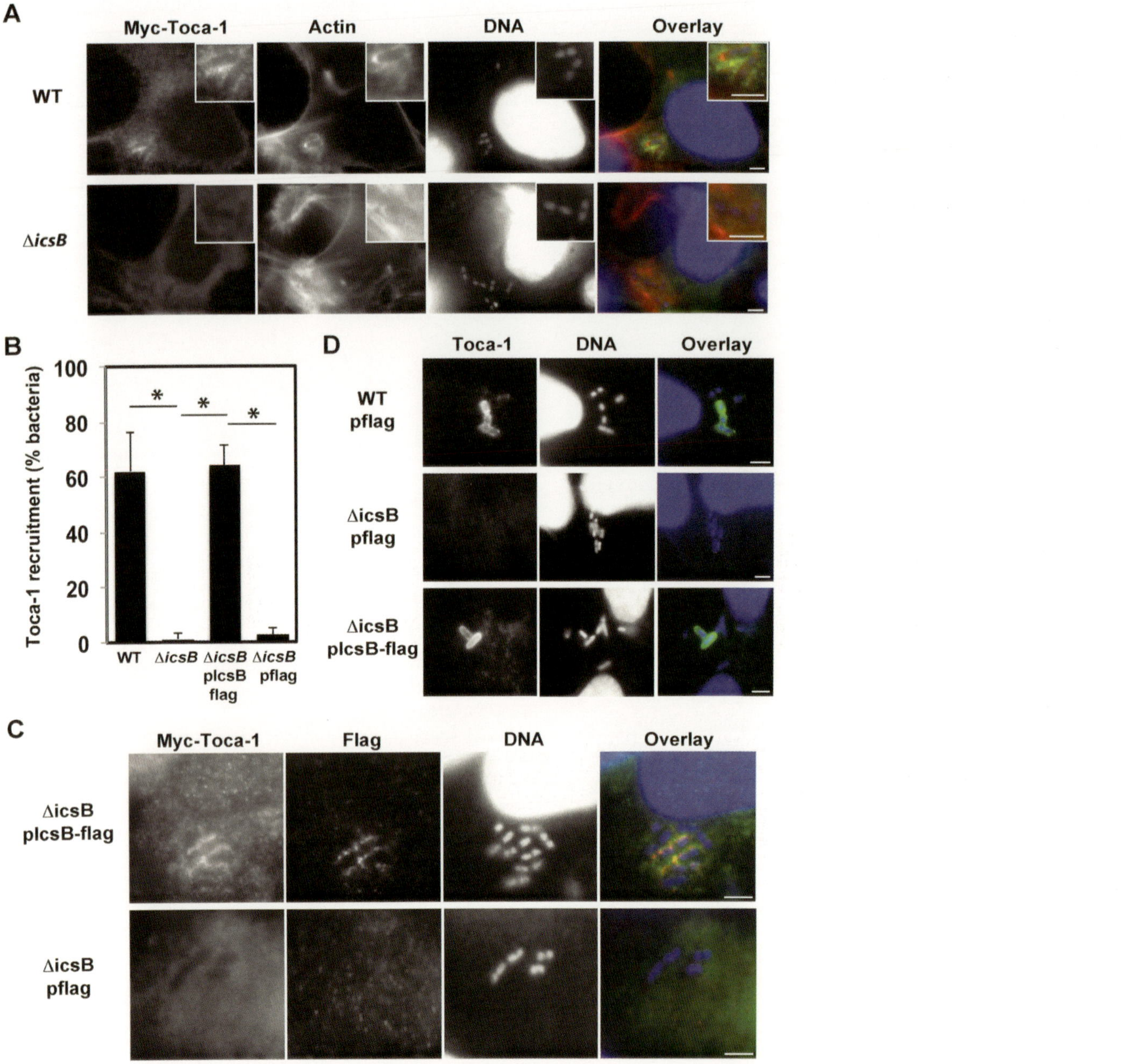

Figure 1. IcsB is required for recruitment of Toca-1. (A) Wild-type (WT) or Δ*icsB S. flexneri* infection (40 min.) of HeLa cells that had been transfected with Myc-Toca-1, with immunofluorescence using antibody to Myc and staining with phalloidin (polymerized actin) and DAPI (DNA). (B) Association with Myc-Toca-1 with intracellular wild-type (WT) or Δ*icsB S. flexneri* and complemented strains. Data represent the mean ± S.D. of three independent experiments. *P<0.05. (C) Infection (40 min.) by Δ*icsB S. flexneri* and IcsB-flag complemented strain of HeLa cells that had been transfected with Myc-Toca-1, with immunofluorescence using antibodies to Myc and flag. (D) Infection (40 min.) by Δ*icsB S. flexneri* and IcsB-flag complemented strain of HeLa cells, with immunofluorescence using antibody to Toca-1 and stained with DAPI. Scale bars, 5 μm.

experiments with three exceptions (Toca-1$_{105-373}$, Toca-1$_{245-373}$, and Toca$_{245-547}$). Toca-1$_{105-373}$ and Toca-1$_{245-373}$ interacted by precipitation, but failed to be recruited in the context of infection; these discrepancies are likely due to non-native tertiary structure or the requirement for an additional host protein to promote localization to intracellular bacteria.

In addition, Toca$_{245-547}$ reproducibly bound poorly in vitro, but localized well to *S. flexneri* in cells (Fig. 2D and S3). Whereas we do not understand these findings, we speculate that in this construct, the Toca-1 SH3 domain may partially interfere with binding to IcsB under the *in vitro* conditions, but not inside cells, where perhaps another interaction prevents the interference. Consistent with this possibility is that Toca-1 constructs that contain the core IcsB binding domain (residues 245–477) and lack the SH3 domain were generally precipitated better by IcsB than the corresponding constructs that contain the SH3 domain.

To test whether the interaction between IcsB and Toca-1 is dependent on other *S. flexneri* or other mammalian proteins, we performed co-precipitation analysis in *E. coli*. In this system, MBP-IcsB and a truncation mutant of Toca-1 that was still recruited to

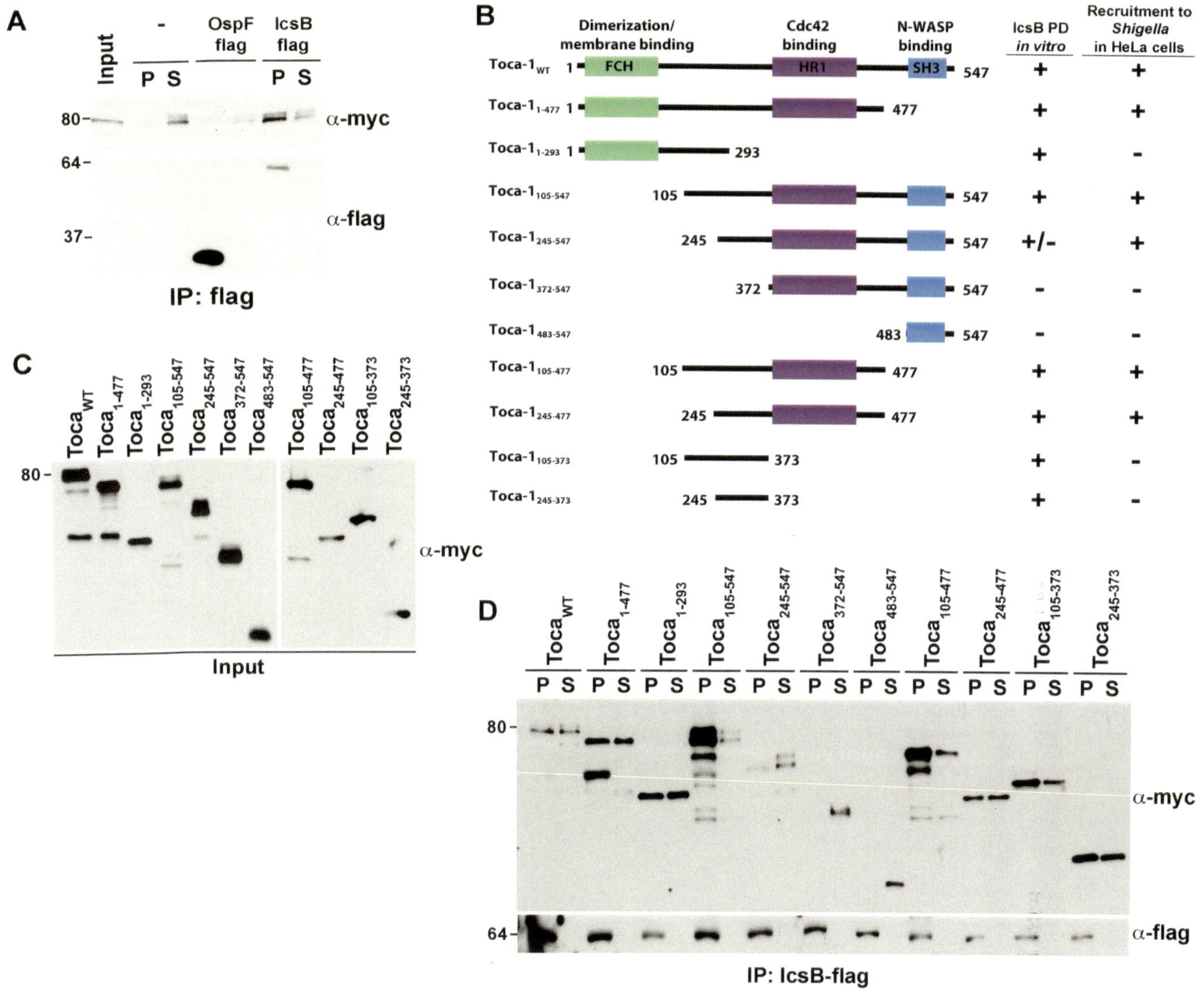

Figure 2. IcsB interacts with the HR1 and adjacent coiled coil region of Toca-1. (A) Immunoprecipitation of Myc-Toca-1 with IcsB-flag. Proteins secreted by *S. flexneri* strains carrying no plasmid, IcsB-flag, or OspF-flag were bound to anti-flag beads, which were then used to precipitate Myc-Toca-1 from cell lysates. Western blot analysis. Input, cell lysate. (B) Schematic of Toca-1 domain structure and truncation mutants, indicating pull down by IcsB *in vitro* and recruitment to wild type *S. flexneri* in cells. (C and D) Immunoprecipitation of Myc-Toca-1 and its truncation mutants with IcsB-flag, as in panel (A). (C) Input. Panels are from the same blot. (D) Precipitated proteins. Western blot analysis. P, pellet; S, supernatant.

intracellular *S. flexneri* (Toca-$1_{105-477}$) reciprocally interacted by co-precipitation (Fig. 3). The interaction was specific, since when MBP was produced with Toca-1, no interaction was observed (Fig. 3). These results indicate that the interaction between IcsB and Toca-1 is independent of *S. flexneri* and other mammalian proteins.

IcsB is associated with decreased early LC3 recruitment

Since IcsB is implicated in inhibition of autophagy at late time points (4–6 hr) during *S. flexneri* infection [15], we considered whether IcsB recruitment of Toca-1 early during infection might alter autophagy related processes at that time. Recognition of cytosolic bacteria by the autophagy pathway (anti-bacterial autophagy) may involve ubiquitination of bacterial surface proteins or signaling via pattern-recognition molecules, including Toll-like receptors (TLRs), NOD-like receptors (NLRs), and/or diacylglycerol (DAG) [23,24]. Specificity is provided by receptors that function as adaptor proteins, referred to as sequestrosome 1/P62-like receptors (SLRs) [25], including NDP52 and P62 [26]. These receptor/adaptor proteins recognize ubiquitin and other markers of cargo and in turn activate recruitment of the lipidated form of Atg8, LC3 II (LC3), a canonical marker of autophagosomal membranes.

To test whether IcsB altered the recruitment of these markers early in infection, we measured the prevalence of recruitment of LC3, NDP52, P62, and ubiquitin in the vicinity of intracellular *S. flexneri* in the presence or absence of IcsB at 40 min. post-invasion (Fig. 4A). In the absence of IcsB, recruitment of LC3 and NDP52 was significantly increased, and recruitment of P62 and ubiquitin was increased, albeit not to statistical significance. These data indicate that, soon after bacterial entry into host cells, IcsB can

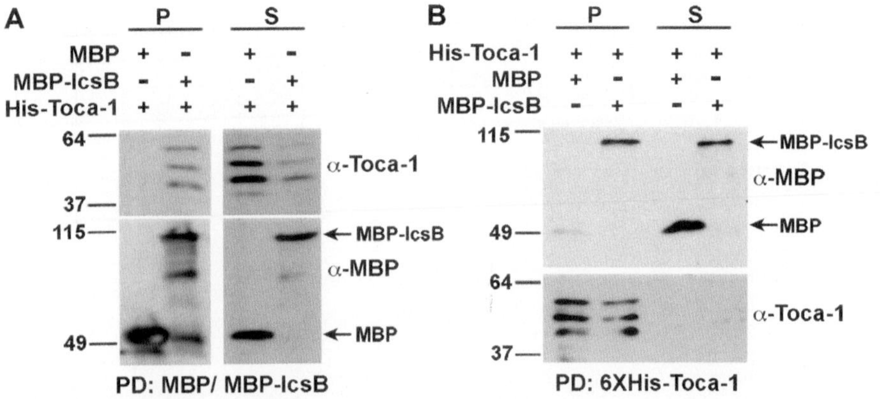

Figure 3. Toca-1 and IcsB reciprocally co-precipitate. Reciprocal co-precipitation of His-Toca-$1_{105-477}$ and MBP-IcsB from soluble fractions of *E. coli* BL21 DE3 that co-express the two proteins or the relevant controls, using amylose (for MBP, panel A) or cobalt (for His, panel B) resin. Western blot analysis. The apparent degradation observed for the Toca-1 construct was independent of IcsB. Apparent molecular weights in kilodaltons are indicated to the left of the blots. P, pellet; S, supernatant.

limit recruitment of these autophagy-related proteins to the vicinity of intracellular bacteria.

Escape from the uptake vacuole and actin tail formation are independent of IcsB

In addition to being critical to the process of autophagy, components of the macroautophagy pathway participate in innate immune responses that are distinct from autophagy. Of particular interest here is LC3-associated phagocytosis, a process that occurs early upon uptake of pathogens and other cargo, involves several components of the classical autophagy pathway, and promotes phagosome maturation [16–18]. LC3-associated phagocytosis has been described for both phagocytic cells and non-phagocytic cells and is notably not associated with decreased pathogen survival [27–29]. Alternatively, LC3 has been observed at early times during *S. flexneri* infection associated with vacuolar membrane remnants [30], which similarly has not been shown to be associated with decreased pathogen survival. The presence of LC3 and NDP52 around a subset of intracellular *S. flexneri* at 40 min. of infection raised the possibility that LC3 recruitment was occurring in the process of LC3-mediated phagocytosis and/ or associated with recognition of vacuolar membrane remnants.

In previous descriptions of LC3-associated phagocytosis, LC3 accumulates on phagosomal membranes. During *S. flexneri* infection of HeLa cells, bacteria lyse the phagosome beginning as early as 15 min. after bacterial contact with the cell, and essentially all phagosomes are lysed by 30 min. [31], whereas at 40 min. after contact, we observed LC3 around 15–20% of wild type and 35–40% of Δ*icsB* mutant bacteria (Fig. 4A). This raised the possibility that if LC3 was associated with the phagosomal membrane, the absence of IcsB caused a delay in lysis of the phagosome. To test this, we compared the recruitment of galectin-3 around the *icsB* mutant to that around the wild type strain at 40 min. of infection; since galectins bind β-galactosides on the luminal face of vesicles [32], galectin-3 serves as a marker of vacuolar lysis by *S. flexneri* [30,33,34]. At 40 min. of infection, galectin-3 was present around an equivalent percentage of Δ*icsB* mutant and wild type bacteria (Fig. 4B), suggesting that the absence of IcsB had no impact on phagosomal escape and that the differences in LC3 recruitment to the Δ*icsB* and the wild type strain were independent of phagosomal escape *per se*.

Since actin tails can only form after bacteria access the cytoplasm, the efficiency of actin tail formation can serve as an additional marker of access to the cytoplasm. Moreover, Toca-1 is required for efficient initiation of actin tail formation by intracellular *Shigella* [11]. Toca-1, which is recruited to intracellular bacteria prior to actin tail formation, relieves auto-inhibition of N-WASP, thereby activating N-WASP and enabling N-WASP-mediated actin polymerization. Based on this, we considered whether IcsB-mediated recruitment of Toca-1 to the bacteria might be required for initiation of actin tail formation. At 40 min. of infection, actin tail formation was similar for the Δ*icsB* mutant and the wild type strain (Fig. 4C, left graph). The same was also true at 1–2 hr. of infection (Fig. 4C, right graph). These results are consistent with the galectin-3 data indicating that phagosomal escape was similar for the Δ*icsB* mutant and the wild type strains. They also indicate that actin tail formation occurs independently of IcsB. Together with our previously published results [11], this observation demonstrates that for actin tails to form efficiently, Toca-1 must be present in the cell, but need not be enriched around bacteria. Thus, the relatively lower concentration of Toca-1 that is present diffusely in the cytosol is sufficient for efficient actin tail initiation.

Early IcsB-dependent repression of LC3 recruitment is independent of IcsA

The IcsB-mediated inhibition of autophagy that occurs at later times during infection (4–6 hr) involves IcsB binding to the *Shigella* surface protein IcsA, which blocks IcsA recognition by the pro-autophagy factor Atg5 [15]. This pathway is dependent on IcsA, since at 4 hrs of infection, LC3 recruitment to an *icsA* mutant is minimal [15].

To test whether early IcsB-dependent repression of LC3 recruitment was dependent on IcsA, we compared LC3 recruitment in the vicinity of strains containing or lacking IcsA at early and late infection times. At 40 min., whether or not IcsA was present, the prevalence of LC3 recruitment significantly increased in the absence of IcsB (Fig. 5A and B), indicating that this early process is independent of IcsA. Moreover, Toca-1 recruitment was independent of *icsA* (Fig. 5C). In contrast, at 4 hrs of infection, levels of autophagy were significantly lower in each strain that lacked IcsA compared to the IcsA+ strains (Fig. 5D; †, $P<0.05$), confirming the previous observation that at late times, an IcsA-dependent autophagy inhibition mechanism predominates [15]. Thus, *Shigella* IcsB interferes with two distinct processes, an early

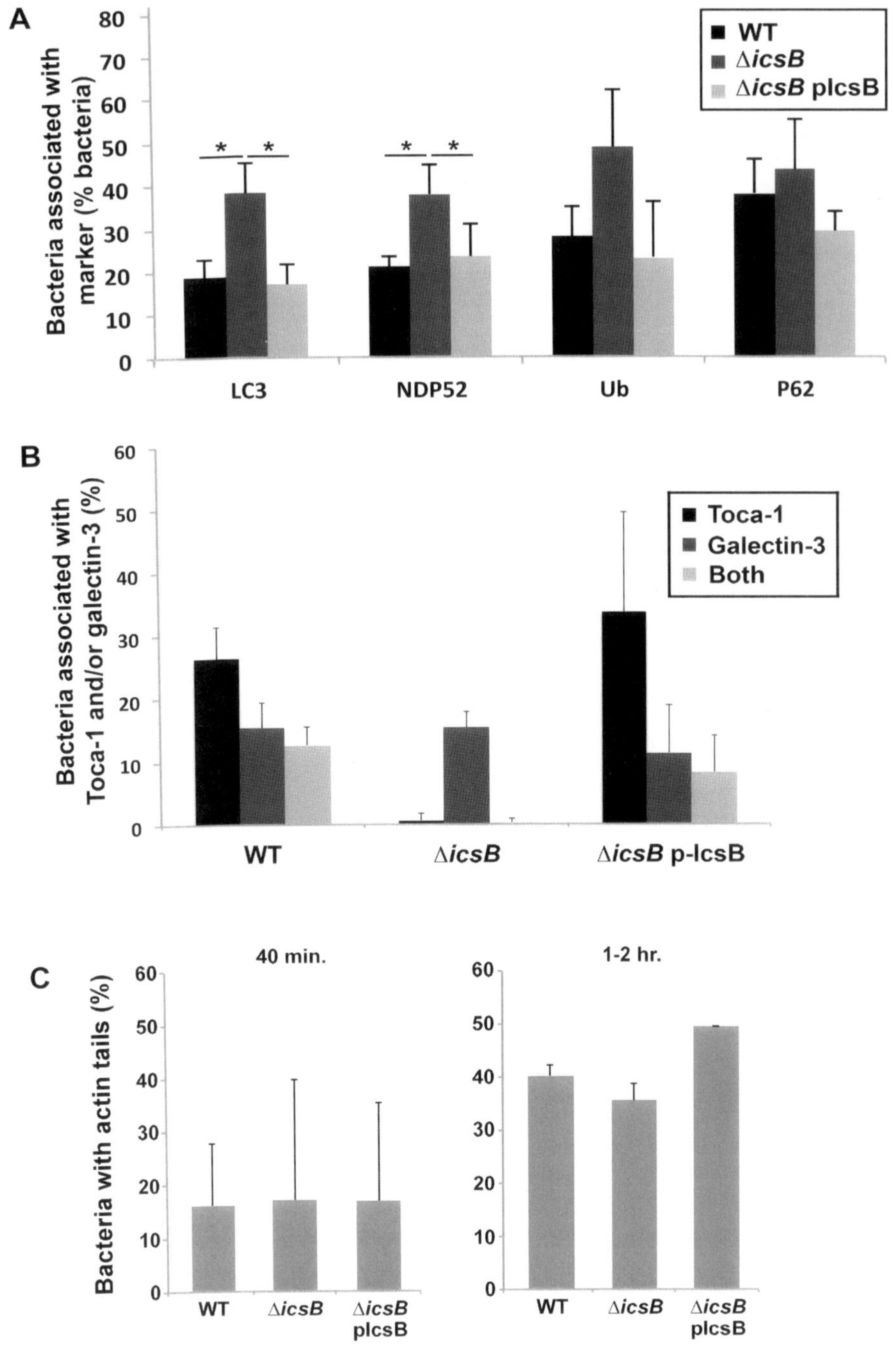

Figure 4. IcsB inhibits early recruitment of LC3 around *S. flexneri* that are cytoplasmic. (A) LC3, NDP52, ubiquitin and P62 recruitment in the vicinity of wild-type pflag (WT), Δ*icsB* pflag, or Δ*icsB* pIcsB-flag *S. flexneri*, at 40 min. of infection of HeLa cells that had been transfected with LC3-GFP or labeled with antibodies to other autophagy markers. *P<0.05. (B) Prevalence of galectin-3, Toca-1, or both around intracellular wild-type *S. flexneri* at 40 min. of infection. (C) Formation of actin tails at 40 min. (left graph) or 1-2 hr. (right graph) of infection by wild type (WT), Δ*icsB S. flexneri*, or Δ*icsB S. flexneri* complemented with pflag-IcsB. Data represent the mean ± S.D. of three independent experiments. Within each panel, the P value for each pair of data is >0.1. Data represent mean ± S.D. of three independent experiments.

one that is IcsA-independent, and a late autophagy pathway that is IcsA-dependent.

When present, the pattern of LC3 recruitment was notably distinct at the two times we analyzed (Fig. 5E and data not shown). At early times (40 min.), LC3 appeared fragmented with punctate foci adjacent to bacteria, while at late times (4 hr.), LC3 appeared as a continuous signal that completely surrounded bacteria (Fig. 5E and data not shown). The pattern of LC3 observed at early times was reminiscent of that directed against membrane remnants [30], leading us to speculate that LC3 may be localized to membrane remnants as a result of either LC3-associated phagocytosis or autophagy triggered by membrane remnants. Indeed, galectin-3 and cholesterol, a membrane component, localized with Toca-1 in the vicinity of intracellular *S. flexneri* at this early infection time (Figs. 4B and S4).

Relationship of Toca-1 to early LC3 recruitment

The requirement of IcsB for both Toca-1 recruitment and repression of LC3 recruitment raised the possibility that Toca-1 participated in limiting LC3 recruitment. Indeed, we found that the subpopulation of bacteria associated with Toca-1 was non-overlapping with the subpopulation associated with LC3. Two ±1% of intracellular bacteria were associated with both LC3 and Toca-1, compared with 17±3% associated with LC3 only and 32±7% with Toca-1 only (Fig. 6A and 6E).

Since Toca-1 recruitment anti-correlated with LC3 recruitment, we examined whether other autophagy-related factors were also anti-correlated with Toca-1 recruitment early during *S. flexneri* infection. We compared the subpopulation of bacteria associated with NDP52, p62, or ubiquitin to that associated with Toca-1. Very few intracellular bacteria were associated with both Toca-1 and NDP52 (5±1%; Fig. 6B and 6F). Moreover, in the cases of P62 and ubiquitin, whereas more than half of the bacteria associated with P62 or ubiquitin also displayed Toca-1 recruitment (Fig. 6C-D and 6G–H), a closer examination of individual bacteria exhibiting recruitment of both Toca-1 and an autophagy-associated protein revealed that the two proteins were restricted to distinct, non-overlapping microdomains around the bacteria (Fig. 6I–M). For more than 75% of the bacteria that were associated with both Toca-1 and another autophagy associated protein, the two signals were restricted to non-overlapping microdomains (Fig. 6M). Thus, even when Toca-1 and an autophagy-associated factor were recruited to the same bacterium, they were not co-localized.

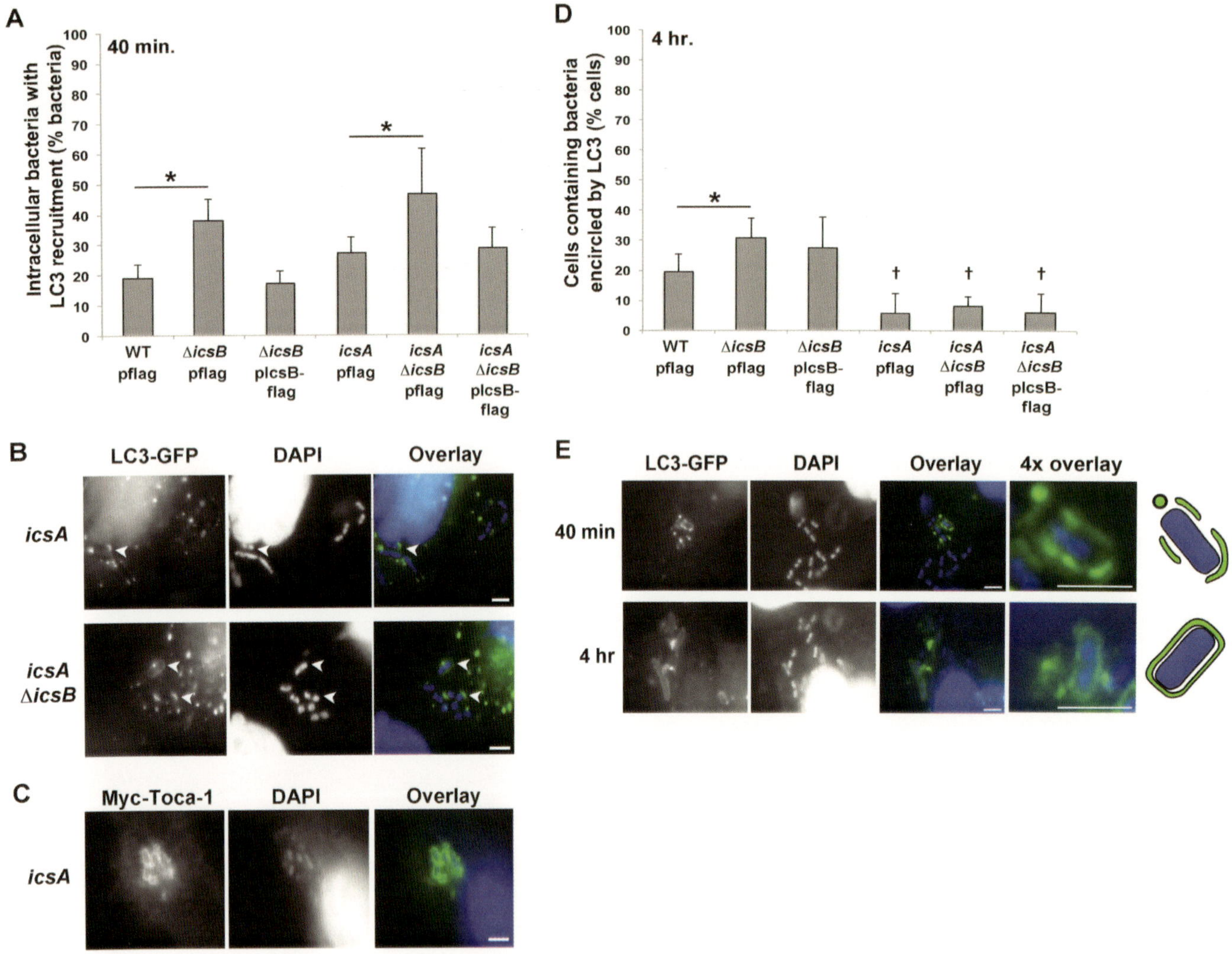

Figure 5. Early repression of LC3 recruitment is independent of IcsA. (A) LC3 recruitment to the vicinity of wild-type (WT), Δ*icsB*, or *icsA* Δ*icsB* *S. flexneri*, complemented or not with plcsB-flag, at 40 min. of infection of HeLa cells that had been transfected with LC3-GFP. (B) Representative images corresponding to (A). Arrowheads, bacteria with LC3 recruitment. (C) Toca-1 recruitment to *icsA S. flexneri* at 40 min. of infection of HeLa cells that had been transfected with Myc-Toca-1, with immunofluorescence using antibody to Myc and staining with DAPI. (D) Cells containing LC3 encircling WT, Δ*icsB*, *icsA*, or *icsA* Δ*icsB S. flexneri*, complemented or not with plcsB-flag, at 4 hr of infection of MEFs that had been transfected with LC3-GFP. (E) Distinctive LC3 distribution patterns around WT *S. flexneri* at early (40 min., top panels) and late (4 hr., bottom panels) times after infection. Data represent the mean ± S.D. of three independent experiments. *$P<0.05$. Images are representative. †, each bar was statistically different from bars for isogenic strain that contains *icsA*. Scale bars, 5 µm.

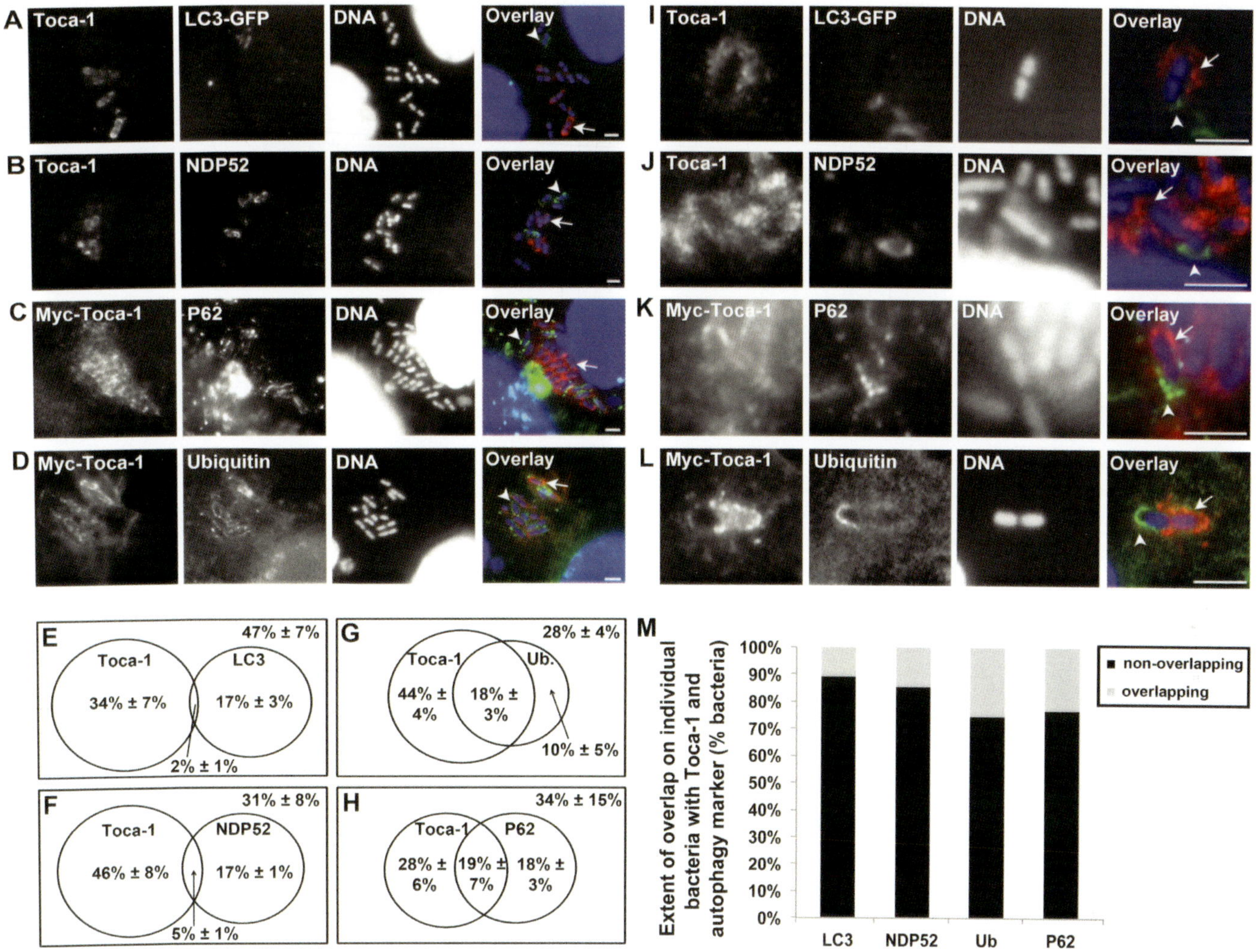

Figure 6. Toca-1 recruitment around wild-type bacteria is associated with decreased recruitment of LC3 and autophagy markers. A–D. Wild-type *S. flexneri* infection (40 min.) of HeLa cells that were untransfected or had been transfected with Myc-Toca-1 or LC3-GFP (A), with immunofluorescence using antibody to Toca-1 or Myc and to NDP52 (B), P62 (C) and ubiquitin (D). Arrowheads, bacteria exhibiting recruitment of autophagy-associated proteins. Arrows, bacteria exhibiting recruitment of Toca-1. (E–H) Venn diagrams of the distribution of Toca-1 and autophagy markers around individual intracellular bacteria for experiments shown in panels A-D. Numbers in the upper right corners of the rectangles represent the percentage of bacteria that were surrounded by neither marker. Data represent the mean ± S.D. of three independent experiments. (I–L) Magnified images of individual bacteria that were surrounded by both Toca-1 and LC3 (I), NDP52 (J), P62 (K), or ubiquitin (L). Distribution of Toca-1 (arrow) and autophagy marker (arrowhead) to distinct non-overlapping microdomains around each bacterium. (M) Quantification of overlap of signal around individual bacteria that exhibited recruitment of both Toca-1 and an autophagy protein. Data represent the mean of three independent experiments. Images are representative. Scale bars, 5 µm.

The pro-autophagy activity of Toca-1 observed during infection with *S.* Typhimurium is absent early during *S. flexneri* infection

These findings suggested that the function of Toca-1 might be very different in the setting of *S. flexneri* infection from its role in supporting autophagy of intracellular *S.* Typhimurium. During *S.* Typhimurium infection, Toca-1 co-localizes with LC3 around a subset of intracellular bacteria and promotes anti-bacterial autophagy [35]. We postulated that in the context of *S. flexneri* infection, rather than functioning to promote LC3 recruitment, Toca-1 was either neutral or inhibitory in this function. We tested the role of Toca-1 in LC3 recruitment by comparing LC3 association with bacteria at 40 min. of infection in the presence or absence of Toca-1 (Fig. 7A), using cells stably transfected with a short hairpin RNA (shRNA) directed against Toca-1 or, as a control, an empty lentiviral vector. During *S.* Typhimurium infection, the absence of Toca-1 was associated with a significant decrease in LC3 recruitment (Fig. 7B, left graph), as described previously [35]. So as to control for any effect actin tail formation might have on this process, in addition to examining LC3 recruitment around wild type *S. flexneri*, we examined its recruitment around the *icsA* mutant. The absence of Toca-1 was associated with an increase in LC3 recruitment that reached significance for the *icsA* mutant and was a trend for the wild-type strain (Fig. 7B, right and middle graphs, respectively). Complementation of the Toca-1 depletion using an shRNA-resistant form of Toca-1 rescued repression of LC3 recruitment by the *icsA* mutant (Fig. 7C), indicating that the increase in LC3 recruitment observed was due to the absence of Toca-1 *per se*. These data indicate that in the context of *Shigella* infection, Toca-1 does not promote LC3 recruitment, but rather is neutral in this respect, and in the absence of *Shigella* actin tail formation, represses it.

We demonstrated above that early during infection, IcsB is required both for Toca-1 recruitment (Figs. 1 and S1) and for repression of LC3 recruitment (Fig. 4A–B) around intracellular *S. flexneri*. To test whether the role of IcsB in limiting LC3 recruitment depends on Toca-1, we compared LC3 recruitment around strains expressing or lacking IcsB in cells containing or lacking Toca-1. In both the wild type and the *icsA* mutant background, IcsB played a role in limiting LC3 recruitment only in the presence of Toca-1 (Fig. 8A).

As in Fig. 7B, the increase in LC3 recruitment that occurred in the absence of Toca-1 reached statistical significance for the *icsA* mutant and was a trend for the wild-type strain (Fig. 8). The differences observed for the wild type and the *icsA* mutant may be a result of functional overlap between actin tail formation and repression of LC3 recruitment around stationary bacteria. We postulate that in the presence of IcsA, bacteria can escape LC3 recruitment either by forming actin tails, which would enable them to move away from LC3-studded membrane fragments, or via IcsB-mediated repression of LC3; wild type bacteria are able to form actin tails independent of whether they secrete sufficient IcsB to repress LC3 recruitment. For the *icsA* mutant, actin tail formation does not occur, so that IcsB-mediated repression of LC3 is the only option for escape from being marked with LC3; thus, the *icsA* mutant serves as a tool for evaluating IcsB-mediated repression of LC3 in relative isolation. Consistent with this possibility, under each condition, the percentage of bacteria associated with LC3 trended higher for the *icsA* mutant than for the wild-type strain (Fig. 8A).

It seemed unlikely that LC3 recruitment to intracellular *S. flexneri* early during infection was associated with an autophagy pathway targeting bacterial survival, since the absence of IcsB led to significant increases in LC3 recruitment (Fig. 4A), yet the absence of IcsB has no effect on bacterial survival up to 3 hr of infection [15]. To further explore whether LC3 recruitment to *S. flexneri* at these early times might be associated with autophagy, we determined the impact of Toca-1-associated repression of LC3 recruitment on *S. flexneri* survival. At 2–1/2 hr of infection, we found no difference in bacterial survival in the Toca-1 KD versus Toca-1$^{+/+}$ cells for either the wild type or the Δ*icsB* strain (Fig. 8B), indicating that absence of Toca-1 does not alter *Shigella* survival and lending support to the possibility that LC3 recruitment early during infection may be indicative of either LC3-associated phagocytosis or an autophagy pathway directed against membrane remnants that does not target bacteria directly for destruction.

Discussion

The host protein LC3 is best described for the role of the lipidated form in the formation of autophagosomes during autophagy. However, a distinct yet critical role for lipidated LC3 is in LC3-associated phagocytosis, wherein it marks phagosomal membranes in a process that is independent of

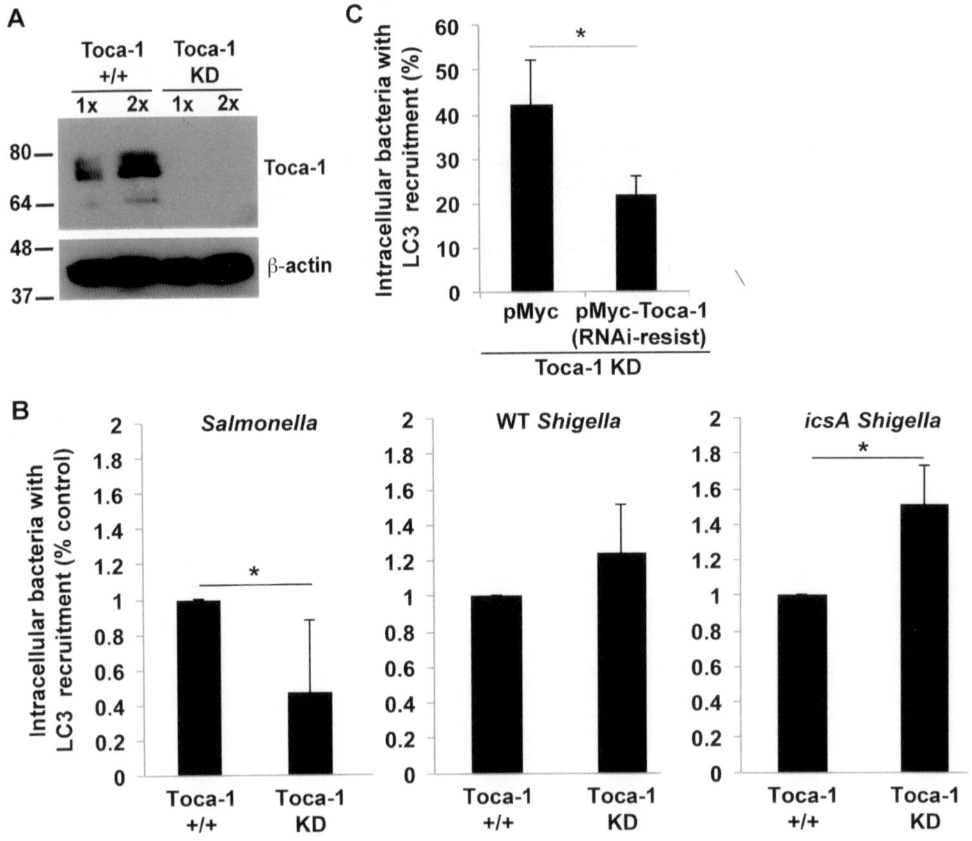

Figure 7. The pro-autophagy activity of Toca-1 observed during infection with *Salmonella* Typhimurium is absent in the setting of *S. flexneri* infection. (A) Levels of Toca-1 in stable Toca-1 KD or control (Toca-1$^{+/+}$) cells by western blot. 1x and 2x, relative loading. (B) LC3 recruitment around *S.* Typhimurium or WT or *icsA S. flexneri* at 40 min. of infection of Toca-1$^{+/+}$ or Toca-1 KD cells. For each strain, the values are normalized to LC3 recruitment in the presence of Toca-1. (C) LC3 recruitment around *icsA S. flexneri* at 40 min. of infection of Toca-1 KD cells complemented with Myc-tagged shRNA-resistant Toca-1 [pMyc-Toca-1 (RNAi-resist)] or Myc alone. Data represent the mean ± S.D. of three independent experiments. $^{*}P<0.05$.

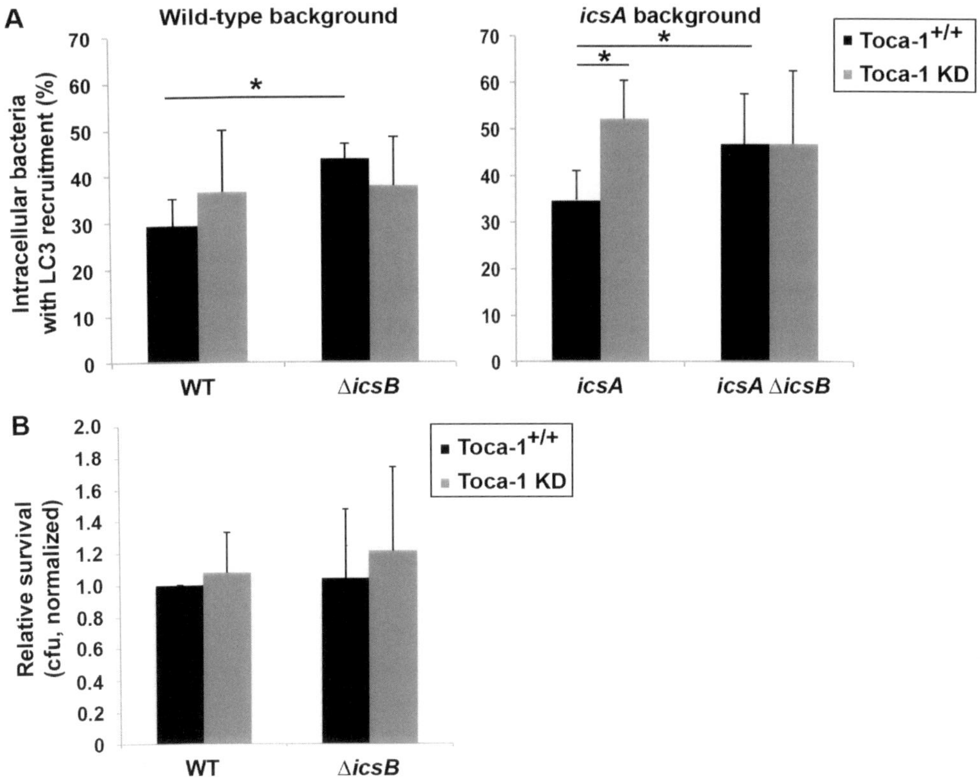

Figure 8. IcsB mediates repression of LC3 recruitment and increased survival independent of IcsA in the presence of Toca-1. (A) LC3 recruitment around wild-type (WT) versus Δ*icsB* (left graph) or around *icsA* versus *icsA* Δ*icsB* (right graph) *S. flexneri* at 40 min. of infection of Toca-1$^{+/+}$ or Toca-1 KD cells. (B) Survival of wild type or Δ*icsB S. flexneri* at 2.5 hrs. of infection by gentamicin protection assay in Toca-1$^{+/+}$ or Toca-1 KD cells. Data represent the mean ± S.D. of three independent experiments. *P<0.05.

autophagy [16]. We describe LC3 recruitment around a subset of *S. flexneri* soon after entry into MEFs and other non-phagocytic mammalian cells. LC3 recruitment around *S. flexneri* at this time appears to be unrelated to autophagy targeting bacteria for destruction, as conditions that lead to significant changes in the level of LC3 recruitment did not lead to reductions in bacterial survival (Figs. 4A and 8, and [15]). Moreover, *Shigella* IcsB, which we show represses LC3 recruitment (Fig. 1), does not contribute to inhibition of autophagy-related killing of *S. flexneri* at these early infection times [15]. Given evidence that recruitment of LC3 around *S. flexneri* at 40 min. of infection is not promoting bacterial killing, we conclude that it likely represents either LC3-associated phagocytosis or activation of autophagy targeting membrane remnants that serves a purpose other than destruction of intracellular bacteria.

LC3-associated phagocytosis is a poorly understood process that is characterized by LC3 studding of membranes of intact phagosomes [16,17]. At least in some cases, the process promotes maturation of the phagosome [16–18]. Several features described in this manuscript suggest that the process we observe is distinct from classical descriptions of LC3-associated phagocytosis in that, at the time we characterize (40 min. after bacterial contact with the cell), the bacterial cargo is no longer within intact phagosomes, but rather that LC3 is associated with phagosomal membrane fragments that surround cytoplasmic bacteria. First, recruitment of Toca-1 is initiated during bacterial uptake into cells (Fig. S2), concurrent with the formation of membrane ruffles that will constitute phagosomes that engulf entering bacteria. Within minutes of uptake, *Shigella* lyse the phagosome, and phagosomal membrane remnants surround intracellular *S. flexneri* at early infection times [30,34,36–38]. It seems likely that Toca-1 and IcsB remain associated with the phagosomal remnants after uptake and phagosomal lysis has occurred. Secondly, galectin-3, a marker of damaged or lysed vacuolar membranes, and cholesterol, a component of the membrane, are enriched in the vicinity of bacteria associated with Toca-1 (Figs. 4B and S4). And thirdly, at this early infection time, LC3 is typically distributed in fragments adjacent to and partially surrounding bacteria (Fig. 5E), a pattern strikingly similar to that observed for membrane remnants early after *S. flexneri* entry [30,34]. This suggests that assembly of LC3-associated machinery occurs during the process of cargo engulfment. These findings also suggest that LC3-mediated phagocytosis does not impede *Shigella* lysis of the phagosomal membrane and that the LC3-associated machinery does not immediately dissociate from the phagosomal membrane upon its fragmentation. Whether the LC3-associated phagocytosis machinery contributes to recycling of phagosomal membrane fragments during *S. flexneri* infection, as suggested by other studies [30], will require additional investigation.

Several cellular factors have been shown to be required for LC3-associated phagocytosis, including Atg5, Atg7, and Beclin-1, PI3 kinase activity and the generation of reactive oxygen species [16–18,27,28]. In distinct cellular circumstances, each of these also participates in autophagy, highlighting the overlap of LC3-associated phagocytosis with autophagy pathways. Dupont et al. [30] have described LC3 recruitment to vacuolar membrane remnants around a subset of intracellular *S. flexneri* early during infection. LC3 recruitment in this case may be promoting autophagy of membrane remnants in a manner that is independent of autophagy of the bacteria *per se*. Indeed, previous descriptions of recruitment of autophagy markers to vacuolar membrane remnants during *Shigella* infection have not demonstrated a role for autophagy marker recruitment in bacterial survival *per se* [23,30,34]. In the case of *Shigella* infection, since membrane remnants are derived from the phagocytic vacuole, the recruitment of LC3 to these membrane remnants may be the same process LC3-associated phagocytosis.

We found that LC3 recruitment to intracellular *S. flexneri* is inhibited by IcsB (Fig. 1). LC3-associated phagocytosis has been described for the intracellular pathogen *Burkholderia pseudomallei* [39]. Of note, the *B. pseudomallei* type three secreted effector BopA, a homolog of IcsB, inhibits LC3 recruitment to *B. pseudomallei* phagosomes [39]. This lends further support to our conclusion that the process described herein represents IcsB inhibition of an LC3-associated phagocytosis-like process and provides support to the idea that, during infection by *Shigella*, *Burkholderia*, and possibly other pathogens, LC3-associated phagocytosis may be the same process as LC3 recognition of vacuolar membrane remnants. A notable difference in the function of these two proteins is that whereas BopA contributes to lysis of the phagosome [39], we found no evidence that IcsB altered phagosome lysis (Fig. 4B–C).

Our findings together with these published results identify IcsB and BopA as a conserved family of type three effectors proteins that inhibit recruitment of LC3 to pathogen-associated phagosomal structures. In addition, they identify IcsB is a bacterial factor that modulates early recruitment of LC3 to *Shigella*. BopA and IcsB are the only bacterial factors reported thus far as inhibitors of this process.

Travassos et al. [23] examined LC3 recruitment around intracellular *S. flexneri* at slightly later infection times. At that time, LC3 was present around a subset of intracellular bacteria, and the number of bacteria associated with LC3 was increased for an *icsB* mutant, suggesting that for at least some bacteria, the association of bacteria with LC3 that we observed persists. LC3 recruitment was defective in the absence of the pattern-recognition molecule Nod1. In addition, the autophagy protein Atg16 was recruited to bacterial entry sites, dependent on the Nod1 and Nod2 [23]. An effect of Nod1 on survival of *S. flexneri* was documented only at 6 hr of infection, raising the possibility that the events described by these authors early during infection are part of the same process we describe here.

Previous work has shown that at later times during *S. flexneri* infection (4–5 hr), IcsB inhibits anti-bacterial autophagy by blocking Atg5 recognition of IcsA at the bacterial surface [15,40]. Of note, whereas IcsB inhibition of autophagy depends on IcsA [15], we found here that IcsB inhibition of LC3 recruitment is independent of IcsA (Fig. 5A). Moreover, the absence of IcsA had no effect on the recruitment and localization of Toca-1 or IcsB. Together, these results suggest that IcsB inhibits innate immune responses in two distinct ways, first, by inhibiting LC3-associated phagocytosis and/or LC3 recruitment to vacuolar membrane fragments early during infection, and second, by inhibiting autophagy late during infection.

We observed that at early infection times (40 min.), IcsB recruited the host protein Toca-1 to intracellular bacteria (Fig. 1). This raised the possibility that Toca-1 would be required for inhibition of LC3 recruitment. Since Toca-1 is required for efficient formation of actin tails by *S. flexneri* [11], and actin tail formation likely enhances bacterial movement away from phagosomal membrane remnants, to test the role of Toca-1 in early LC3 recruitment *per se*, we examined LC3 recruitment for *icsA* mutant bacteria, which are unable to form actin tails [41,42]. We found that Toca-1, like IcsB (Fig. 5A), is required for inhibition of LC3 recruitment around intracellular *S. flexneri* (Fig. 7B, right panel), thus identifying Toca-1 as a protein that modulates early LC3 recruitment.

Toca-1 is an F-BAR domain containing protein implicated in integration of regulation of the actin cytoskeleton with membrane trafficking [12,43–45]. F-BAR domains are membrane-binding scaffolds that typically sense and promote positive curvature membrane deformation that leads to inward invagination of the membrane [46]. Toca-1 functions both in activation of the actin nucleation-promoting factor N-WASP and in autophagy [12,35]. Indeed, we have shown previously that Toca-1 is required for efficient initiation of actin tail formation by *S. flexneri* [11]. Our finding here that Toca-1 is required for inhibition of LC3 recruitment identifies it as a cellular factor that likely modulates LC3-associated phagocytosis and/or LC3 recognition of membrane fragments. Moreover, the observation that Toca-1 recruitment is mutually exclusive with ubiquitination and recruitment of autophagy adaptor proteins raises the possibility that Toca-1 may be interfering with an early step in pathogen recognition. Our findings add Toca-1 to the list of factors that likely function both in LC3-associated phagocytosis and in autophagy. Under the conditions of our investigations described herein, Toca-1 appears to inhibit, rather than promote, LC3-associated phagocytosis and/or LC3 recognition of membrane fragments. Moreover, the contrasting function of Toca-1 during infection with *S.* Typhimurium [35] raises the possibility that Toca-1 plays opposing functions at different stages of bacterial infection and/or in the context of different pathogens.

Supporting Information

Figure S1 Recruitment of Toca-1 to intracellular bacteria lacking individual type three-secreted effector proteins. Infection for 40 min. of HeLa cells that had been transfected with Myc-Toca-1 by a panel of 21 isogenic *S. flexneri* strains, each harboring a deletion of a single gene encoding a type three effector protein, followed by immunofluorescence using antibody to Myc. Images are representative. Arrowheads, bacteria with Toca-1 recruitment.

Figure S2 Localization of Toca-1 to membrane ruffles. Localization of Toca-1 around bacteria in membrane ruffles during entry (40 min. after contact) of wild-type *S. flexneri* into HeLa cells that had been transfected with Myc-Toca-1. Immunofluorescence using antibody to Myc, phalloidin staining of polymerized actin, and DAPI staining of DNA. Images are representative. Size bar, 5 μm.

Figure S3 Recruitment of Toca-1 truncation mutants to intracellular *S. flexneri*. *S. flexneri* infection for 40 min. of HeLa cells transfected with full length Myc-Toca-1 or one of the ten Myc-Toca-1 truncation mutants, followed by immunofluorescence with antibody to Myc and staining with phalloidin (polymerized actin) and DAPI (DNA). The residues included in each truncation mutant are indicated to the left. Scale bars, 5 μM.

Figure S4 Localization of galectin-3 and cholesterol around *S. flexneri* early in infection. Wild-type *S. flexneri* infection (40 min) of HeLa cells that had been transfected with Myc-Toca-1, followed by labeling of galectin-3 and Myc by immunofluorescence and staining of cholesterol with filipin and of

DNA with DAPI. In overlays, Myc-Toca-1 is green, cholesterol and DAPI are blue, and galectin-3 is red. Size bars, 5 μm. Images are representative.

Acknowledgments

We are grateful to Marc Kirschner, Andrew Craig, Giorgio Scita, Noboru Mizushima, Cammie Lesser, and David Sacks for their contributions of reagents, to Serge Mostowy for helpful discussion, and to Jeremy Rock, Soo Young Lee, and Zaoping Li for critical reading of the manuscript.

Author Contributions

Conceived and designed the experiments: LAB MBG. Performed the experiments: LAB. Analyzed the data: LAB MBG. Contributed reagents/materials/analysis tools: LAB MBG. Wrote the paper: LAB MBG.

References

1. Mead PS, Slutsker L, Dietz V, McCaig LF, Bresee JS, et al. (1999) Food-related illness and death in the United States. Emerg Infect Dis 5: 607–625.
2. Kotloff KL, Winickoff JP, Ivanoff B, Clemens JD, Swerdlow DL, et al. (1999) Global burden of Shigella infections: implications for vaccine development and implementation of control strategies. Bulletin of the World Health Organization 77: 651–666.
3. Kotloff KL, Nataro JP, Blackwelder WC, Nasrin D, Farag TH, et al. (2013) Burden and aetiology of diarrhoeal disease in infants and young children in developing countries (the Global Enteric Multicenter Study, GEMS): a prospective, case-control study. Lancet 382: 209–222.
4. Clerc P, Sansonetti PJ (1987) Entry of Shigella flexneri into HeLa cells: evidence for directed phagocytosis involving actin polymerization and myosin accumulation. Infect Immun 55: 2681–2688.
5. Menard R, Sansonetti P, Parsot C (1994) The secretion of the Shigella flexneri Ipa invasins is activated by epithelial cells and controlled by IpaB and IpaD. EMBO J 13: 5293–5302.
6. Goldberg MB (2001) Actin-based motility of intracellular microbial pathogens. Microbiol Mol Biol Rev 65: 595–626.
7. Lommel S, Benesch S, Rottner K, Franz T, Wehland J, et al. (2001) Actin pedestal formation by enteropathogenic Escherichia coli and intracellular motility of Shigella flexneri are abolished in N-WASP-defective cells. EMBO Rep 2: 850–857.
8. Snapper SB, Takeshima F, Anton I, Liu CH, Thomas SM, et al. (2001) N-WASP deficiency reveals distinct pathways for cell surface projections and microbial actin-based motility. Nat Cell Biol 3: 897–904.
9. Egile C, Loisel TP, Laurent V, Li R, Pantaloni D, et al. (1999) Activation of the CDC42 effector N-WASP by the Shigella flexneri IcsA protein promotes actin nucleation by Arp2/3 complex and bacterial actin-based motility. J Cell Biol 146: 1319–1332.
10. Suzuki T, Miki H, Takenawa T, Sasakawa C (1998) Neural Wiskott-Aldrich syndrome protein is implicated in the actin-based motility of Shigella flexneri. EMBO J 17: 2767–2776.
11. Leung Y, Ally S, Goldberg MB (2008) Bacterial actin assembly requires toca-1 to relieve N-wasp autoinhibition. Cell Host Microbe 3: 39–47.
12. Ho HY, Rohatgi R, Lebensohn AM, Le M, Li J, et al. (2004) Toca-1 mediates Cdc42-dependent actin nucleation by activating the N-WASP-WIP complex. Cell 118: 203–216.
13. Bompard G, Caron E (2004) Regulation of WASP/WAVE proteins: making a long story short. J Cell Biol 166: 957–962.
14. Baxt LA, Garza-Mayers AC, Goldberg MB (2013) Bacterial subversion of host innate immune pathways. Science 340: 697–701.
15. Ogawa M, Yoshimori T, Suzuki T, Sagara H, Mizushima N, et al. (2005) Escape of intracellular Shigella from autophagy. Science 307: 727–731.
16. Sanjuan MA, Dillon CP, Tait SW, Moshiach S, Dorsey F, et al. (2007) Toll-like receptor signalling in macrophages links the autophagy pathway to phagocytosis. Nature 450: 1253–1257.
17. Lam GY, Cemma M, Muise AM, Higgins DE, Brumell JH (2013) Host and bacterial factors that regulate LC3 recruitment to Listeria monocytogenes during the early stages of macrophage infection. Autophagy 9: 985–995.
18. Martinez J, Almendinger J, Oberst A, Ness R, Dillon CP, et al. (2011) Microtubule-associated protein 1 light chain 3 alpha (LC3)-associated phagocytosis is required for the efficient clearance of dead cells. Proc Natl Acad Sci U S A 108: 17396–17401.
19. Datsenko KA, Wanner BL (2000) One-step inactivation of chromosomal genes in Escherichia coli K-12 using PCR products. Proc Natl Acad Sci U S A 97: 6640–6645.
20. Giard DJ, Aaronson SA, Todaro GJ, Arnstein P, Kersey JH, et al. (1973) In vitro cultivation of human tumors: establishment of cell lines derived from a series of solid tumors. J Natl Cancer Inst 51: 1417–1423.
21. Hu J, Mukhopadhyay A, Craig AW (2011) Transducer of Cdc42-dependent actin assembly promotes epidermal growth factor-induced cell motility and invasiveness. J Biol Chem 286: 2261–2272.
22. Ren JG, Li Z, Sacks DB (2007) IQGAP1 modulates activation of B-Raf. Proc Natl Acad Sci U S A 104: 10465–10469.
23. Travassos LH, Carneiro LA, Ramjeet M, Hussey S, Kim YG, et al. (2010) Nod1 and Nod2 direct autophagy by recruiting ATG16L1 to the plasma membrane at the site of bacterial entry. Nat Immunol 11: 55–62.
24. Shahnazari S, Yen WL, Birmingham CL, Shiu J, Namolovan A, et al. (2010) A diacylglycerol-dependent signaling pathway contributes to regulation of antibacterial autophagy. Cell Host Microbe 8: 137–146.
25. Deretic V (2012) Autophagy: an emerging immunological paradigm. J Immunology 189: 15–20.
26. Boyle KB, Randow F (2013) The role of 'eat-me' signals and autophagy cargo receptors in innate immunity. Curr Opin Microbiol.
27. Cullinane M, Gong L, Li X, Lazar-Adler N, Tra T, et al. (2008) Stimulation of autophagy suppresses the intracellular survival of Burkholderia pseudomallei in mammalian cell lines. Autophagy 4: 744–753.
28. Huang J, Canadien V, Lam GY, Steinberg BE, Dinauer MC, et al. (2009) Activation of antibacterial autophagy by NADPH oxidases. Proc Natl Acad Sci U S A 106: 6226–6231.
29. Meyer-Morse N, Robbins JR, Rae CS, Mochegova SN, Swanson MS, et al. (2010) Listeriolysin O is necessary and sufficient to induce autophagy during Listeria monocytogenes infection. PLoS One 5: e8610.
30. Dupont N, Lacas-Gervais S, Bertout J, Paz I, Freche B, et al. (2009) Shigella phagocytic vacuolar membrane remnants participate in the cellular response to pathogen invasion and are regulated by autophagy. Cell Host Microbe 6: 137–149.
31. Sansonetti PJ, Ryter A, Clerc P, Maurelli AT, Mounier J (1986) Multiplication of Shigella flexneri within HeLa cells: lysis of the phagocytic vacuole and plasmid-mediated contact hemolysis. Infect Immun 51: 461–469.
32. Leffler H, Carlsson S, Hedlund M, Qian Y, Poirier F (2004) Introduction to galectins. Glycoconj J 19: 433–440.
33. Paz I, Sachse M, Dupont N, Mounier J, Cederfur C, et al. (2010) Galectin-3, a marker for vacuole lysis by invasive pathogens. Cell Microbiol 12: 530–544.
34. Thurston TL, Wandel MP, von Muhlinen N, Foeglein A, Randow F (2012) Galectin 8 targets damaged vesicles for autophagy to defend cells against bacterial invasion. Nature 482: 414–418.
35. Huett A, Ng A, Cao Z, Kuballa P, Komatsu M, et al. (2009) A novel hybrid yeast-human network analysis reveals an essential role for FNBP1L in antibacterial autophagy. J Immunol 182: 4917–4930.
36. Ivanov SS, Roy CR (2009) Modulation of ubiquitin dynamics and suppression of DALIS formation by the Legionella pneumophila Dot/Icm system. Cell Microbiol 11: 261–278.
37. Mesquita FS, Thomas M, Sachse M, Santos AJ, Figueira R, et al. (2012) The Salmonella deubiquitinase SseL inhibits selective autophagy of cytosolic aggregates. PLoS Pathogens 8: e1002743.
38. Tattoli I, Sorbara MT, Vuckovic D, Ling A, Soares F, et al. (2012) Amino acid starvation induced by invasive bacterial pathogens triggers an innate host defense program. Cell Host Microbe 11: 563–575.
39. Gong L, Cullinane M, Treerat P, Ramm G, Prescott M, et al. (2011) The Burkholderia pseudomallei type III secretion system and BopA are required for evasion of LC3-associated phagocytosis. PLoS One 6: e17852.
40. Ogawa M, Yoshikawa Y, Kobayashi T, Mimuro H, Fukumatsu M, et al. (2011) A Tecpr1-dependent selective autophagy pathway targets bacterial pathogens. Cell Host Microbe 9: 376–389.
41. Bernardini ML, Mounier J, d'Hauteville H, Coquis-Rondon M, Sansonetti PJ (1989) Identification of icsA, a plasmid locus of Shigella flexneri that governs bacterial intra- and intercellular spread through interaction with F-actin. Proc Natl Acad Sci U S A 86: 3867–3871.
42. Lett M-C, Sasakawa C, Okada N, Sakai T, Makino S, et al. (1989) *virG*, a plasmid-coded virulence gene of *Shigella flexneri*: identification of the *virG* protein and determination of the complete coding sequence. J Bacteriol 171: 353–359.
43. Giuliani C, Troglio F, Bai Z, Patel FB, Zucconi A, et al. (2009) Requirements for F-BAR proteins TOCA-1 and TOCA-2 in actin dynamics and membrane trafficking during Caenorhabditis elegans oocyte growth and embryonic epidermal morphogenesis. PLoS Genetics 5: e1000675.
44. Yan S, Lv Z, Winterhoff M, Wenzl C, Zobel T, et al. (2013) The F-BAR protein Cip4/Toca-1 antagonizes the formin Diaphanous in membrane stabilization and compartmentalization. J Cell Sci 126: 1796–1805.
45. Fricke R, Gohl C, Dharmalingam E, Grevelhorster A, Zahedi B, et al. (2009) Drosophila Cip4/Toca-1 integrates membrane trafficking and actin dynamics through WASP and SCAR/WAVE. Curr Biol 19: 1429–1437.
46. Chen Y, Aardema J, Corey SJ (2013) Biochemical and functional significance of F-BAR domain proteins interaction with WASP/N-WASP. Sem Cell Dev Biol 24: 280–286.

47. Labrec EH, Schneider H, Magnani TJ, Formal SB (1964) Epithelial Cell Penetration as an Essential Step in the Pathogenesis of Bacillary Dysentery. J Bacteriol 88: 1503–1518.
48. Steinhauer J, Agha R, Pham T, Varga AW, Goldberg MB (1999) The unipolar Shigella surface protein IcsA is targeted directly to the bacterial old pole: IcsP cleavage of IcsA occurs over the entire bacterial surface. Mol Microbiol 32: 367–377.
49. Kabeya Y, Mizushima N, Ueno T, Yamamoto A, Kirisako T, et al. (2000) LC3, a mammalian homologue of yeast Apg8p, is localized in autophagosome membranes after processing. EMBO J 19: 5720–5728.

11

Investigation of Key Interventions for Shigellosis Outbreak Control in China

Tianmu Chen[1]◆, Ross Ka-kit Leung[2]◆, Zi Zhou[3], Ruchun Liu[1], Xixing Zhang[1], Lijie Zhang[4]*

1 Office for Disease Control and Emergency Response, Changsha Center for Disease Control and Prevention, Changsha, The People's Republic of China, **2** Stanley Ho Centre for Emerging Infectious Diseases, The Chinese University of Hong Kong, Shatin, New Territories, Hong Kong SAR, The People's Republic of China, **3** School of Public Health, Xiamen University, Xiamen, The People's Republic of China, **4** Chinese Field Epidemiology Training Program, Chinese Center for Disease Control and Prevention, Beijing, The People's Republic of China

Abstract

Shigellosis is a major public health concern in China, where waterborne disease outbreaks are common. Shigellosis-containing strategies, mostly single or multiple interventions, are implemented by primary-level health departments. Systematic assessment of the effectiveness of these measures is scarce. To estimate the efficacy of commonly used intervention strategies, we developed a Susceptible–Exposed–Infectious/Asymptomatic–Recovered–Water model. No intervention was predicted to result in a total attack rate (TAR) of 90% of the affected population (95% confidence interval [CI]: 86.65–92.80) and duration of outbreak (DO) of 89 days, and the use of single-intervention strategies can be futile or even counter-productive. Prophylactics and water disinfection did not improve TAR or DO. School closure for up to 3 weeks did not help but only increased DO. Isolation alone significantly increased DO. Only antibiotics treatment could shorten the DO to 35 days with TAR unaffected. We observed that these intervention effects were additive when in combined usage under most circumstances. Combined intervention "Isolation+antibiotics+prophylactics+water disinfection" was predicted to result in the lowest TAR (41.9%, 95%CI: 36.97–47.04%) and shortest DO (28 days). Our actual Shigellosis control implementation that also included school closure for 1 week, attained comparable results and the modeling produced an epidemic curve of Shigellosis highly similar to our actual outbreak data. This lends a strong support to the reality of our model that provides a possible reference for public health professionals to evaluate their strategies towards Shigellosis control.

Editor: Hiroshi Nishiura, The University of Tokyo, Japan

Funding: This work was partially supported by the Scientific Research Program of Health Depatrment of Hunan Province (B2012-138, http://www.21hospital.com/) and by the Scientific Research Program of Changsha Science and Technology Bureau (K1205028-31, http://www.cssti.cn/html/cskjw/index.html). The funders had no role in study design, data collection and analysis, decision to publish, or preparation of the manuscript.

Competing Interests: The authors have declared that no competing interests exist.

* E-mail: cfetpzlj@126.com

◆ These authors contributed equally to this work.

Introduction

Shigellosis (bacillary dysentery), the result of infection with *Shigella*, is an enteric infectious disease responsible for approximately 1,100,000 deaths per year worldwide [1]. As approximately two-thirds of those who die from shigellosis are children under 5 years of age, it is one of the most common diarrhea-related causes of morbidity and mortality in children in developing countries [2]. Shigellosis epidemics usually occur in areas with crowding and poor sanitary conditions, where person-to-person transmission or contamination of food or water by the organism is common [3–8]. In China, many private wells supplying water to schools are built in close proximity to sources of pollution, including toilets, septic tanks, sewer ditches, and lakes and ponds into which sewage is discharged. As water from these wells is often not treated before being piped into schools, waterborne outbreaks of *Shigella* frequently occur [6], with devastating effects on students, their families, and schools.

Many outbreak control strategies developed by primary-level health departments in China are empirically-driven. This can be attributed to a lack of data regarding the rate of morbidity in the absence of intervention, making it difficult to estimate whether the efficacy of a single or combined intervention could be decreased if implemented using traditional methods. In these circumstances, researchers often perform mathematical modeling to estimate the total attack rate (TAR), an indicator of the extent of an outbreak [9–13]. A bacillary dysentery model with seasonal fluctuation was formulated and studied by Bai et al. [14], in which a simple Susceptible–Infectious–Recovered–Susceptible framework was employed that could not clarify the person–water–person transmission pathways.

Fortunately, a waterborne pathogen model termed the Susceptible–Infectious–Recovered–Water (SIRW) model can be used to examine disease outbreaks that occur via multiple transmission pathways [15], such as shigellosis. The SIRW model is a simple ordinary differential equation model that extends the classic SIR framework by adding a compartment (W) that tracks the pathogen concentration in water. Infected individuals shed the pathogen into water compartments, and new infections arise both through exposure to contaminated water as well as by the classic SIR person–person transmission pathway. Combining the characteristics of the SIRW model with those of shigellosis, we developed a

Susceptible–Exposed–Infectious/Asymptomatic–Recovered–Water (SEIARW) model to examine the efficacy of different intervention strategies in controlling an outbreak of shigellosis at a primary school in Changsha City, China.

Materials and Methods

Ethics Statement

Each shigellosis case was required to be notified for epidemiologic surveillance. These surveillance data were used in this study, without the need for the collection of additional information (e.g. demographics) for the research. This study was approved by Medical Ethics Committee of Changsha Center for Disease Control and Prevention. Consent requirement, either verbal or written, was waived by Medical Ethics Committee of Changsha Center for Disease Control and Prevention Center for Disease Control and Prevention on the following grounds: (1) only anonymized records were used without the need for direct involvement nor active participation of patients; (2) neither medical intervention nor biological samples were involved; (3) study procedures and results would not affect clinical management of patients in any form.

Data Collection and Analysis

On October 19, 2012, a local branch of the Center for Disease Control and Prevention (CDC) reported an outbreak of shigellosis in a primary school in a rural area. As the longest incubation period is 9 days, subsequent immediate investigation between October 3 and 31, reflecting identification of the first and final cases on October 11 and 23, respectively, permitted data collection for 134 cases. However, no case was found to be chronic or fatal, and 7 anal swab samples were collected from healthy individuals from the school, and no culture was positive for *Shigella sonnei*. The 2 primary transmission routes were identified as person–to-person and person–water–person; *Shigella sonnei* was identified as the pathogen responsible for the outbreak. The definition of a case in this investigation followed that specified in "Diagnostic criteria for bacillary and amoebic dysentery (WS 287–2008)," a report published by the Ministry of Health of China in 2008 based on a shigellosis outbreak investigation conducted by He et al. [6]. A probable case of shigellosis was identified in a teacher or a student of the primary school or in a resident who lived in close proximity to the school between October 5 and 28, if the affected individual experienced diarrhea ≥3 times per day in addition to ≥1 of the following symptoms: fever ≥37.5°C, vomiting, and/or abdominal pain. A confirmed case was identified when culture confirmation of *Shigella* infection was obtained from a stool specimen or rectal swab from an individual who had been identified as a suspected case.

This outbreak was used as an example for modeling the use of combined strategies for containing a shigellosis outbreak, including 4 major measures (case isolation, medical intervention, school closure, and water disinfection) and 3 supplementary measures (environmental disinfection, health education, and hand hygiene). As the supplementary measures were difficult to quantify, a combination of the resulting in 22 strategy options, including single and combined-intervention strategies was simulated.

We collected the basic information of the school and the data of cases. The former included the number of students and faculty and staff, and the number of classes. The later included name, sex, age,class of each case, and the date of illness onset, the date of medical intervention implemented, the date of recovered, and the symptoms (such as fever, headache or dizziness, times of diarrhea per day, stool texture, abdominal pain, vomit, etc.) of each case. From this data, we can analyze the temporal distribution of each case and the infectious period with medical intervention or not.

No Intervention

A deterministic model was developed on the basis of the following conditions:

(1) Transmission occurs via either a person–person or a person–water–person route.
(2) Although fatal cases (albeit a low number) have been identified in previous shigellosis epidemic, it was not identified in the outbreak investigated here. Thus, fatal cases were not included in the model.
(3) We also considered asymptomatic cases in the model since asymptomatic carriers have been identified in previous outbreaks.
(4) Infection during an outbreak confers permanent immunity.
(5) The transmission of shigellosis during a school outbreak occurs within a closed system, defined as a system with no migration in or out; adjustment for births and natural deaths was not included in the model.
(6) The county in which the affected school is located contains 33 towns and a population of more than 1.37 million. Despite these numbers, only 8 cases of shigellosis were reported among individuals who were not affiliated with the school, indicating a low probability of infection among them. Thus, the model did not consider the probability of infection in the wider community.

Figure 1 depicts the flow diagram for the development of the SEIARW model, where individuals are characterized according to their epidemiological status as susceptible (S), exposed (E, infected but not yet fully contagious), infectious (I), asymptomatic (A), and recovered (R); W denotes the reservoir (water) compartment. The definitions of the 6 epidemiological classes are summarized in Table 1.

As illustrated in Figure 1, susceptible individuals become infected (i.e., move from S to E) by contact with either infected/asymptomatic individuals or contaminated water at rates of βSI, βkSA and $\beta_W SW$ respectively, where β and β_W are the probability of transmission per contact, k is the relative transmissibility of asymptomatic to symptomatic individuals. As exposed individuals become infectious after an incubation period, they move from E to I at a rate of $(1-p)\omega E$ and E to A at a rate of $p\omega E$, where $1/\omega$ is the incubation period of the disease and p is the proportion of asymptomatic individuals. After the infectious period has passed, infectious and asymptomatic individuals may move to R at a rate of γI and $\gamma' A$ respectively, where $1/\gamma$ and $1/\gamma'$ are the infectious period of the I and A. Infectious and asymptomatic individuals can

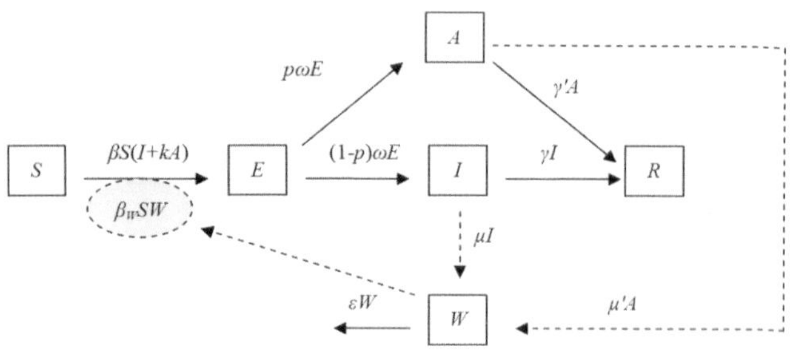

Figure 1. Flowchart of development of the SEIARW model (1).

Table 1. Variables within the SEIARW model (1).

Variable	Description	Unit
S	Susceptible individual density	Individuals·km^{-2}
E	Exposed individual density	Individuals·km^{-2}
I	Infectious individual density	Individuals·km^{-2}
A	Asymptomatic individual density	Individuals·km^{-2}
R	Recovered/removed individual density	Individuals·km^{-2}
N	Total population density	Individuals·km^{-2}
W	Pathogen concentration in water reservoir	Cells·mL^{-3}

in turn contaminate the water compartment by shedding the pathogen into W at a shedding rate of μI and $\mu' A$, where μ and μ' are the shedding coefficients. The pathogen in W will subsequently leave the water compartment at a rate of εW, where $1/\varepsilon$ is the lifetime of the pathogen. The corresponding model equations are as follows:

$$\begin{cases} dS/dt = -\beta S(I+kA) - \beta_W SW \\ dE/dt = \beta S(I+kA) + \beta_W SW - \omega E \\ dI/dt = (1-p)\omega E - \gamma I \\ dA/dt = p\omega E - \gamma' A \\ dR/dt = \gamma I + \gamma' A \\ dW/dt = \mu I + \mu' A - \varepsilon W \end{cases} \quad (1)$$

It would be instructive to consider a rescaling of model (1) using dimensionless variables. If N is assumed to denote the total population size and $s = S/N$, $e = E/N$, $i = I/N$, $a = I/A$, $r = R/N$, $w = \varepsilon W/\mu N$, $\mu' = c\mu$, $b = \beta N$, and $b_W = \mu\beta_W N/\varepsilon$, the following rescaled model can be developed:

$$\begin{cases} ds/dt = -bs(i+ka) - b_W sw \\ de/dt = bs(i+ka) + b_W sw - \omega e \\ di/dt = (1-p)\omega e - \gamma i \\ da/dt = p\omega e - \gamma' a \\ dr/dt = \gamma i + \gamma' a \\ dw/dt = \varepsilon(i + ca - w) \end{cases} \quad (2)$$

As the SEIAR model assumes that transmission occurs via daily contact, it assumes that transmission occurs solely via the person–person route. The corresponding model equation is thus:

$$\begin{cases} ds/dt = -bs(i+ka) \\ de/dt = bs(i+ka) - \omega e \\ di/dt = (1-p)\omega e - \gamma i \\ da/dt = p\omega e - \gamma' a \\ dr/dt = \gamma i + \gamma' a \end{cases} \quad (3)$$

Case Isolation

In practice, milder shigellosis cases were requested to stay home. Dedicated staff paid visits to ensure adherence, hygiene and proper disinfection. More severe cases were hospitalized and isolated. Both cases received a full course of antibiotics treatment and were discharged two days since the day they have been free of symptoms. In the case isolation model, neither the reservoir-to-person nor the person–to-person routes are viable means of transmission. Nevertheless, individuals in compartment S could become infected via the reservoir–to-person and asymptomatic-susceptible routes, leading to development of the following rescaled model:

$$\begin{cases} ds/dt = -b_W sw - bksa \\ de/dt = b_W sw + bksa - \omega e \\ di/dt = (1-p)\omega e - \gamma i \\ da/dt = p\omega e - \gamma' a \\ dr/dt = \gamma i + \gamma' a \\ dw/dt = \varepsilon(ca - w) \end{cases} \quad (4)$$

Medical Intervention

Medical interventions including therapeutics and prophylactic, were both simulated in our model. For therapeutics, several antibiotics, including ampicillin-sulbactam sodium, ceftazidime pentahydrate, cefixime, and cefaclor, had all been used in exactly the same manner for different individuals during the outbreak; we used drug sensitivity tests to determine their effectiveness against *S. sonnei*. If a case of shigellosis is treated with a standard course of antibiotics from the date of illness onset, the mean infectious period can be reduced by η, which ranges from 0 to 1 (Figure 2).

For prophylactic, berberine hydrochloride was targeted at individuals other than recovered (R) or infectious (I), so susceptible (S), exposed (E), asymptomatic (A) individuals were all targeted. We assumed that given a standard course (3 days) of berberine hydrochloride, a susceptible individual cannot be infected by *S. sonnei* for 3 days, an exposed individual will become recovered (R) directly, and the transmissibility of asymptomatic individual will be discounted by f, where f ranges from 0 to 1.

Water Disinfection

We have been following the guidelines of "Technical Standard For Disinfection (The 2002 Edition)" issued by the Chinese National Health and Family Planning Commission and chlorine-releasing agents, such as chlorinated lime and calcium hypochlorite have been being used for disinfection. According to a previous study conducted by Wu et al [16], no *S. sonnei* was found in

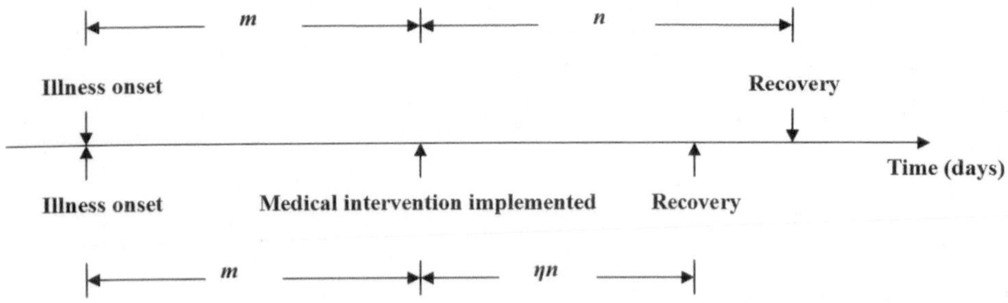

Figure 2. Infectious period of a typical shigellosis case with or without medical intervention. *m+n*: Infectious period with no medical intervention; *m+ηn*: infectious period with partial medical intervention, which is equivalent to part of the infectious period with no medical intervention (*m*) and part of the infectious period with medical intervention (*ηn*); *η*(*m+n*): infectious period with a medical intervention that had been implemented on the date of illness onset.

chlorinated water. Therefore, the variables W, ε, and b_W are removed from the water disinfection model.

School Closure

During a school closure, all the people in a school return home. Person–to-person and reservoir–to-person contacts are severed, making both b and b_W become zero in effect in the school closure model. We simulated the school closure of 1, 2, or 3 weeks, to examine the effects.

Combined-Intervention Strategies

We simulated the following 17 combined interventions to examine their impact: AW, antibiotics+water disinfection; IA, isolation+antibiotics; IW, isolation+water disinfection; S_{1w}I, school closure (1 week)+isolation; S_{1w}W, school closure (1 week)+water disinfection; S_{1w}A, school closure (1 week)+antibiotics; APW, antibiotics+prophylactic+water disinfection; IAP, isolation+antibiotics+prophylactic; IPW, isolation+prophylactic+water disinfection; S_{1w}IP, school closure (1 week)+isolation+prophylactic; S_{1w}PW, school closure (1 week)+prophylactic+water disinfection; S_{1w}AP, school closure (1 week)+antibiotics+prophylactic; IAPW, isolation+antibiotics+prophylactic+water disinfection; S_{1w}IPW, school closure (1 week)+isolation+prophylactic+water disinfection; S_{1w}IAP, school closure (1 week)+isolation+antibiotics+prophylactic; S_{1w}APW, school closure (1 week)+antibiotics+prophylactic+ water disinfection; S_{1w}IAPW, school closure (1 week)+isolation+ antibiotics+prophylactic+water disinfection.

Estimation of Parameters

Of b, b_W, k, ω, p, γ, γ', c, ε, f, and η, the 11 parameters in the model (Table 2), γ and η could be estimated by reviewing data regarding the outbreak. According to the reports from the Department of Health, Victorian State Government, North Dakota Department of Health Division of Disease Control and New Mexico Department of Health Epidemiology and Response Division Infectious Disease Epidemiology Bureau, asymptomatic individuals can shed the bacteria for at least 4 weeks. Here we simulated 5 weeks in our model, thus $\gamma' = 0.0286$.

Several studies have found that although *S. sonnei* can survive from several to 170 days and can even grow well in food [17,18], its die-off rate (half-time) in well water is only 24.5 h [19], meaning that only 50% of the *S. sonnei* present at the beginning of a study period ($t = 0$) remains after 1 day ($t = 1$). According to the SEIARW model, the die-off rate of *S. sonnei* in well water can be represented by the following equation:

$$dw/dt = -\varepsilon w \quad (5)$$

Thus, $\varepsilon = 0.6931$ under the conditions described above.

In our data, a typical case of diarrhea was about 3.2 times (range 3–12 times) per day but an asymptomatic individual only shedding stool once per day. Thus $\mu' = c\mu$, $c = 0.3125$. Due to reduction of shedding frequency, the relative transmissibility of asymptomatic individual (k) was modeled to be a reduced quantity (0.3125). The proportions of asymptomatic individuals were reported to range from 0.0037 to 0.27 [20–22]. We set $p = 0.1$ in SEIARW model.

Although the incubation period of shigellosis ranges from 7 h to 9 days and is typically 1 to 3 days [23,24], ω cannot be obtained from analysis of the collected data. The parameters b and ω were therefore estimated by curve fitting using outbreak data collected from October 11 to 15 in the SEIAR model, the parameter b_W using outbreak data collected from October 16 to 19 in the SEIARW model, and the parameter f using outbreak data collected from October 19 to 28 in the SEIARW model.

Strategy Assessment Indicators

We estimated TAR and duration of outbreak (DO) to assess the efficacy of the strategies for controlling the outbreak (Table 3). Epidemic curves were compared to evaluate the efficacy of using the containing strategies as compared to no intervention and to the actual combined strategies implemented by the health and education departments.

Simulation Methods

Berkeley Madonna 8.3.18 and Microsoft Office Excel 2003 software were employed for model simulation and figure development, respectively. The Runge-Kutta method of order 4 with the tolerance set at 0.001 was used to perform curve fitting. While the curve fit is in progress, Berkeley Madonna displays the root mean square (RMS) deviation between the data and best run so far.

Sensitivity Analysis

Since two parameters, p and γ', were estimated by references, there was some uncertainty about them which might impact the results of models we built. In our study, sensitivity was tested by varying the two parameters which were split into 1000 values ranging from 0.0037 to 0.27 and from 0.0036 to 0.0357 (which

Table 2. Parameter definitions and values.

Parameter	Description	Unit	Value	Method
β	Person–to-person contact rate	$km^2 \cdot individuals^{-1} \cdot day^{-1}$	–	–
b	Scaled person– to-person contact rate	day^{-1}	1.1240	Curve fitting
β_W	Reservoir– to-person contact rate	$mL^3 \cdot cells^{-1} \cdot day^{-1}$	–	–
b_W	Scaled reservoir– to-person contact rate	day^{-1}	1.1289	Curve fitting
k	Relative transmissibility rate of asymptomatic to symptomatic individuals	1	0.3125	Analysis of outbreak data
ω	Incubation relative rate	day^{-1}	1	Curve fitting
p	Proportion of the asymptomatic	1	0.1	References[20–22]
γ	Recovery rate of the infectious	day^{-1}	0.0741	Analysis of outbreak data
γ'	Recovery rate of the asymptomatic	day^{-1}	0.0286	See text
ε	Pathogen lifetime relative rate	day^{-1}	0.6931	Calculation using Equation (5)
μ	Person–to-reservoir contact rate ("shedding" by Infectious)	$cells \cdot mL^{-3} \cdot day^{-1} \cdot km^2 \cdot individuals^{-1}$	–	–
μ'	Person–to-reservoir contact rate ("shedding" by Asymptomatic)	$cells \cdot mL^{-3} \cdot day^{-1} \cdot km^2 \cdot individuals^{-1}$	–	–
c	Shedding rate of the asymptomatic comparing to the infectious	1	0.3125	Analysis of outbreak data
η	Efficacy of medical intervention [antibiotics]	1	0.3111	Analysis of outbreak data
f	Efficacy of medical intervention [prophylactic]	1	5.7221×10^{-7}	Curve fitting

means asymptomatic individuals can shed the bacteria from 4 weeks to 40 weeks) respectively.

Results

Timing of Outbreak

Among the 348 students and 17 faculty and staff present at the school when the outbreak occurred, we identified 134 cases of shigellosis, of which 59 were suspected, 55 probable, and 20 confirmed, yielding a TAR of 36.71%. After the first case had been identified on October 11, the number of cases increased gradually, peaking between October 12 and 14, and then beginning to decrease on October 15. However, after a rainstorm on October 16 resulted in contamination of the shallow school well by sewage containing the feces of the cases, as identified using laboratory detection methods, the number of cases began to increase rapidly, peaking on October 19 before beginning to decrease after the local CDC initiated an investigation on the same day until the last case was identified on October 23. Field epidemiological study revealed that the 2 primary routes of transmission corresponded to the 2 epidemic peaks in terms of temporal distribution, with the first peak resulting from primarily person–to-person transmission, and the second from both person–water–person and person–to-person transmission (Figure 3).

Analysis of all data collected revealed that the mean infectious period of all cases provided with partial medical intervention ($m+\eta n$) was 5.1 (2.4 SD) days (range 1–12 days) (Figure 4A), with $m = 1.3$ (Figure 4C), whereas the mean infectious period of all cases with full intervention ($\eta[m+n]$) was 4.2 (1.9 SD) days (range 1–8 days) (Figure 4B). As no chronic cases were identified, the mean infectious period of all cases provided with no medical intervention ($m+n$) was 13.5 days, with $\eta = 0.3111$.

Curve fitting analysis revealed that the daily prevalence of the outbreak fit the data to the greatest extent when $b = 1.1240$, $b_W = 1.1289$, $\omega = 1$, and $f = 5.7221 \times 10^{-7}$ (Figure 5). The model thus reproduced the typical epidemic curve observed for a shigellosis outbreak in a school population.

Efficacy of Interventions

Table 3 lists the results regarding analysis of the efficacy of the 22 intervention strategies. In the absence of any intervention, the model predicted that all exposed individuals would become infected and sick, yielding a TAR of 90% (95% confidence interval [CI]: 86.65–92.79) and a DO of 89 days. We note that the TAR only includes observable cases (i.e. it does not include asymptomatic cases). Single-intervention options were predicted to result in high TAR. Specifically, strategy antibiotics had a TAR of 90% (95% CI: 86.65–92.79), but a relatively brief DO of 35 days. While strategy water disinfection also had a TAR of 90% (95% CI: 86.65–92.79), it had a much longer DO of 90 days. Likewise, the 3 school closure options (1 week, 2 weeks, and 3 weeks) all had a TAR of 90% (95% CI: 86.65–92.79) and a DO of 94, 100, and 107 days, respectively, all of which were longer than the DO of no intervention. Strategy prophylactics had no effects as if there was no intervention at all. Although strategy isolation was predicted to reduce the TAR slightly to 85.3% (95% CI: 81.20–88.48), the cost was a DO of 147 days.

Combined-intervention strategies that consist of only 2 single intervention options had little improvement over the single-intervention options. Among these 6 options, IW was the most effective, reducing the TAR to 70.8% (95% CI: 66.10–75.38) but a DO of 180 days, followed by, in descending order of efficacy, $S_{1w}I$, IA, AW, $S_{1w}A$, and $S_{1w}W$. Combined-intervention strategies that consist of 3 single intervention options had better efficacy. Among these 6 options, IPW was the most effective, reducing the TAR to 41.9% (95% CI: 36.97–47.04) and the DO to 70 days, followed by $S_{1w}IP$, IAP, APW, $S_{1w}AP$, and $S_{1w}PW$.

The 5 combined-intervention options that each included 4 or 5 different single options had the best efficacy. IAPW, $S_{1w}IAP$, and $S_{1w}IAPW$ had almost the same efficacy, specifically a TAR of

Table 3. Results of simulation of effectiveness of shigellosis interventions implemented on October 19.

	TAR (%)		
Intervention	**%**	**95% CI**	**DO (days)**
None	90.0	86.65–92.79	89
Antibiotics	90.0	86.65–92.79	35
Prophylactics	90.0	86.65–92.79	89
Water disinfection	90.0	86.65–92.79	90
Isolation	85.3	81.20–88.48	147
School closure			
1 week	90.0	86.65–92.79	94
2 weeks	90.0	86.65–92.79	100
3 weeks	90.0	86.65–92.79	107
AW	89.6	86.03–92.32	37
IA	84.5	80.30–87.74	93
IW	70.8	66.10–75.38	180
S1wI	83.4	79.41–87.01	175
S1wW	90.0	86.65–92.79	95
S1wA	90.0	86.65–92.79	37
APW	87.7	83.90–90.66	46
IAP	44.5	39.37–49.51	38
IPW	41.9	36.97–47.04	70
S1wIP	42.1	37.23–47.31	73
S1wPW	90	86.65–92.79	94
S1wAP	89.8	86.34–92.55	46
IAPW	41.9	36.97–47.04	28
S1wIPW	41.9	36.97–47.04	70
S1wIAP	41.9	36.97–47.04	28
S1wAPW	86.7	82.70–89.70	58
S1wIAPW	41.9	36.97–47.04	28

TAR, Total attack rate; CI, confidence interval as calculated by binomial distribution; DO, duration of outbreak.

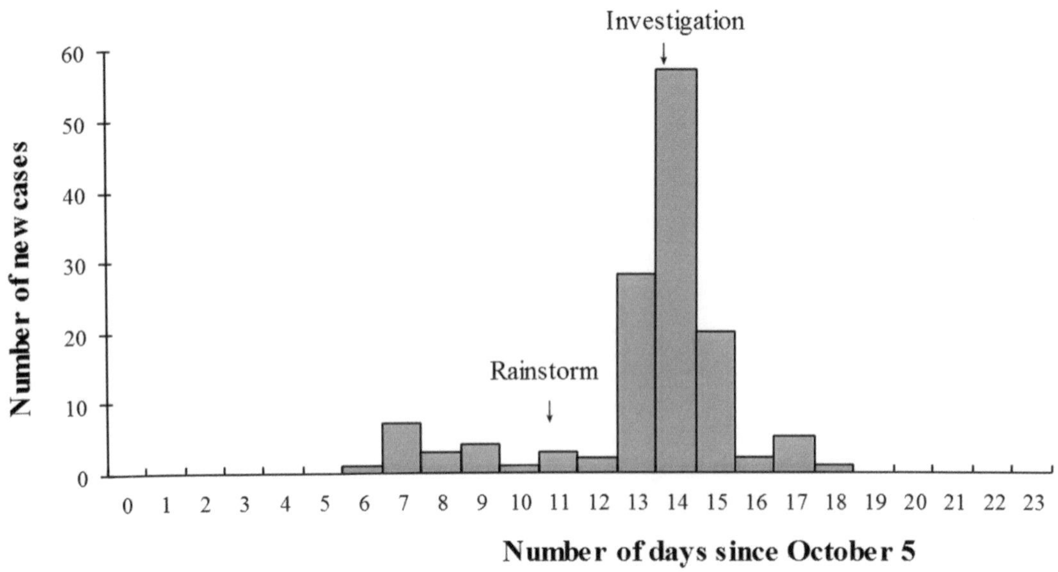

Figure 3. Temporal distribution of shigellosis new cases in a primary school since October 5.

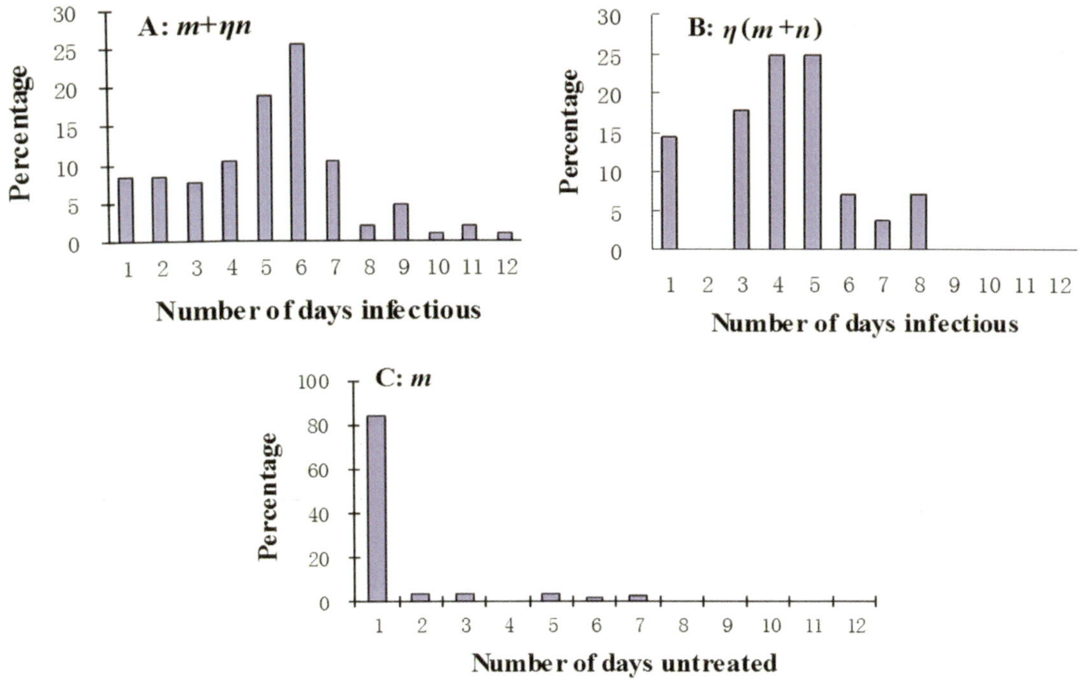

Figure 4. Infectious periods of all cases. A, Distribution of cases provided with fractional medical intervention ($m+\eta n$) during infectious period; B, distribution of cases provided with combined intervention ($\eta[m+n]$) during infectious period; C, distribution of part of the infectious period with no medical intervention (m).

41.9% (95% CI: 36.97–47.04) and a DO of only 28 days. Although S_{1w}IPW had a similar TAR to IAPW, its DO was longer, and S_{1w}APW had a longer DO and higher TAR than IAPW.

Figure 6 depicts the epidemic curve of the outbreak without intervention or with each intervention strategy. As can be observed, the curve of the single-intervention strategy water disinfection is most similar to that of the curve of no intervention; the curve of S_{1w}IAPW is almost the same and most similar to the curve of the data of this outbreak in which actual combined strategies had been implemented.

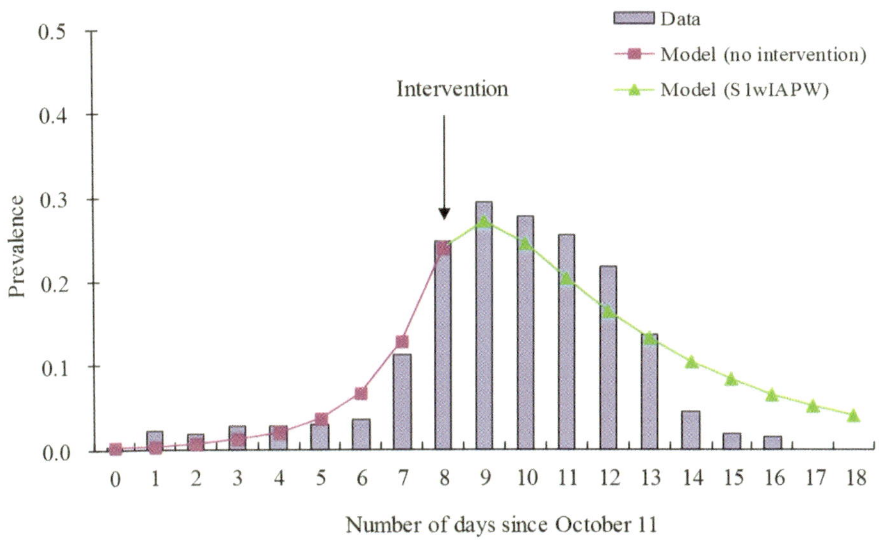

Figure 5. Curve fitting of data from the baseline of the outbreak simulation from October 11 to 29. Since the local CDC investigated and implemented the actual combined strategies at day 8 in this outbreak, SEIARW model with no intervention was employed for curve fitting during 0~8 days (pink line), and SEIARW model with combined strategies of S1wIAPW was employed for curve fitting for the days thereafter (green line). Prevalence = $I/N = i$, where I is the infectious and N is the total number of persons.

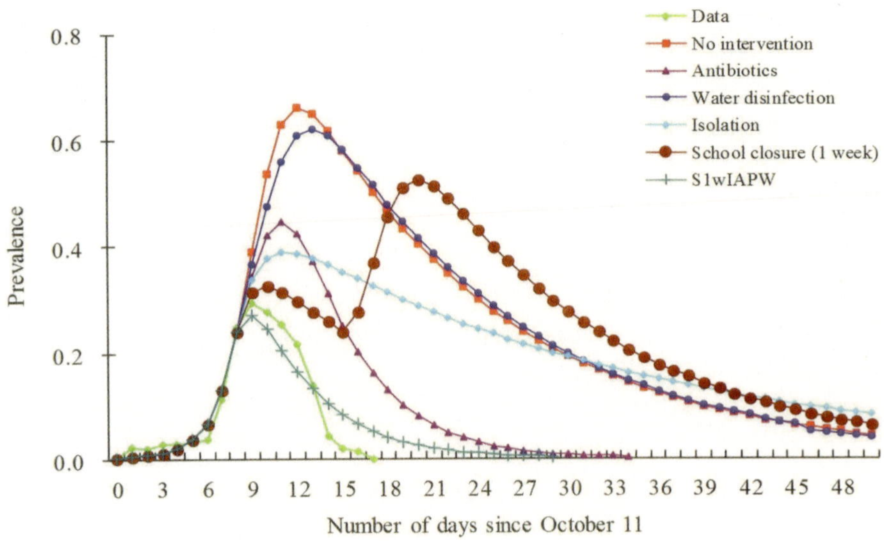

Figure 6. Results of simulation of efficacy of main intervention strategy options for controlling shigellosis outbreak. Prevalence = $I/N = i$, where I is the infectious and N is the total number of persons.

Sensitivity Analysis

Our model is only slightly sensitive to the parameter p, the value which we set in our model ($p = 0.1$) lead to the same prevalence to the mean value of sensitivity analysis based on the 1000 of the model ran (Figure 7). The model is not sensitive to the parameter γ', the prevalence are the same to the mean value, mean-sd, mean+sd, and the value we set (figure 8).

Discussion

In China, cooperation between local health departments (i.e., local CDC branches), which develop outbreak control and intervention strategies, and education departments (i.e., schools), which implement the strategies, is necessary for controlling outbreaks, especially at the primary school level. It is crucial to determine whether these strategies are likely to be effective before adopted. To aid in fulfilling the need for such an estimation, we developed models to estimate the effectiveness of a variety of strategies in controlling an outbreak of shigellosis, yielding findings that will be of great importance for controlling future outbreaks.

Our results revealed that the effectiveness of single-intervention strategies in containing outbreaks would be limited, whereas that of combined-intervention strategies would be significantly greater. Specifically, the strategies IAPW, $S_{1w}IAP$, and $S_{1w}IAPW$, all of which had a TAR of 41.9% (95% CI: 36.97–47.04) and a DO of 28 days, thus reflecting the efficacy of the actual combined strategies most closely, would be the most effective.

Currently, school closure is the most common strategy used by primary-level health departments in China to control infectious disease outbreaks. However, this strategy has several negative effects on students, especially those who are about to graduate from primary or junior high school, their families, and the entire school. It has been demonstrated that closing schools during an epidemic may impose substantial costs on society, particularly the loss of productivity and the necessity of childcare, that far

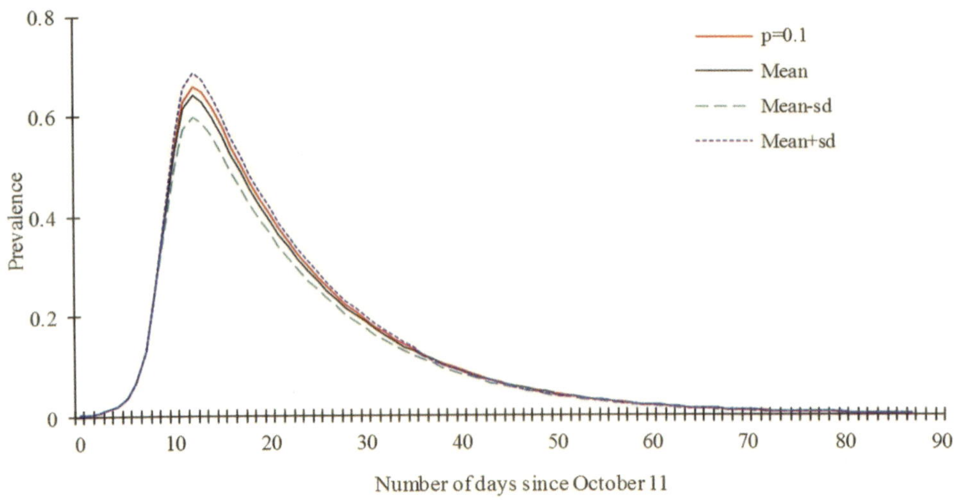

Figure 7. Sensitivity analysis to p based on the 1000 runs of the SEIARW model where p ranges from 0.0037 to 0.27.

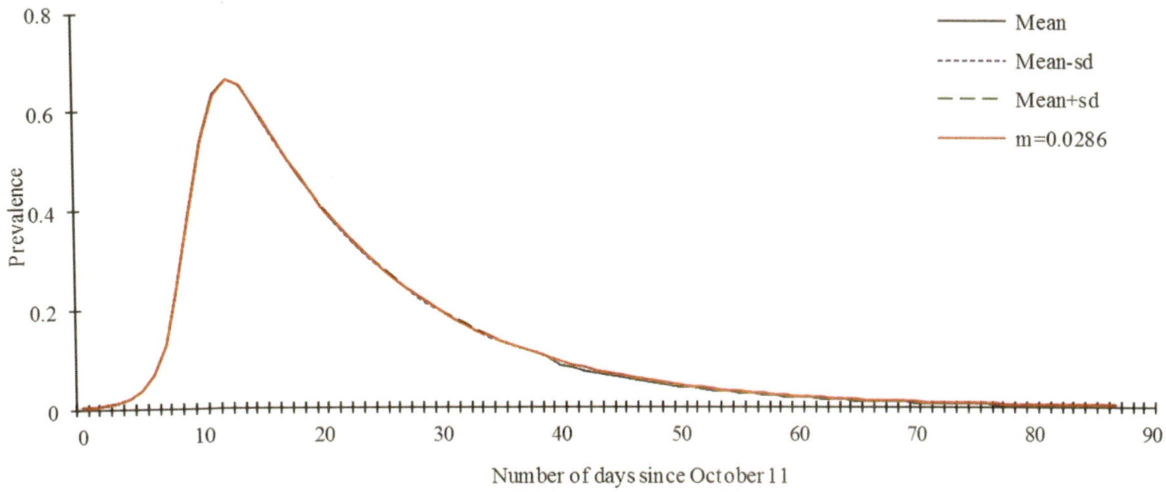

Figure 8. Sensitivity analysis to γ' based on the 1000 runs of the SEIARW model where γ' ranges from 0.0036 to 0.0357.

outweigh the cost savings in preventing infection [25]. Moreover, our results indicate that school closure, whether as a single strategy or in combination with other strategies, may not be effective, or may even exacerbate an outbreak. As our results indicate that the most effective strategy for controlling an outbreak of shigellosis is a combined strategy of case isolation, antibiotic administration, and water disinfection, this, rather than a school closure–based strategy, should be used to control future outbreaks. A similar observation was also identified in water disinfection, which was predicted to add marginal benefit in the shigellosis control. A single isolation intervention might do more harm than good. All these pieces of information point to the need for attention to careful design and evaluation of strategies before implementation.

Acknowledgments

The authors would like to thank the Stanley Ho Centre for Emerging Infectious Diseases, Faculty of Medicine, The Chinese University of Hong Kong for supporting this research. The authors would also like to thank the anonymous reviewers who provide invaluable comments that help convey more important and clear messages to wider audience.

Author Contributions

Conceived and designed the experiments: TC RKL ZZ LZ. Performed the experiments: TC RL XZ. Analyzed the data: TC RKL RL. Contributed reagents/materials/analysis tools: TC RKL. Wrote the paper: TC RKL ZZ RL XZ LZ.

References

1. Kotloff KL, Winickoff JP, Ivanoff B, Clemens JD, Swerdlow DL, et al. (1999) Global burden of *Shigella* infections: Implications for vaccine development and implementation of control strategies. Bull World Health Organ 77: 651–666.
2. Chiou CS, Hsu WB, Wei HL, Chen JH (2001) Molecular epidemiology of a *Shigella flexneri* outbreak in a mountainous township in Taiwan, Republic of China. J Clin Microbiol 39: 1048–1056.
3. Martin DL, Gustafson TL, Pelosi JW, Suarez L, Pierce GV (1986) Contaminated produce, a common source for two outbreaks of *Shigella* gastroenteritis. Am J Epidemiol 124: 299–305.
4. Samonis G, Elting L, Skoulika E, Maraki S, Tselentis Y (1994) An outbreak of diarrhoeal disease attributed to *Shigella sonnei*. Epidemiol Infect 112: 235–245.
5. Swaddiwudhipong W, Karintraratana S, Kavinum S (1995) A common-source outbreak of shigellosis involving a piped public water supply in northern Thai communities. J Trop Med Hyg 98: 145–150.
6. He F, Han K, Liu L, Sun W, Zhang L, et al. (2012) Shigellosis outbreak associated with contaminated well water in a rural elementary school: Sichuan Province, China, June 7–16, 2009. PLoS ONE 7: e47239.
7. Mead PS, Slutsker L, Dietz V, McCaig LF, Bresee JS, et al. (1999) Food-related illness and death in the United States. Emerg Infect Dis 5: 607–625.
8. Dupont HL (2000) *Shigella* species (bacillary dysentery). In: Mandell GL, Bennett JE, Dolin R, editors. Principles and practices of infectious diseases. 5th ed. Philadelphia: Churchill Livingstone. 2363–2368.
9. Wu JT, Cowling BJ (2011) The use of mathematical models to inform influenza pandemic preparedness and response. Exp Biol Med (Maywood) 236: 955–961.
10. Longini IM Jr, Nizam A, Xu S, Ungchusak K, Hanshaoworakul W, et al. (2005) Containing pandemic influenza at the source. Science 309: 1083–1087.
11. Yang Y, Sugimoto JD, Halloran ME, Basta NE, Chao DL, et al. (2009) The transmissibility and control of pandemic influenza A (H1N1) virus. Science 326: 729–733.
12. Tang S, Xiao Y, Yang Y, Zhou Y, Wu J, et al. (2010) Community-based measures for mitigating the 2009 H1N1 pandemic in China. PLoS ONE 5: e10911.
13. Gojovic MZ, Sander B, Fisman D, Krahn MD, Bauch CT (2009) Modelling mitigation strategies for pandemic (H1N1) 2009. CMAJ 181: 673–680.
14. Bai ZG, Zhou YC (2011) Threshold dynamics of a bacillary dysentery model with seasonal fluctuation. Discrete Continuous Dyn Syst Ser B 15: 1–14.
15. Tien JH, Earn DJD (2010) Multiple transmission pathways and disease dynamics in a waterborne pathogen model. Bull Math Biol 72: 1506–1533.
16. Wu FM, Doyle MP, Beuchat LR, Wells JG, Mintz ED, et al. (2000) Fate of Shigella sonnei on parsley and methods of disinfection. J Food Prot 63: 568–72.
17. Taylor BC, Nakamura M (1964) Survival of shigellae in food. J Hyg Camb 62: 303–311.
18. Islam MS, Hasan MK, Khan SI (1993) Growth and survival of *Shigella flexneri* in common Bangladeshi food under various conditions of time and temperature. Appl Environ Microbiol 59: 652–654.
19. Mcfeters GA, Bissonnette GK, Jezeski JJ, Thomson CA, Stuart DG (1974) Comparative survival of indicator bacteria and enteric pathogens in well water. Appl Microbiol 27: 823–829.
20. Qadri MH, Ai-Gamdi MA, Al-Harfi RA (1995) Asymptomatic Salmonella, Shigella and Intestinal Parasites Among Primary School Children in the Eastern Province. J Family Community Med 2: 36–40.
21. Bovée L, Whelan J, Sonder GJ, van Dam AP, van den Hoek A (2012) Risk factors for secondary transmission of Shigella infection within households: implications for current prevention policy. BMC Infect Dis 12: 347.
22. Khan AI, Talukder KA, Huq S, Mondal D, Malek MA, et al. (2006) Detection of intra-familial transmission of shigella infection using conventional serotyping and pulsed-field gel electrophoresis. Epidemiol Infect 134: 605–611.
23. Xiao GG, Fan J, Deng JJ, Chen CH, Zhou W, et al. (2012) A school outbreak of *Shigella sonnei* infection in China: Clinical features, antibiotic susceptibility and molecular epidemiology. Indian Pediatr 49: 287–290.
24. World Health Organization (2008) Foodborne disease outbreaks: Guidelines for investigation and control. Geneva: World Health Organization. 84 p.
25. Brown ST, Tai JH, Bailey RR, Cooley PC, Wheaton WD, et al. (2011) Would school closure for the 2009 H1N1 influenza epidemic have been worth the cost?: A computational simulation of Pennsylvania. BMC Public Health 11: 353.

Shigella flexneri Infection in *Caenorhabditis elegans:* Cytopathological Examination and Identification of Host Responses

Divya T. George[1], Carolyn A. Behm[1], David H. Hall[2], Ulrike Mathesius[3], Melanie Rug[4], Ken C. Q. Nguyen[2], Naresh K. Verma[1]*

1 Division of Biomedical Science and Biochemistry, Research School of Biology, The Australian National University, Canberra, Australia, **2** Center for *C. elegans* Anatomy, Department of Neuroscience, Albert Einstein College of Medicine, Bronx, New York, United States of America, **3** Division of Plant Science, Research School of Biology, The Australian National University, Canberra, Australia, **4** Centre for Advanced Microscopy, The Australian National University, Canberra, Australia

Abstract

The Gram-negative bacterium *Shigella flexneri* is the causative agent of shigellosis, a diarrhoeal disease also known as bacillary dysentery. *S. flexneri* infects the colonic and rectal epithelia of its primate host and induces a cascade of inflammatory responses that culminates in the destruction of the host intestinal lining. Molecular characterization of host-pathogen interactions in this infection has been challenging due to the host specificity of *S. flexneri* strains, as it strictly infects humans and non-human primates. Recent studies have shown that *S. flexneri* infects the soil dwelling nematode *Caenorhabditis elegans,* however, the interactions between *S. flexneri* and *C. elegans* at the cellular level and the cause of nematode death are unknown. Here we attempt to gain insight into the complex host-pathogen interactions between *S. flexneri* and *C. elegans.* Using transmission electron microscopy, we show that live *S. flexneri* cells accumulate in the nematode intestinal lumen, produce outer membrane vesicles and invade nematode intestinal cells. Using two-dimensional differential in-gel electrophoresis we identified host proteins that are differentially expressed in response to *S. flexneri* infection. Four of the identified genes, *aco-1, cct-2, daf-19* and *hsp-60,* were knocked down using RNAi and ACO-1, CCT-2 and DAF-19, which were identified as up-regulated in response to *S. flexneri* infection, were found to be involved in the infection process. *aco-1* RNAi worms were more resistant to *S. flexneri* infection, suggesting *S. flexneri*-mediated disruption of host iron homeostasis. *cct-2* and *daf-19* RNAi worms were more susceptible to infection, suggesting that these genes are induced as a protective mechanism by *C. elegans.* These observations further our understanding of the processes involved in *S. flexneri* infection of *C. elegans,* which is immensely beneficial to the routine use of this new *in vivo* model to study *S. flexneri* pathogenesis.

Editor: Nicholas J. Mantis, New York State Dept. Health, United States of America

Funding: DH gratefully acknowledges support of the NIH grant (NIH OD010943). The funders had no role in study design, data collection and analysis, decision to publish, or preparation of the manuscript.

Competing Interests: The authors have declared that no competing interests exist.

* Email: Naresh.Verma@anu.edu.au

Introduction

Shigellosis, more commonly known as bacillary dysentery, is caused by enteric bacteria belonging to the genus *Shigella. Shigella flexneri* strains most frequently associated with the disease invade the colonic and rectal epithelia of their host and induce a strong inflammatory response that culminates in severe tissue damage; this manifests in a spectrum of clinical symptoms ranging from watery diarrhoea to severe dysentery characterized by fever, abdominal cramping and bloody, mucoid stool [1]. *S. flexneri* is highly contagious, with as few as 10–100 bacterial cells capable of causing infection [2]. The low infection dose, coupled with the emergence of numerous multidrug resistant strains of *S. flexneri,* has escalated the need to develop effective preventive and therapeutic measures to reduce the global burden of shigellosis.

S. flexneri has a very narrow host range and only infects human and non-human primate hosts, as a result of which there is no simple intestinal small-animal model available. The lack of a relevant *in vivo* model of shigellosis has been one of the major impediments to the development of preventive and therapeutic measures. A number of alternative animal models have been identified which use mucosal surfaces other than the colon as sites of infection. The most commonly used *in vivo* models are the murine pulmonary model of shigellosis [3–5] and the guinea pig keratoconjunctivitis model [6], however both these *in vivo* models lack clinical relevance as the site of *S. flexneri* infection and symptoms produced do not mirror infection in humans.

In recent years, the soil-dwelling roundworm, *Caenorhabditis elegans,* has been used extensively to study host-pathogen interactions *in vivo,* uncovering a wealth of information about microbial virulence factors and host defense responses [7]. *C. elegans* has been identified as a valuable *in vivo* model to study host-pathogen interactions on account of innumerable experimental advantages [8,9]. This *in vivo* model is particularly useful to study enteric pathogens, as nematode intestinal cells share morphological similarities with human intestinal cells, including apical, finger-like microvilli anchored into a cytoskeletal terminal web composed of actin and intermediate filaments. In addition, the human innate immune system shares many characteristics with that of *C. elegans* and thus mechanisms of bacterial and nematode responses may be similar in mammalian cells [10]. A range of bacterial virulence factors have been shown to be required for both nematode and mammalian pathogenesis [8,9,11–14], further validating the use of *C. elegans* as a relevant *in vivo* model to study host-pathogen interactions. On account of these characteristics, the list of bacterial pathogens that are known to infect *C. elegans* is growing and includes prominent human pathogens such as *Salmonella enterica, Pseudomonas aeruginosa* and *Serratia marcescens* [15–17].

In the past decade, two independent groups have provided preliminary evidence to suggest that *C. elegans* can potentially be used as an *in vivo* model for shigellosis [18,19]. These studies demonstrate that *S. flexneri* kills *C. elegans* in an infection-like process that requires live bacterial cells harboring intact virulence plasmids. Both studies also show that *S. flexneri* accumulates in the *C. elegans* intestine and kills the nematodes on solid media and in liquid culture. However, *C. elegans* as a model for shigellosis has not been completely understood, as the *S. flexneri*-mediated killing response and the nematode responses to *S. flexneri* infection remain unknown. This study aims to further our understanding of the interactions between *S. flexneri* and *C. elegans* in order to establish this *in vivo* model as a viable alternative to study *S. flexneri* pathogenesis. Here we report for the first time, the cytopathological changes induced in the nematode intestines during *S. flexneri* infection and identify novel host genes that are induced in response to *S. flexneri* infection.

Results

Wild type *S. flexneri* serotype 3b kills *C. elegans* and killing requires the expression of bacterial virulence plasmid-encoded genes

Previously, Burton *et al.* [18] and Kesika *et al.* [19] have shown that wild type strains of *S. flexneri* serotypes 2a and 2b kill *C. elegans*. In this study, we chose to use the *S. flexneri* serotype 3b strain (SFL1520), identified to be virulent in the murine pulmonary model of shigellosis, to characterize the pathogenesis of this strain in *C. elegans*. Using liquid infection assays [19], we compared the survival rates of nematodes fed *S. flexneri* serotype 3b (SFL1520), an avirulent *S. flexneri* strain (which does not carry the virulence plasmid harboring genes required for adherence and invasion of host tissues) (SFL1223) and *E. coli* OP50 for 48 hours. Liquid killing assays were not carried out beyond 48 hours with N2 *C. elegans* due to the large number of L1/L2 progeny produced after 48 hours which masked the adults, thereby making scoring of survival rates difficult. Future studies using temperature-sensitive fertility mutants of *C. elegans* as hosts will allow investigation of the course of the infection beyond 48 hours. Results of the liquid killing assays with N2 worms showed that *S. flexneri* serotype 3b kills nematodes ($TD_{50} = 46 \pm 1$ h, where TD_{50} is the time taken to kill 50% of the initial worm population) much faster than control worms fed *E. coli* OP50 (<50% killing in 48 h) (Figure 1). Consistent with previous studies, we found that *S. flexneri* requires the virulence plasmid-encoded factors for *C. elegans* killing, as the survival of worms fed SFL1520 (carrying an intact virulence plasmid) was significantly reduced compared with worms fed SFL1223 (Figure 1).

Wild type *S. flexneri* accumulates in the nematode intestinal lumen

Burton and colleagues [18] have previously shown that virulent *S. flexneri* serotype 2a cells accumulate in the intestinal lumen of nematodes, while avirulent *S. flexneri* strains are digested. To confirm that the *S. flexneri* serotype 3b strain also accumulates in the nematode intestinal lumen, we performed bacterial accumulation assays using wild type *S. flexneri* 3b (SFL1520), avirulent *S. flexneri* (SFL 1223), and *E. coli* OP50 as a negative control. The results of bacterial accumulation assays confirmed that *S. flexneri* serotype 3b-mediated killing of nematodes is associated with bacterial accumulation in the intestinal lumen (Figure 2.A). Using GFP^+-tagged bacterial strains (bacterial strains transformed with plasmid pCR2.1, expressing GFP^+), we further confirmed that wild type *S. flexneri* serotype 3b (SFL1520) accumulates in the nematode intestinal lumen while the avirulent strain (SFL1223) and *E. coli* OP50 are digested (Figure 2.B).

A recent study showed that fluorescence produced by live and dead bacteria in the nematode intestinal lumen is indistinguishable [20]. Furthermore, the bacterial accumulation assays fail to distinguish between live bacterial accumulation in the pharynx and bacterial cells that have progressed past the grinder in the terminal bulb. Thus, the results of bacterial accumulation observed using the accumulation assay and fluorescence assays fail to confirm that live bacterial cells evade grinding by the nematode grinder and accumulate in the intestinal lumen. We therefore used transmission electron microscopy (TEM) to compare the intestinal lumen of nematodes fed avirulent *S. flexneri* SFL1223 and wild type *S. flexneri* serotype 3b (SFL1520) over three time points, 24, 96 and 144 hours post infection. Using this approach we confirmed the presence of intact *S. flexneri* serotype 3b (SFL1520) cells in the intestinal lumina of infected nematodes, with the bacterial load increasing over time (Figure 3D, F and H). No intact bacterial cells were observed in the intestinal lumina of nematodes fed the avirulent strain (Figure 3C, E and G). These observations clearly suggest that virulent *S. flexneri* cells escape the grinder-mediated breakdown and accumulate in the *C. elegans* intestinal lumen.

Intraluminal *S. flexneri* cells produce putative outer membrane vesicles (OMVs) and invade *C. elegans* intestinal cells

TEM micrographs revealed that *S. flexneri* serotype 3b cells within the nematode intestinal lumen produce putative outer membrane vesicles (OMVs) (Figure 4.A and B). OMVs are secreted elements produced by Gram-negative bacteria as part of a bacterial stress response induced during infection of host tissues [21]. *S. flexneri* OMVs contain the invasion protein antigens - Ipa proteins (IpaB, C & D) that are required for bacterial adherence, invasion and survival within infected tissues. It has been shown that the production of OMVs by *S. flexneri* cells provides a mechanism for the delivery of virulence factors to host tissues [22]. The identification of *S. flexneri* OMVs in the *C. elegans* intestinal lumen therefore suggests a potential mechanism for the delivery of bacterial virulence factors to host cells.

Using TEM, intracellular *S. flexneri* cells were observed 96 and 144 hours post infection (Figure 4.C and D). These observations indicated that virulent *S. flexneri* cells cross the protective, apical microvilli boundary of nematode intestinal cells and enter the intestinal cell cytoplasm. We also found evidence suggesting that intraluminal *S. flexneri* cells degrade the microvilli (Figure 4.E). These findings are extremely significant as, although several studies have shown that intracellular mammalian pathogens kill *C.*

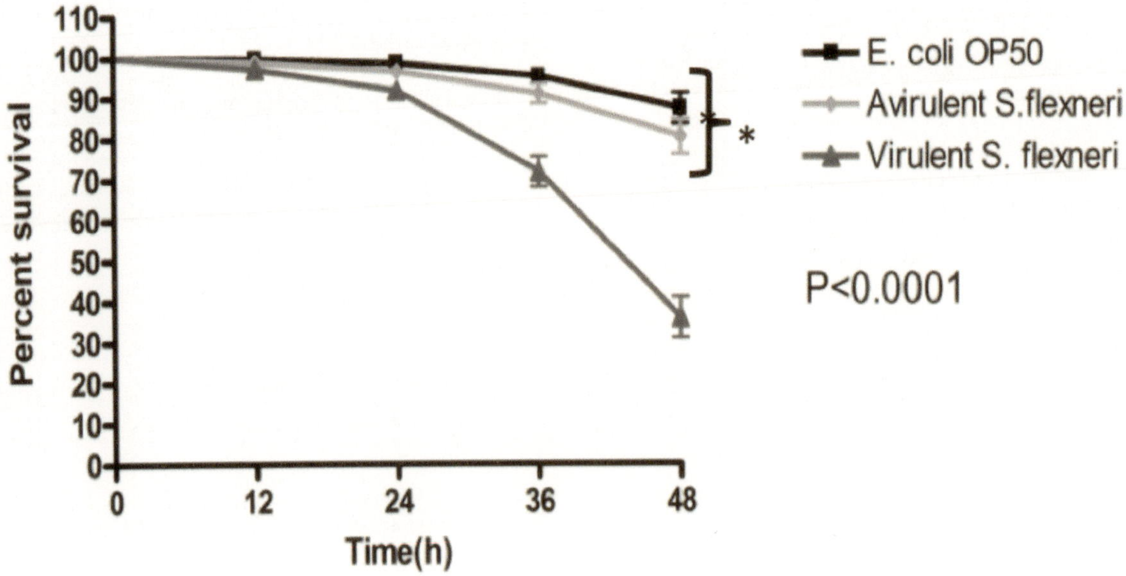

Figure 1. ***S. flexneri*** **is pathogenic to** ***C. elegans.*** Survival of wild-type N2 nematodes when fed *E. coli* OP50, an avirulent *S. flexneri* strain (virulence plasmid-cured *S. flexneri*-SFL1223), and virulent *S. flexneri* serotype 3b strain (SFL1520) ($p<0.0001$, Log rank test). Survival curve represents the means of data from three independent experiments with standard error (error bars), each using 20 nematodes. Asterisks indicate statistically significant differences.

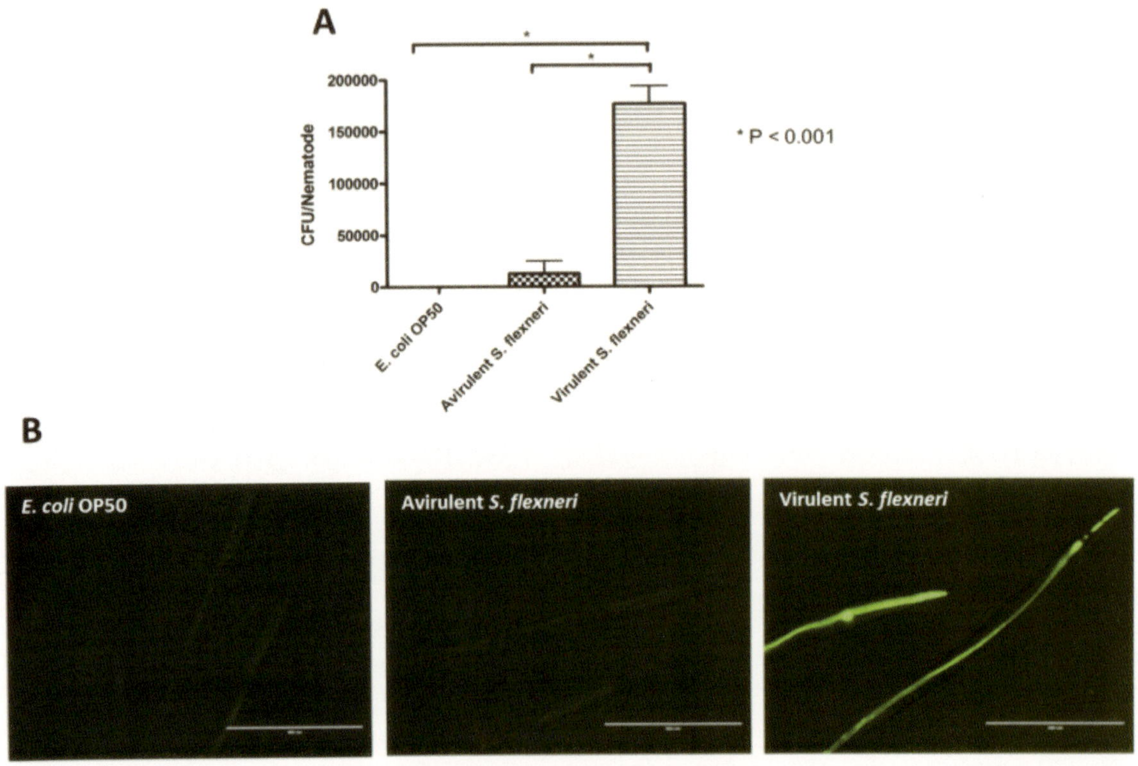

Figure 2. Virulent ***S. flexneri*** **serotype 3b accumulates in** ***C. elegans*** **intestinal lumen 24 hours post infection. A:** Young adult hermaphrodite N2 nematodes were fed either *E. coli* OP50, avirulent *S. flexneri* (SFL1223) or virulent *S. flexneri* 3b (SFL1520) for 24 hours at 22°C. 20 worms were picked off each bacterial lawn, disrupted using glass beads and appropriate dilutions of each lysate were plated on LB agar to obtain bacterial counts. Wild type *S. flexneri* 3b (SFL1520) accumulated in the intestinal lumen while the plasmid-cured *S. flexneri* strain (SFL1223) and OP50 were digested ($p<0.001$, One way ANOVA). Results represent the means of three independent experimental repeats with standard errors (error bars). **B:** Young adult hermaphrodite N2 nematodes were fed on lawns of *E. coli* OP50, avirulent *S. flexneri* (SFL1223) or virulent *S. flexneri* 3b (SFL1520) tagged with GFP^{+} for 24 h and fluorescence was observed using an EVOS digital inverted microscope (AMG). Scale bar = 400 μm.

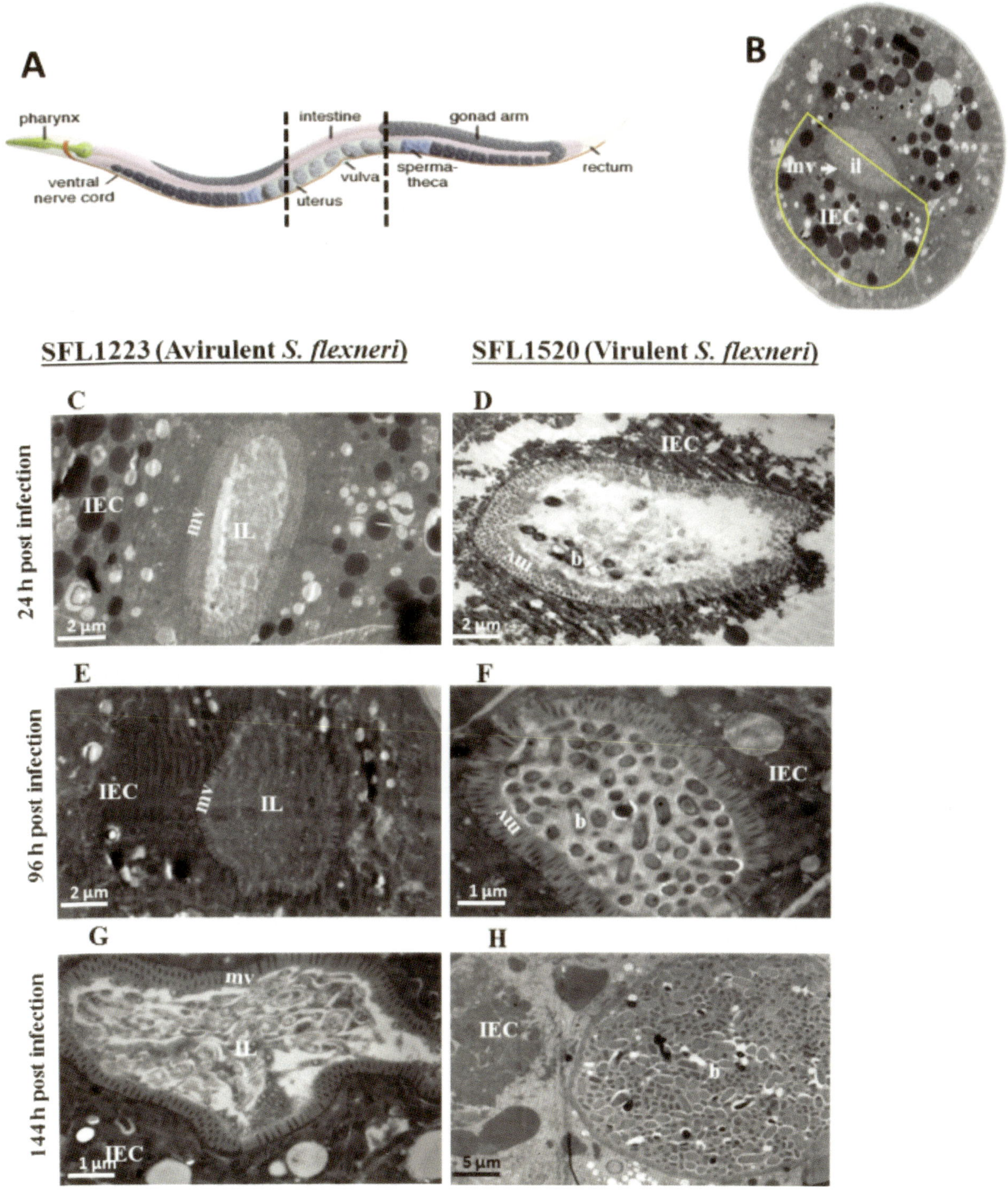

Figure 3. Virulent *S. flexneri* cells escape pharyngeal grinding and accumulate in the *C. elegans* intestinal lumen. A: Schematic representation of the *C. elegans* body plan with the plane of sections highlighted (artwork by Altun and Hall, © Wormatlas). **B:** Transverse section of the mid body of a healthy nematode with the intestinal cell highlighted in yellow. **C–H:** Transmission electron microscopy micrographs of transverse mid body sections of animals feeding on plasmid-cured, avirulent *S. flexneri* (SFL1223) (**C, E, G**) and virulent *S. flexneri* serotype 3b (SFL1520) (**D, F, H**) for 24 h (**C, D**), 96 h (**E, F**) and 144 h (**G, H**). IEC-intestinal epithelial cell; mv-microvilli; IL-intestinal lumen; b-intact *S. flexneri* cells.

elegans by persistently colonizing the intestinal lumen, most of these pathogens remain extracellular and fail to invade the nematode intestinal cells [23].

Identification of nematode responses to *S. flexneri* infection using two dimensional differential in-gel electrophoresis

Two dimensional differential in-gel electrophoresis (DIGE) was performed to gain insight into *S. flexneri*-induced responses in *C.*

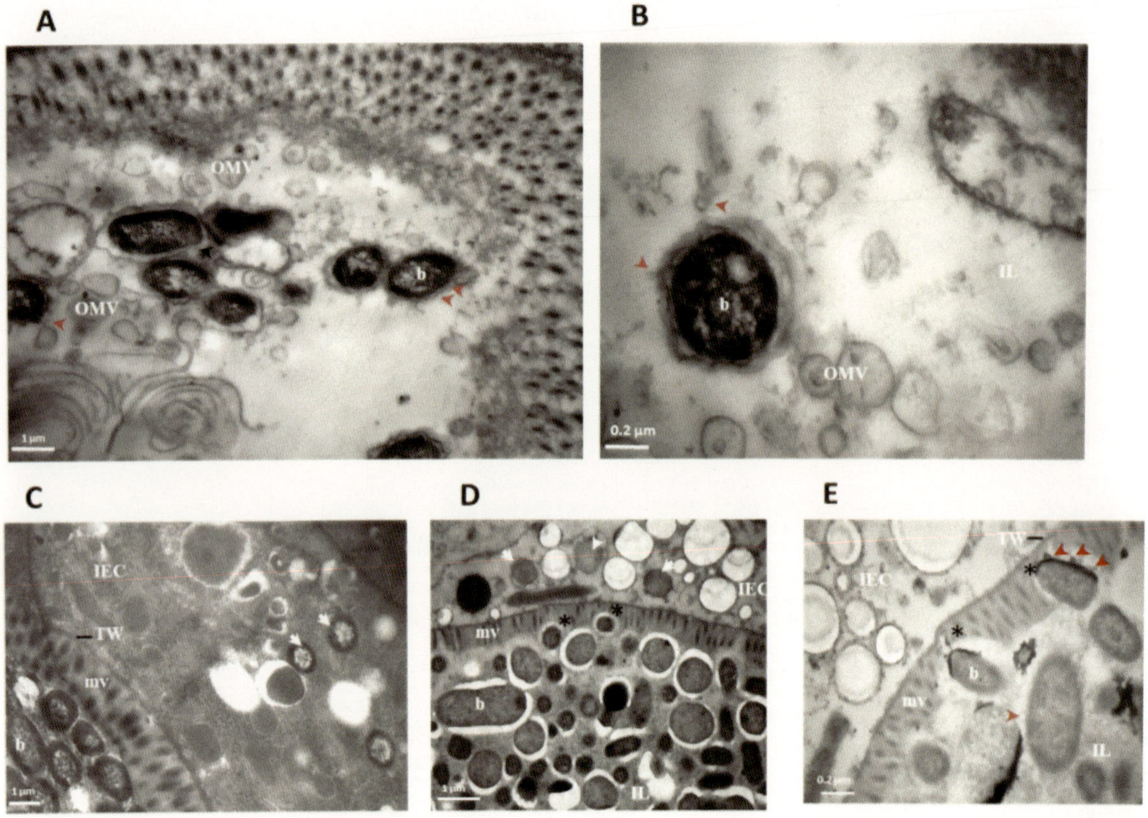

Figure 4. Intraluminal *S. flexneri* cells produce putative outer membrane vesicles and invade *C. elegans* intestinal cells. A–E: TEM micrographs of transverse mid body sections of young adult nematodes infected with wild type *S. flexneri* serotype 3b (SFL1520) for 24 h (**A, B**), 96 h (**C**) and 144 h (**D, E**). **A, B:** Intraluminal bacterial cells produce outer membrane vesicles (OMV), red arrowheads indicate OMV shedding from bacterial cells. **C, D:** White arrowheads indicate intracellular bacterial cells that have penetrated the ciliated epithelial barrier of the intestinal cell, 96 and 144 h post infection. **E:** Intraluminal *S. flexneri* cells degrading the apical microvilli boundary (asterisk) of the *C. elegans* intestinal cells. IEC- intestinal epithelial cells; mv-microvilli; IL-intestinal lumen; TW-terminal web; b-intraluminal bacterial cells; OMV-outer membrane vesicles.

elegans. Total protein was isolated from nematodes infected with *S. flexneri* serotype 3b and *E. coli* OP50 for 24 hours. We decided to use a 24 hour infection period as we observed significant accumulation of *S. flexneri* in the worm intestine at this time point (Figure 2). 2 mg of total protein, isolated from four independent experiments, was used to perform DIGE. Analysis of DIGE results identified 41 *S. flexneri*-induced nematode proteins (37 up-regulated and 4 down-regulated) (Figure S1). All 41 identified spots were excised from the gels for identification by peptide sequencing using liquid chromatography mass spectrometry (LC-MS), following which, proteins were identified using the MASCOT database (Matrix Science).

MASCOT searches using stringent search parameters (mass tolerance between 0.3 and 0.1 Da), only identified 7 proteins out of 41 predicted protein spots (Figure S1 and Table 1). The low success rate of protein identification could be due to insufficient protein in the spots excised from the DIGE gels. Since MASCOT searches only identified 7 out of 41 potential *S. flexneri*-induced nematode proteins, the stringency of the search parameters was decreased in an attempt to identify the remaining proteins. Using low stringency MASCOT search parameters (mass tolerance between 0.8 Da and 0.6 Da), we identified significant hits for 39 out of the 41 identified spots, with many spots corresponding to more than one protein (Table S1). Some of these proteins (UNC-22, NHR-77 and C10C6.6) were identified more than once in different locations on the gel and thus represent different isoforms, which could be the result of post-translational modifications or different splice variants of the same protein. Theoretical molecular weights (Mwt) and pI values of identified proteins were compared with the Mwt and pI of spots on the DIGE gels; peptide coverage and distribution were also taken into account to eliminate false positive hits.

Proteins identified as potential *S. flexneri*-induced nematode responses were subdivided into different categories based on their biological functions (Figure S2). Most of the nematode proteins induced by *S. flexneri* infection were involved in transcription and translation, followed closely by proteins required for locomotion and pharyngeal pumping.

Quantitative real-time reverse-transcriptase PCR (qRT-PCR) to confirm the results of DIGE analysis

Quantitative real-time reverse transcription polymerase chain reaction (qRT-PCR) was used to compare mRNA levels of the seven proteins identified using high stringency MASCOT search parameters (ACO-1, CCT-2, EEF-2, DAF-19, HSP-60, UNC-54 and UNC-41). The *C. elegans act-2* gene, which encodes actin, was used as a control gene to normalize all reactions, as the mRNA levels of *act-2* were expected to remain constant in both healthy and infected worms. Consistent with our DIGE analysis, qRT-PCR revealed a significant increase in the transcript levels of *cct-2, daf-19, hsp-60* and *unc-54* and a decrease in the level of *unc-41* in worms infected with *S. flexneri* serotype 3b (Figure 5).

Table 1. Predicted *S. flexneri*-induced *C. elegans* responses using DIGE analysis.

Identified protein	Gene name	*Shigella*-induced change in expression	Description	Predicted pI/Mwt (kDa)	Observed pI/Mwt (kDa)	Peptide Coverage (%)	No of peptides Matched	Score	P value (One Way ANOVA)
Putative stoned B-like protein	*unc-41*	Down-regulated	Potential adapter protein, which may be involved in endocytic vesicle recycling of synaptic vesicles	4.81/190.58	4.8/~94.00	3	7	27	0.029
Myosin-4	*unc-54*	Up-regulated	Encodes a muscle myosin class II heavy chain (MHC B). Expressed in the intestine. Involved in pharyngeal pumping and egg laying	5.59/225.958	5.2/96.00	8	5	134	0.038
Probable cytoplasmic aconitate hydratase	*aco-1*	Up-regulated	Enzyme that catalyzes the isomerization of citrate to isocitrate via cis-aconitate. Required for iron homeostasis	5.49/97.11	5.5/95.00	14	5	86	0.022
Elongation factor 2	*eef-2*	Up-regulated	Catalyzes the GTP-dependent ribosomal translocation step during translation elongation. Required for embryogenesis	6.1/95.47	5.5/95.00	18	8	72	0.022
RFX-like transcription factor	*daf-19*	Up-regulated	A transcription factor that regulates genes of ciliated sensory neurons. *daf-19* mutants are defective in their ability to taste or smell and are susceptible to bacterial infection!	5.97/91.42	5.1/86.00	2	3	24	0.040
Chaperonin homolog Hsp-60	*hsp*-60	Up-regulated	Heat shock protein implicated in mitochondrial protein import and macromolecular assembly. Required for response to oxidative stress	5.31/60.24	5.1/68.00	49	20	1446	0.040
T-complex protein 1 subunit beta	*cct-2*	Up-regulated	Molecular chaperone; assists the folding of proteins upon ATP hydrolysis.	5.65/53.38	5.6/67.5	6	2	41	0.047

No statistically significant differences were observed in the transcript levels of *aco-1* in infected and control worms. *aco-1* encodes aconitase, an enzyme whose expression is regulated post-translationally by iron levels [24]. This would explain why the elevated levels of ACO-1 protein observed in response to *S. flexneri* infection were not reflected by the mRNA levels in infected versus uninfected worms. Contrary to the DIGE analysis, the transcription of *eef-2* appeared to be down-regulated, suggesting that the EEF-2 protein levels in infected worms may also be regulated post-transcriptionally. The changes in protein and transcript expression observed in the DIGE and qRT-PCR experiments described above should ideally be confirmed by Western analysis when suitable antibody preparations become available.

RNAi-mediated knock down of *aco-1, cct-2, daf-19* and *hsp-60*

RNAi nematodes for *aco-1, cct-2, daf-19, hsp-60* and pCB19 (RNAi control) were prepared using the feeding protocol as described in materials and methods. Target genes were silenced in nematodes from the L1 stage using the appropriate RNAi constructs. Nematodes were maintained on *E. coli* lawns harboring the appropriate RNAi constructs until they reached the L4 stage, following which the RNAi worms were infected with *S. flexneri* serotype 3b (SFL1520), avirulent *S. flexneri* (SFL1223) and *E. coli* OP50 for 24–48 hours. Liquid killing (Figure 6.A-E) and bacterial accumulation (Figure 7.A–F) assays were performed to determine whether these *S. flexneri*-induced genes play a role in protecting nematodes against *S. flexneri* infection.

aco-1 RNAi nematodes fed *S. flexneri* serotype 3b showed a significant increase in survival rates (with less that 50% killing in 48 h) compared with the RNAi control worms ($TD_{50} = 46 \pm 1$ h) (Figure 6.B). This enhanced resistance to *S. flexneri* serotype 3b infection correlated with decreased bacterial accumulation (Figure 7.A and C). These observations suggest that *aco-1* acts as a negative regulator of host responses to *S. flexneri* serotype 3b infection.

cct-2 RNAi nematodes fed *S. flexneri* serotype 3b were more susceptible to *S. flexneri* infection (TD_{50} 38±2 h compared with $TD_{50} = 46 \pm 1$ h of control worms, $p<0.0001$, Log rank test) (Figure 6.C). The increased killing of *cct*-2 RNAi worms correlates with increased bacterial accumulation (Figure 7.A and D). These observations suggest that CCT-2 induces or contributes to host protective mechanisms.

daf-19 RNAi worms showed increased bacterial accumulation (Figure 7.A and E) and significantly enhanced susceptibility to *S. flexneri*-mediated killing at earlier time points when compared with RNAi control worms (24 and 36 hours, $p<0.0001$, Log rank

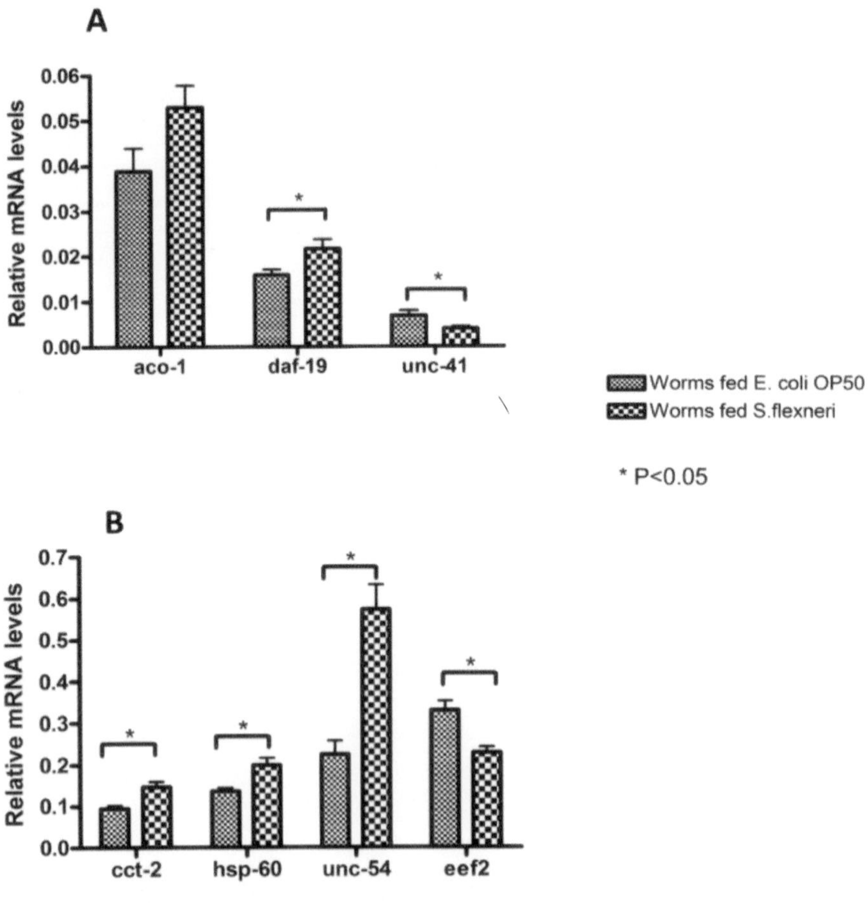

Figure 5. Reverse transcription quantitative PCR (qRT-PCR) analysis of *S. flexneri*-induced genes predicted by DIGE analysis. Transcript levels of *aco-1, daf-19* and *unc-41* (**A**), *cct-2, hsp-60, unc-54* and *eef-2* (**B**) were measured in synchronized young adult wild type animals feeding on *E. coli* OP50 or infected with *S. flexneri* serotype 3b for 24 h. Data represent the means of three biological replicates, each replicate measured in triplicate and normalized to the control gene, *act*-2, expressed as the ratio of the corresponding *S. flexneri*-induced levels and the basal *E. coli* OP50 levels. Asterisks indicate statistically significant differences identified using unpaired Student's *t*-tests and error bars represent standard error.

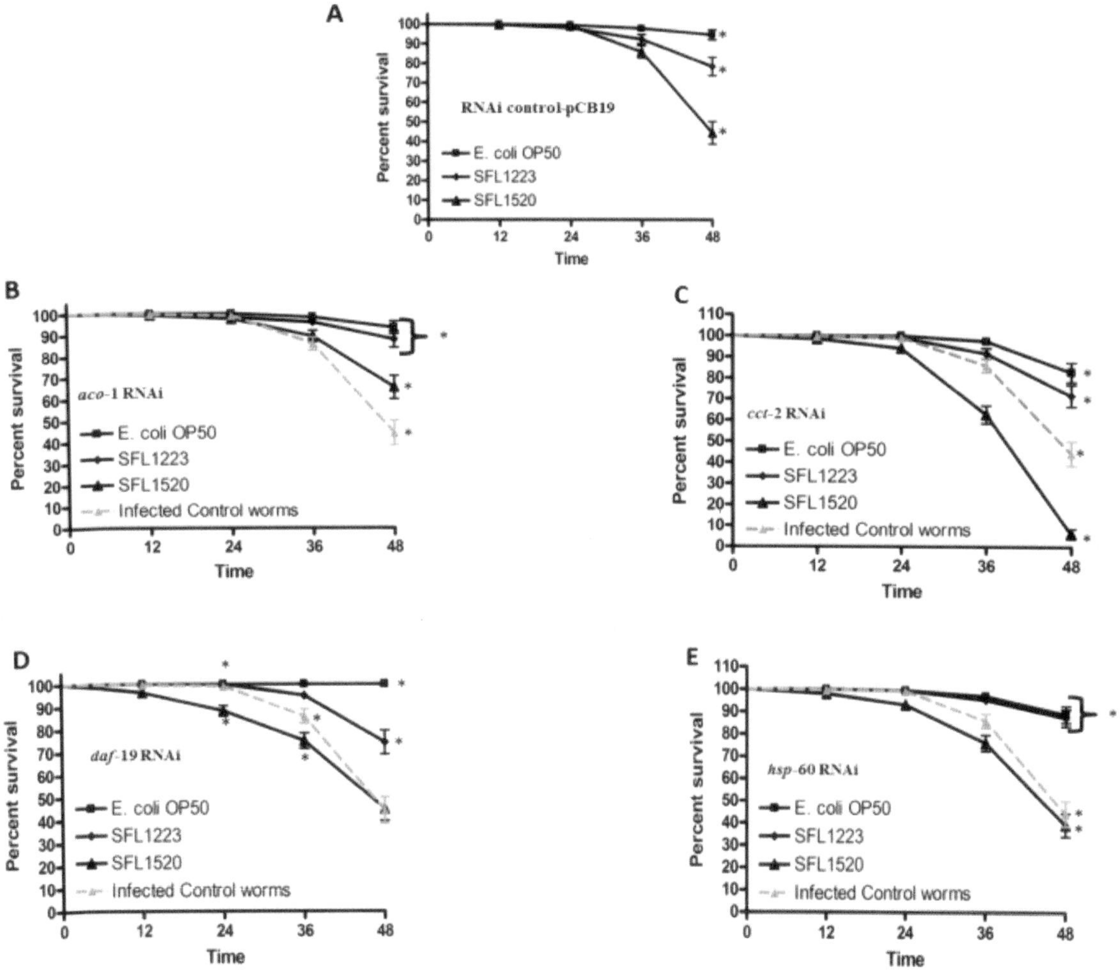

Figure 6. Effects of knockdown of *S. flexneri*-induced host response genes on nematode survival. After RNAi knockdown of *S. flexneri*-induced genes *aco*-1 (**B**), *cct*-2 (**C**), *daf*-19 (**D**) and *hsp*-60 (**E**), young adult hermaphrodites were transferred onto lawns of either *E. coli* OP50, avirulent *S. flexneri* (SFL1223) or virulent *S. flexneri* serotype 3b (SFL1520) and scored at 12 hour intervals for survival. **A:** Nematodes treated with pCB19 (RNAi control vector) were used as a non-specific ds-RNA control. Survival curve represents data from three independent experiments, each using 20 nematodes. The survival curves of RNAi worms infected with *S. flexneri* serotype 3b were compared with RNAi control-pCB19 worms infected with *S. flexneri* serotype 3b (grey, dashed curves); and asterisks indicate statistically significant difference in survival curves ($p<0.05$) identified using Log rank tests.

test) (Figure 6. D). These observations suggest that DAF-19 is involved in the initial nematode protective mechanisms. *hsp-60* RNAi worms were slightly more susceptible to *S. flexneri*-mediated killing (TD_{50} 45±1) compared with control worms (TD_{50} 46±1 h, $p<0.0416$), however no significant differences were observed in *S. flexneri* accumulation in *hsp*-60 RNAi and control worms (Figure 7.A and F).

Discussion

Virulent *S. flexneri* cells ingested by *C. elegans*, evade pharyngeal grinding, accumulate in the nematode intestinal lumen and invade the intestinal cells

Consistent with previous reports, here we confirmed that a virulent *S. flexneri* serotype 3b strain kills nematodes and nematode killing was associated with bacterial accumulation within the intestinal lumen. TEM micrographs obtained in this study show the presence of intact *S. flexneri* cells within the intestinal lumina of infected worms, with the bacterial load increasing over time (Figure 3). These results suggest that *S. flexneri* cells evade pharyngeal grinding. The *C. elegans* grinder crushes ingested bacterial cells and is therefore the worm's primary defense against invading pathogens. The presence of intact *S. flexneri* cells within the nematode intestinal lumen suggests that *S. flexneri* cells overcome this nematode defense mechanism.

Worms infected with virulent *S. flexneri* are sluggish, show impaired grinding of ingested food, and fail to lay eggs as efficiently as control worms [19]. All these symptoms correlate with an overall loss of energy and defective neuromuscular functions. Results of our DIGE analysis identified several nematode proteins involved in locomotion (UNC-22, UNC-41, UNC-54, UNC-79 and UNC-89) and pharyngeal pumping (UNC-54, SLO-1 and HSP-6) as differentially expressed in response to *S. flexneri* infection. These observations suggest that *S. flexneri* infection potentially induces an overall systemic neuromuscular defect in infected nematodes, leading to defective grinder activity.

TEM micrographs obtained in this study show that live *S. flexneri* cells within the nematode intestinal lumen produce outer membrane vesicles (OMVs) (Figure 4.A and B). OMVs produced

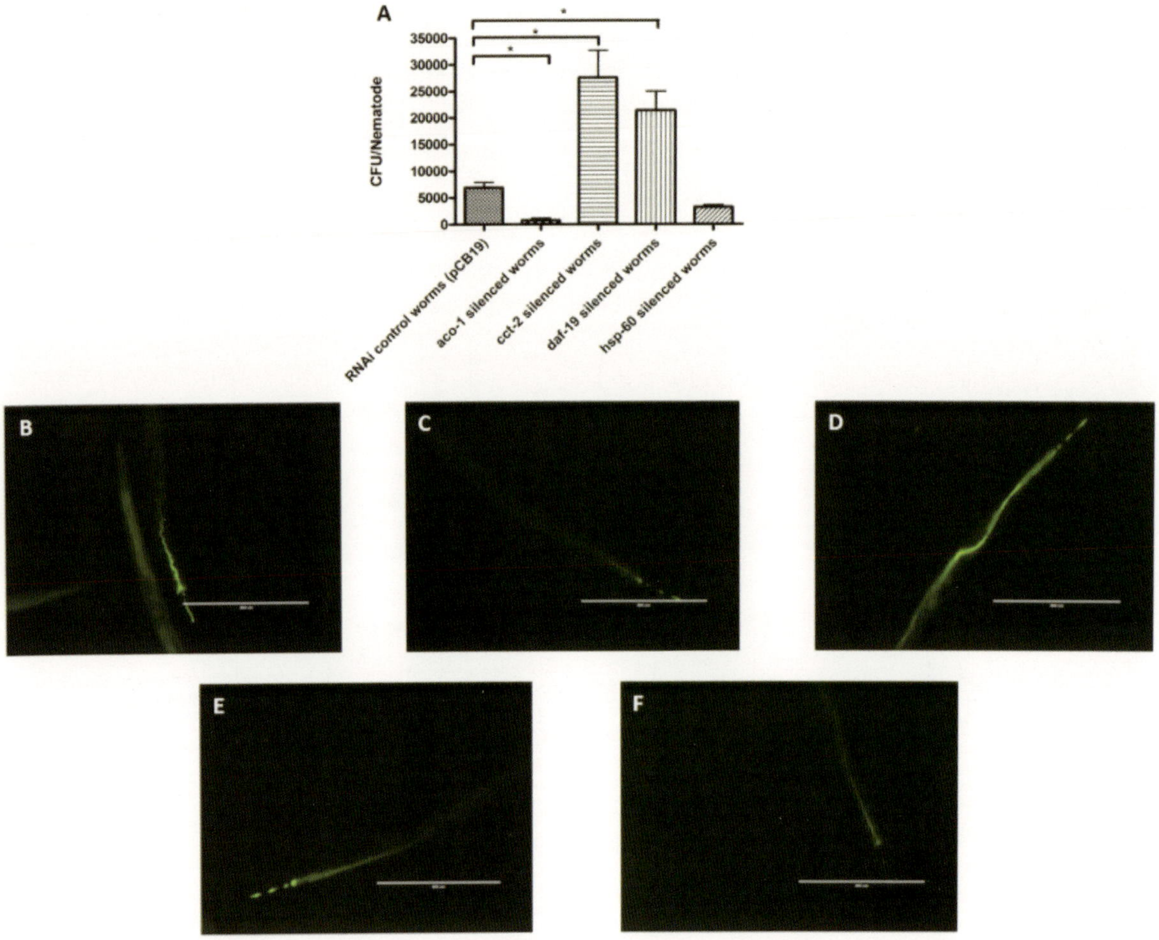

Figure 7. Effects of knockdown of *S. flexneri*-induced host response genes on bacterial accumulation. After RNAi knockdown of *S. flexneri*-induced genes, *aco-1, daf-19, hsp-60,* plus pCB19 as an RNAi negative control, young adult hermaphrodites were transferred onto lawns of virulent *S. flexneri* (SFL1520) for 24 h. **A:** 20 worms were picked off bacterial lawns and disrupted following which appropriate dilutions of each lysate was plated onto LB agar to obtain the bacterial counts. Results represent the means of three independent experimental repeats with standard error (error bars), asterisks indicate statistically significant differences ($p<0.005$, unpaired *t*-tests). pCB19 (**B**), *aco-1* (**C**), *cct-2* (**D**), *daf-19* (**E**) and *hsp-60* (**F**) RNAi knockdown animals were transferred onto GFP^+-tagged SFL1520 for 24 h. Fluorescence was observed using the EVOS digital inverted microscope (AMG) and representative images are shown. Scale bar = 400 µm.

by pathogenic bacteria contain biologically active proteins, including virulence factors, proteases and immunomodulatory compounds required for infection [25–31]. OMV production therefore constitutes a mechanism used by pathogenic bacteria to deliver virulence factors to host cells [32–36]. *S. flexneri* OMVs contain the invasion protein antigens-Ipa proteins (IpaB, C and D) that are required for bacterial adherence, invasion and survival within infected tissues [22]. OMVs produced by *S. flexneri* have been shown to adhere to and invade mammalian cells [22]. The identification of *S. flexneri* OMV in the *C. elegans* intestinal lumen therefore suggests a potential mechanism for the delivery of *S. flexneri* virulence factors to the nematode intestinal cells. This will be tested further by investigating the effects of exposing *C. elegans* to isolated *S. flexneri* OMVs.

TEM analysis also indicates that *S. flexneri* cells cross the protective apical microvilli brush border lining and invade the nematode intestinal cells. This finding is highly significant: while several intracellular bacterial pathogens have been shown to infect *C. elegans,* they remain extracellular throughout nematode infection, in contrast to the infection in mammals [23]. During human infection, *S. flexneri* cells exploit the transcytotic properties of specialized M cells to gain access into the sub-epithelial space, and invade the colonic and rectal epithelial cells through their less-protected basolateral surfaces [37]. *C. elegans* lacks specialized M cells and the results of this study suggest that *S. flexneri* possibly invade the nematode intestinal cells through the apical side by degrading the protective microvilli (Figure 4.E). A similar bacterial attack on intestinal microvilli (but without cytoplasmic invasion) has previously been noted in very old nematodes [38], perhaps due to changes in OP50 when they are allowed to continue growing in this environment, or due to a loss of innate immunity or structural integrity in extreme aging.

The ability of *S. flexneri* to invade the *C. elegans* intestinal cells makes this animal model a promising alternative to study shigellosis. Outside of Macaque monkeys, none of the current animal models of shigellosis show bacterial invasion of intestinal cells following oral infection.

S. flexneri may disrupt iron homeostasis in infected cells and potentially induces a hypoxic response, resulting in nematode death

ACO-1 was shown to be up-regulated in response to *S. flexneri* infection. RNAi-mediated silencing of *aco-1* indicated that on knocking down this gene, worms showed enhanced resistance to *S. flexneri* infection. These results suggest that the up-regulation of ACO-1 in response to *S. flexneri* infection contributes to nematode death. *aco-1* encodes aconitase, an enzyme whose expression is negatively regulated post-translationally by iron levels [39]. In *C. elegans, aco-1* is expressed in the cytosol of cells of the hypodermis and intestine [24]. Its mammalian homologue, iron regulatory protein 1 (IRP-1), expressed in the brain and intestinal cells, plays a central role in iron homeostasis. The up-regulation of ACO-1 in response to *S. flexneri* infection therefore suggests that *S. flexneri* potentially disrupts iron homeostasis in *C. elegans*.

A recent study showed that *Pseudomonas aeruginosa* infection disrupts iron homeostasis in *C. elegans*, causing a *hif-1*-mediated hypoxic response leading to nematode death [40]. Similarly, *S. flexneri* could potentially kill nematodes by disrupting iron homeostasis, leading to the up-regulation of ACO-1 and the induction of a hypoxic response. Results of our DIGE analysis also identified the nematode MTSS1 protein (Table S1, spot no. 32) as down-regulated in response to *S. flexneri* infection. MTSS1 is a mitochondrial single stranded DNA binding protein that is essential for mitochondrial DNA replication [41]. RNAi knock down of MTSS1 results in the transcriptional alterations leading to the induction of hypoxia responses [41]. The up-regulation of ACO-1 and down-regulation of MTSS1 in response to *S. flexneri* suggests that *S. flexneri* potentially disrupts nematode iron homeostasis which potentially induces a hypoxic response culminating in death.

Nematode innate immune responses to *S. flexneri* infection

RNAi experiments clearly indicated that *cct-2* and *daf-19* knock down worms show enhanced susceptibility to *S. flexneri* infection (Figures 6.C, D and 7.D, E), suggesting that these responses form part of the nematode protective mechanism. The chaperonin CCT-2 has been predicted to interact with DAF-16, which forms part of the nematode DAF-2/DAF-16 insulin signaling pathway; RNAi knock down of *cct-2* inhibits the nuclear localization of DAF-16 in intestinal cells [42], suggesting that CCT-2 is required for the nuclear translocation of DAF-16. DAF-16 is a transcription factor that has been associated with the expression of several antimicrobial genes [43]. The increased susceptibility of *cct-2* RNAi worms to *S. flexneri* infection could therefore be due to the decreased expression of antimicrobial peptides on account of defective nuclear translocation of DAF-16. The up-regulation of CCT-2 in response to *S. flexneri* and the increased susceptibility of *cct-2* RNAi worms suggest that *S. flexneri* infection activates the DAF-2/DAF-16 insulin signaling pathway.

DAF-19 is a transcription factor that has recently been shown to play a role in the p38 mitogen activated protein kinase (MAPK) pathway in *C. elegans* [44]. DAF-19 mutant worms display enhanced susceptibility to killing by *P. aeruginosa* [44]. DAF-19 is an ortholog of the regulatory factor X (RFX), a transcription factor that is required for human adaptive immunity [45]. The up-regulation of DAF-19 in *S. flexneri* infected worms could therefore be part of the nematode innate immune response at the early stages of *S. flexneri* infection. Furthermore, TIR-1 (Table S1, spot no. 7) was also identified to be up-regulated in response to *S. flexneri* infection using low stringency MASCOT searches. TIR-1 is the toll interleukin 1 receptor domain adaptor protein in *C. elegans* that activates the p38 MAPK innate immune response. During human infection, the multiplication of *S. flexneri* cells within infected intestinal cells activates the MAPK-mediated signaling pathway, thus leading to the production of inflammatory chemokines and cytokines and antimicrobial peptides [46,47]. The up-regulation of both DAF-19 and TIR-1 in infected worms and increased susceptibility of *daf*-19 RNAi worms suggests that the p38 MAPK pathway is potentially induced by *C. elegans* in response to *S. flexneri* infection.

Conclusion

Shigellosis research has been hindered by the lack of an appropriate *in vivo* model. Unlike humans and non-human primates, the small animal models of shigellosis fail to develop intestinal disease upon ingestion of *S. flexneri*. Here we have shown that virulent strains of *S. flexneri* are ingested by the nematode *C. elegans* and that *S. flexneri* cells invade the nematode intestinal cells. This is the first report to investigate the cytopathology and nematode responses to *S. flexneri* infection. DIGE analysis of the nematode proteome induced by *S. flexneri* suggests that both the DAF-2/DAF-16 insulin signaling pathway and the p38 MAPK pathway are induced in response to bacterial infection. Our findings also suggest that *S. flexneri* disrupts iron homeostasis in nematodes and potentially induces a hypoxic response which could lead to death. The results of this study further our understanding of *S. flexneri* infection in *C. elegans*, opening up a new, convenient, economical alternative for screening *Shigella* mutant strains to identify attenuated strains for testing live vaccine strains and for the identification of novel virulence factors.

Materials and Methods

Nematode and bacterial strains

C. elegans strain Bristol N2 [48] obtained from the *Caenorhabditis* Genetic Center (CGC), Minneapolis, MN, was cultured and maintained at 22°C on modified nematode growth medium agar [18] and fed with *E. coli* OP50 as described previously [49]. RNAi of *aco-1, cct-2, daf-19,* and *hsp-60* was performed by feeding as described previously [50]. *E. coli* HT115 (DE3) harboring genes encoding double stranded RNA targeted towards *aco-1* (ZK455.7), *cct-2* (T21B10.7), *eff-2* (F25H5.4) and *hsp-60* (Y22D7AL.5) were obtained from the Ahringer lab library and the *daf-19* (F33H1.1) RNAi construct was obtained from the ORF-RNAi Library v1.1 (Source Bioscience). pCB19 was used as a non-specific dsRNA control, as this vector contains a fragment of the *Arabidopsis thaliana* light harvesting complex gene (LHCB4.3), which shows no homology to *C. elegans*, cloned into the RNAi vector pL4440 [51].

Liquid overnight cultures of bacteria were grown in Luria Bertani (LB) broth, containing ampicillin (100 μg/mL) when necessary. The virulent *S. flexneri* serotype 3b strain-SFL1520 (International Centre for Diarrhoeal Diseases Research Bangladesh-ICDDRB) and virulence plasmid-cured avirulent strain-SFL1223 [52] were used. *S. flexneri* cultures were grown at 30°C overnight for maintenance of the virulence plasmid, following which bacterial cultures were grown to log phase at 37°C to induce expression of the plasmid-based virulence genes.

C. elegans liquid killing assays

Killing assays in liquid culture were performed as described previously [19]. Briefly, a synchronized population of young adult

C. elegans worms was treated with 200 µg/mL gentamycin for 3 hours to eliminate any surface-bound bacteria. Worms were washed thoroughly with S-basal to remove any residual antibiotic. Approximately 20 washed young adults were transferred into each well in a 24-well plate containing 100 µL of appropriate log-phase *S. flexneri* ($OD_{600} = 0.6$) and *E. coli* cultures ($OD_{600} = 0.5$). The volume of solution in each well was adjusted to 500 µL with S-basal and plates were incubated at 22°C. The number of live worms in each well was scored every 12 hours and percentage survival was calculated. Nematodes that showed no pharyngeal pumping and remained immobile on tapping the plate were considered dead. Results are representative of three independent assays, each with triplicates. Survival curves were analysed using the PRISM (version 4.02) software. Kaplan-Meier analysis was used to compare the mean lifespan of *C. elegans*. Logrank tests were used to determine if survival curves were significantly different.

Bacterial accumulation assay

Bacterial strains used for the accumulation assay were grown overnight at 37°C on modified NG agar medium to stimulate expression of virulence plasmid-encoded genes [18]. Plates were cooled to room temperature before they were inoculated with 50–100 synchronized young adult nematodes and incubated at 22°C for 24 hours. 20 worms were picked, treated with 200 mg/mL gentamycin for 3 hours to eliminate surface-bound bacteria and washed thoroughly using S-basal with 1 mM of sodium azide to remove any residual antibiotic. Washed nematodes were suspended in S-basal + 0.1% Triton-X and lysed by mechanical disruption using glass beads as described previously [19]. Appropriate dilutions of the lysates were plated onto LB agar with the appropriate antibiotics, to obtain bacterial counts. In order to visualize the bacterial accumulation within nematode guts, worms were fed *S. flexneri* strains tagged with GFP^+. Following 24 hours of infection bacterial fluorescence was observed using the EVOS digital inverted microscope (AMG).

Transmission electron microscopy

50–100 adult worms were picked off virulent and avirulent *S. flexneri* lawns 24, 96 and 144 hours post infection. For prolonged infection periods, worms were transferred onto fresh *S. flexneri* lawns each day. Worms were transferred into Beem capsules and fixed, rinsed and stained using the microwave-assisted irradiation protocol developed by Hall *et al.* [53]. A Pelco Biowave oven at the Centre of Advanced Microscopy (CAM, ANU), was used for the microwave assisted fixation of worms. Post staining with 0.5% aqueous uranyl acetate, samples were dehydrated at room temperature using the following dehydration cycles; 50% ethanol for 10 minutes, 70% ethanol for 10 minutes, 80% ethanol for 10 minutes, 90% ethanol for 10 minutes, three treatments with 100% ethanol for 10 minutes each. This was followed by infiltration of the sample at room temperature with LR White resin (Pro-SciTech) using the following infiltration regime: 2:1 100% ethanol: LR White; 2 hours, 1:1 100% ethanol: LR White; 2 hours, two treatments with 100% LR White for 2 hours each. LR white was cured at 65°C under nitrogen gas overnight. Thin sections were obtained using a Power Tome XL ultramicrotome (RMC, Boekeler Instruments, Tucson, AZ) at the Albert Einstein College of Medicine (AECOM). Sections were collected on copper slot grids and stained with 2% uranyl acetate in 50% ethanol for 10 minutes and with lead citrate (Reynolds's formulation) for 15 minutes and TEM micrographs were collected on a Phillips CM10 electron microscope at AECOM.

Isolation of total nematode protein

Approximately 500,000 synchronized, young adult nematodes were infected with *E. coli* OP50 (control) and wild type *S. flexneri* 3b (SFL1520) for 24 hours at 22°C. Post infection the nematodes were washed thoroughly using sterile S-basal with 1 mM sodium azide and treated with 200 mg/mL gentamycin for 3 hours to reduce the presence of bacterial spots on the gels. Sucrose flotation [49] was used to separate adult worms from larvae, eggs and bacterial debris. Infected worms were snap-frozen in liquid nitrogen and the frozen pellets were ground to a fine powder using fine glass powder in an ice-cold mortar and pestle and resuspended in solubilisation buffer (7 M urea, 2 M thiourea, 30 mM tris-base, 4% (w/v) CHAPS and Complete Protease Inhibitor (Roche)). The suspensions were homogenized and sonicated. Nematode proteins precipitated using 100% trichloroacetic acid (TCA) were collected by centrifugation, washed thrice using ice-cold acetone, air dried and resuspended in 20–30 µl 0.2 M NaOH and 100–200 µl of solubilization buffer (9 M urea, 4% CHAPS, 1% DTT, 1% ampholytes, 35 mM tris base). Protein concentration was determined using the Bradford method [54] and 2 mg of each sample was labeled with fluorescent dyes Cy3 or Cy5 (GE Healthcare). An internal standard, consisting of 1 mg of each sample, was labeled with Cy2.

2-D electrophoresis

2-D electrophoresis was performed in darkness to maintain the stability of the Cy dyes. Immobiline pH 3–10 NL Drystrips (24 cm, GE Healthcare) were used for the first dimension isoelectric focusing (IEF). The strips were rehydrated overnight in rehydration solution containing, 8 M urea, 0.5% (w/v) CHAPS, 0.2% (w/v) DTT, 0.52% (w/v) bio-ampholytes and 0.6% (w/v) bromophenol blue. Proteins from *S. flexneri* infected and control worms along with internal controls were loaded onto rehydrated Immobiline strips and IEF was carried out in a Multiphor II electrophoresis system (GE Healthcare) at 20°C for a total of 35,000 volt hours [55].

For separation of proteins across the second dimension, self-cast 12.5% SDS-PAGE gels were prepared using the EttanDALTsix system (GE Healthcare). The gels were cast using low fluorescence glass plates, which are compatible with visualizing the CyDyes. Focused first dimension strips were equilibrated as described by [55] and placed on the second dimension gels. SDS-PAGE was carried out at 10°C in SDS running buffer (25 mM Tris, pH 8.0, 192 mM glycine and 0.1% SDS) at 600 V, 10 mA, and 2.5 W per gel for the first hour; 600 V, 40 mA, and 13 W per gel until the bromophenol blue front reached the bottom of the gel.

Gel imaging and image analysis

After the second dimension electrophoresis, DIGE-labeled proteins were visualized using a Typhoon Trio laser scanner (GE Healthcare). Gels were scanned with the specific excitation wavelengths of Cy3 (532-nm laser and a 580-nm band pass 30 emission filter), Cy5 (633-nm laser and a 670-nm band pass 30 emission filter) and Cy2 (488-nm laser and a 580-nm band pass 40 emission filter). Spot detection and analysis was carried out using DeCyder Version 6.5 (GE Healthcare) software followed by careful manual confirmation and rematching of matching errors. Statistics and identification of differentially expressed spots were carried out in the DeCyder DIA and BVA modules (one-way ANOVA).

In-gel trypsin digestion of protein spots and liquid chromatography-mass spectrometry

After analysis of gel images, identified spots of interest were excised from the 2D-DIGE gels using an Ettan spot picker (GE Healthcare). In-gel trypsin digest was carried out as described by Mathesius *et al* [55] with a few modifications. Briefly, excised protein spots were washed four times in acetonitrile: 50 mM ammonium bicarbonate (49.5:49.5, v/v). Spots were dried in 100% acetonitrile for 30 minutes following which they were air-dried to eliminate all acetonitrile. Gel pieces were rehydrated with a trypsin solution (20 units; Promega) and incubated for 2 hours at 4°C followed by overnight incubation at 37°C. Peptides were extracted from the gel pieces using an extraction buffer consisting of acetonitrile: water: trifluoroacetic acid (TFA) (50%:50%:1%, v/v) followed by gentle sonication in a sonic water bath for 40 minutes. Peptides were collected and dried completely to remove all traces of TFA and resuspended in 20 µl of acetonitrile: water: formic acid (10%:89.9%:0.1%, v/v). The peptides were identified at the Mass Spectrometry Facility, The Australian National University, on an Agilent 6530 Q-TOF LC/MS (Santa Clara, CA, USA) with a ChipCube ion source interface (Agilent Technologies, Inc., Palo Alto, CA) containing a liquid chromatographic chip (ProtID-Chip-150(II), separation: 150 mm×75 µm, enrichment: 4 mm 40 nL, packed with 5 µm Zorbax 300SB-C18 particles). The LC separation system included a binary capillary pump operated at a flow rate of 4 µL/min, used for loading the samples, and a nanoflow gradient pump using a linear gradient from 8 to 38% mobile phase B in 47 min at a flow rate of 300 nL/min. The column was then washed with 90% mobile phase B for 5 min. Mobile phase A was 0.1% formic acid and mobile phase B was 90% acetonitrile/water containing 0.1% formic acid.

The spray from the chip was subjected to positive polarity electrospray ionisation (ESI) using the following settings: gas flow rate 4 L/min, gas temperature 300°C, capillary voltage 1900 V, fragmentor 175 V, skimmer 65 V and octopole RF peak 750 V. The instrument was run in extended dynamic range mode with data dependent acquisition switching between MS (*m/z* 100–1700 at 3 spectra/s) and MS/MS (*m/z* 50–1700 at 3 spectra/s), measuring the collision induced dissociation (CID) fragment spectra of the three most intense precursor ions with charge states 2, 3 and ≥3 with a 15 s dynamic exclusion time, within a cycle time of 1.4 s. The collision energy was automatically set by the Agilent MassHunter Acquisition software (slope 3, offset 2). The *m/z* values of all ions present in the mass spectra were corrected against two reference ions (purine, $[MH]^+$ *m/z* 112.985587 and 1H, 1H, 3H tetra(fluoropropoxy)phosphazine, $[MH]^+$ *m/z* 922.0097). Data were acquired and analysed with Agilent Technologies MassHunter software (version B.4.0).

Proteins were identified through peptide sequences using MASCOT (Matrix Science). One missed cleavage per peptide was allowed and a mass tolerance between 0.3 and 0.1 Da was used for high stringency searches and 0.8 and 0.6 Da was used for low stringency searches. Carbamidomethylation of cysteine was set as a fixed modification and oxidation (M) as a variable. We searched the SwissProt database under taxonomy *C. elegans* on the MASCOT database at the Australian Proteomic Computation Facility (APCF).

Quantitative real-time polymerase chain reaction (qRT-PCR)

Approximately 50,000 synchronized young adult worms were infected with either *E. coli* OP50 or *S. flexneri* serotype 3b for 24 h at 22°C. Adult worms were separated from eggs and bacterial debris using sucrose flotation [49]. Infected adult worm pellets were snap frozen in liquid nitrogen and RNA was isolated using Trizol reagent (Invitrogen) according to the manufacturer's instructions. 200 ng of total RNA was used as template in a first strand synthesis using random hexamer primers and SuperScript II (Invitrogen) according to the manufacturer's instructions. cDNA was used to set up qRT-PCRs using the power SYBR Green RT-PCR kit (Applied Biosystems) according to the manufacturer's instructions except that primers were used at a final concentration of 0.4 µM and the final reaction volume was reduced to 10 µl. Results of qRT-PCRs represent 3 independent biological repeats. Reactions were run in a Rotor-Gene Q Real-Time cycler (Qaigen) and data were analysed using the Rota-Gene Q series software package.

Supporting Information

Figure S1 Two-dimensional differential in-gel electrophoresis of the *C. elegans* infected with *S. flexneri*.

Figure S2 Graphical representation of the predicted biological functions of the up- and down-regulated *C. elegans* proteins identified in response to *S. flexneri* infection.

Table S1 Predicted *S. flexneri*-induced responses in *C. elegans* identified through Peptide Mass Fingerprinting using low stringency MASCOT search parameters.

Acknowledgments

We'd like to thank the Australian Microscopy and Microanalysis Research Facility (AMMRF) and the Center for *C. elegans* anatomy (New York, U.S.A) for the use of their facilities and assistance with fixing, staining and sectioning of nematodes. We'd also like to thank Dr. Charles Hocart and Dr. Thy Truong at the Mass Spectrometry Facility, The Australian National University for their assistance with LC-MS.

Author Contributions

Conceived and designed the experiments: DG CB NV. Performed the experiments: DG. Analyzed the data: DG CB DH UM MR NV. Contributed reagents/materials/analysis tools: DG CB DH UM MR KN NV. Wrote the paper: DG CB DH UM MR NV.

References

1. Jennison AV, Verma NK (2004) *Shigella flexneri* infection: pathogenesis and vaccine development. FEMS Microbiol. Revi. 28: 43–58.
2. DuPont HL, Levine MM, Hornick RB, Formal SB (1989) Inoculum size in shigellosis and implications for expected mode of transmission. J. Infect. Dis. 159: 1126–1128.
3. Voino-Yasenetsky MV, Voino-Yasenetskaya MK (1962) Experimental pneumonia caused by bacteria of the *Shigella* group. Acta. Morphol. Acad. Sci. Hung. 11: 439–454.
4. Mallett CP, VanDeVerg L, Collins HH, Hale TL (1993) Evaluation of *Shigella* vaccine safety and efficacy in an intranasally challenged mouse model. Vaccine 11: 190–196.
5. van de Verg LL, Mallett CP, Collins HH, Larsen T, Hammack C, et al (1995) Antibody and cytokine responses in a mouse pulmonary model of *Shigella flexneri* serotype 2a infection. Infect. Immun. 63: 1947–1954.
6. Sereny B (1955) Experimental *Shigella* keratoconjunctivitis; a preliminary report. Acta. Microbiol. Acad. Sci. Hung. 2: 293–296.

7. Kurz CL, Ewbank JJ (2007) Infection in a dish: high-throughput analyses of bacterial pathogenesis. Current Opinion in Microbiology 10: 10–16.
8. Kurz CL, Ewbank JJ (2000) *Caenorhabditis elegans* for the study of host-pathogen interactions. Trends Microbiol. 8: 142–144.
9. Labrousse A, Chauvet S, Couillault C, Kurz CL, Ewbank JJ (2000) *Caenorhabditis elegans* is a model host for *Salmonella typhimurium*. Curr. Biol. 10: 1543–1545.
10. Joshua GW, Karlyshev AV, Smith MP, Isherwood KE, Titball RW, et al (2003) A *Caenorhabditis elegans* model of *Yersinia* infection: biofilm formation on a biotic surface. Microbiol. 149: 3221–3229.
11. Aballay A, Yorgey P, Ausubel FM (2000) *Salmonella typhimurium* proliferates and establishes a persistent infection in the intestine of *Caenorhabditis elegans*. Curr. Biol. 10: 1539–1542.
12. Tan MW, Rahme LG, Sternberg JA, Tompkins RG, Ausubel FM (1999) *Pseudomonas aeruginosa* killing of *Caenorhabditis elegans* used to identify *P. aeruginosa* virulence factors. Proc. Natl. Acad. Sci. U.S.A. 96: 2408–2413.
13. Tan MW, Mahajan-Miklos S, Ausubel FM (1999) Killing of *Caenorhabditis elegans* by *Pseudomonas aeruginosa* used to model mammalian bacterial pathogenesis. Proc. Natl. Acad. Sci. U.S.A. 96: 715–720.
14. Alegado RA, Campbell MC, Chen WC, Slutz SS, Tan MW (2003) Characterization of mediators of microbial virulence and innate immunity using the *Caenorhabditis elegans* host-pathogen model. Cellular Microbiology 5: 435–444.
15. Darby C (2005) Interactions with microbial pathogens. WormBook (Ed) "The C elegans Research Community" (http://www.wormbook.org), 1–15.
16. Sifri CD, Begun J, Ausubel FM (2005) The worm has turned-microbial virulence modeled in *Caenorhabditis elegans*. Trends Microbiol. 13: 119–127.
17. Powell JR, Ausubel FM (2008) Models of *Caenorhabditis elegans* infection by bacterial and fungal pathogens. Methods Mol. Biol. 415: 403–427.
18. Burton EA, Pendergast AM, Aballay M (2006) The *Caenorhabditis elegans* ABL-1 Tyrosine Kinase Is Required for *Shigella flexneri* Pathogenesis. Appl. Environ. Microbiol. 72: 5043–5051.
19. Kesika P, Karutha PS, Balamurugan K (2011) Analysis of *Shigella flexneri*-mediated infections in model organism *Caenorhabditis elegans*. Scand. J. Infect. Dis. 43: 286–295.
20. Hsiao JY, Chen CY, Yang MJ, Ho HC (2013) Live and dead GFP-tagged bacteria showed indistinguishable fluorescence in *Caenorhabditis elegans* gut. J. Microbiol. 51: 367–372.
21. McBroom AJ, MJ Kuehn (2007) Release of outer membrane vesicles by Gram-negative bacteria is a novel envelope stress response. Mol. Microbiol. 63: 545–558.
22. Kadurugamuwa JL, TJ Beveridge (1999) Membrane vesicles derived from *Pseudomonas aeruginosa* and *Shigella flexneri* can be integrated into the surfaces of other gram-negative bacteria. Microbiol. 145: 2051–2060.
23. Balla KM, Troemel ER (2013) *Caenorhabditis elegans* as a model for intracellular pathogen infection. Cell. Microbiol. 15: 1313–1322.
24. Gourley BL, Parker SB, Jones BJ, Zumbrennen KB, Leibold EA (2003) Cytosolic aconitase and ferritin are regulated by iron in *Caenorhabditis elegans*. J. Biol. Chem. 278: 3227–3234.
25. Negrete-Abascal E, Garcia RM, Reyes ME, Godinez D, de la Garza M (2000) Membrane vesicles released by *Actinobacillus pleuropneumoniae* contain proteases and Apx toxins. FEMS Microbiol. Lett. 191: 109–113.
26. Grenier D (1992) Inactivation of human serum bactericidal activity by a trypsinlike protease isolated from *Porphyromonas gingivalis*. Infect. Immun. 60: 1854–1857.
27. Rosen G, Naor R, Rahamim E, Yishai R, Sela MN (1995) Proteases of *Treponema denticola* outer sheath and extracellular vesicles. Infect. Immun. 63: 3973–3979.
28. Dutta S, Iida K, Takade A, Meno Y, Nair GB, et al (2004) Release of Shiga toxin by membrane vesicles in *Shigella dysenteriae* serotype 1 strains and *in vitro* effects of antimicrobials on toxin production and release. Microbiol. Immunol. 48: 965–969.
29. Wai SN, Takade A, Amako K (1995) The release of outer membrane vesicles from the strains of enterotoxigenic *Escherichia coli*. Microbiol. Immunol. 39: 451–456.
30. Wai SN, Westermark M, Oscarsson J, Jass J, Maier E, et al (2003) Characterization of dominantly negative mutant ClyA cytotoxin proteins in *Escherichia coli*. J. Bacteriol. 185: 5491–5499.
31. Fiocca R, Necchi V, Sommi P, Ricci V, Telford J, et al (1999) Release of *Helicobacter pylori* vacuolating cytotoxin by both a specific secretion pathway and budding of outer membrane vesicles. Uptake of released toxin and vesicles by gastric epithelium. J. Pathol. 188: 220–226.
32. Furuta N, Takeuchi H, Amano A (2009) Entry of *Porphyromonas gingivalis* outer membrane vesicles into epithelial cells causes cellular functional impairment. Infect. Immun. 77: 4761–4770.
33. Amano A, Takeuchi H, Furuta N (2010) Outer membrane vesicles function as offensive weapons in host-parasite interactions. Microbes. Infect. 12: 791–798.
34. Kuehn MJ, Kesty NC (2005) Bacterial outer membrane vesicles and the host-pathogen interaction. Genes Dev. 19: 2645–2655.
35. Bomberger JM, Maceachran DP, Coutermarsh BA, Ye S, O'Toole GA, et al (2009) Long-distance delivery of bacterial virulence factors by *Pseudomonas aeruginosa* outer membrane vesicles. PLoS Pathog 5: e1000382.
36. Schertzer JW, Whiteley M (2013) Bacterial outer membrane vesicles in trafficking, communication and the host-pathogen interaction. J. Mol. Microbiol. Biotechnol. 23: 118–130.
37. Wassef JS, Keren DF, Mailloux JL (1989) Role of M cells in initial antigen uptake and in ulcer formation in the rabbit intestinal loop model of shigellosis. Infect. and Immun. 57: 858–863.
38. McGee MD, Weber D, Day N, Vitelli C, Crippen D, et al (2011) Loss of intestinal nuclei and intestinal integrity in aging *C. elegans*. Aging Cell 10: 699–710.
39. Kim YI, Cho JH, Yoo OJ, Ahnn J (2004) Transcriptional regulation and life-span modulation of cytosolic aconitase and ferritin genes in *C. elegans*. J. Mol. Biol. 342: 421–433.
40. Kirienko NV, Kirienko DR, Larkins-Ford J, Wahlby C, Ruvkun G, et al (2013) *Pseudomonas aeruginosa* disrupts *Caenorhabditis elegans* iron homeostasis, causing a hypoxic response and death. Cell Host Microbe 13: 406–416.
41. Sugimoto T, Mori C, Takanami T, Sasagawa Y, Saito R, et al (2008) *Caenorhabditis elegans* par2.1/mtssb-1 is essential for mitochondrial DNA replication and its defect causes comprehensive transcriptional alterations including a hypoxia response. Exp. Cell. Res. 314: 103–114.
42. Wang J, Robida-Stubbs S, Tullet JM, Rual JF, Vidal M, et al (2010) RNAi screening implicates a SKN-1-dependent transcriptional response in stress resistance and longevity deriving from translation inhibition. PLoS Genet 6(8): e1001048.
43. Murphy CT, McCarroll SA, Bargmann CI, Fraser A, Kamath RS, et al (2003) Genes that act downstream of DAF-16 to influence the lifespan of *Caenorhabditis elegans*. Nature 424: 277–283.
44. Xie Y, Moussaif M, Choi S, Xu L, Sze JY (2013) RFX transcription factor DAF-19 regulates 5-HT and innate immune responses to pathogenic bacteria in *Caenorhabditis elegans*. PLoS Genet 9: e1003324.
45. Reith W, Mach B (2001) The bare lymphocyte syndrome and the regulation of MHC expression. Annu. Rev. Immunol. 19: 331–373.
46. Ashida H, Ogawa M, Mimuro H, Sasakawa C (2009) *Shigella infection* of intestinal epithelium and circumvention of the host innate defense system. Curr. Top. Microbiol. Immunol. 337: 231–255.
47. Ogawa M, Handa Y, Ashida H, Suzuki M, Sasakawa C (2008) The versatility of *Shigella* effectors. Nat. Rev. Microbiol. 6: 11–16.
48. Brenner S (1974) Genetics of *Caenorhabditis elegans*. Genetics 77: 71–94.
49. Sulston J, Hodgkin J (1988) Methods: The nematode *Caenorhabditis elegans*; Wood W.B., editor. Cold Spring Harbor, New York: Cold Spring Harbor Laboratory Press.
50. Kamath RS, Ahringer J (2003) Genome-wide RNAi screening in *Caenorhabditis elegans*. Methods 30: 313–321.
51. Fritz JA, Behm CA (2009) CUTI-1: A novel tetraspan protein involved in *C. elegans* CUTicle formation and epithelial integrity. Plos One 4: e5117.
52. Maurelli AT, Blackmon B, Curtiss R (1984) Loss of pigmentation in *Shigella flexneri* 2a is correlated with loss of virulence and virulence-associated plasmid. Infect. Immun. 43: 397–401.
53. Hall DH, Hartwieg E, Nguyen KCQ (2012) Chapter 4 - Modern Electron Microscopy Methods for *C. elegans*. In: Joel H.R., Andrew S., editors. Methods in Cell Biology: Acad. Press. 93–149.
54. Bradford MM (1976) A rapid and sensitive method for the quantitation of microgram quantities of protein utilizing the principle of protein-dye binding. Anal. Biochem. 72: 248–254.
55. Mathesius U (2001) Flavonoids induced in cells undergoing nodule organogenesis in white clover are regulators of auxin breakdown by peroxidase. J. Exp. Bot. 52: 419–426.

13

Cholera and Shigellosis: Different Epidemiology but Similar Responses to Climate Variability

Benjamin A. Cash[1]*, Xavier Rodó[2,3], Michael Emch[4], Md. Yunus[5], Abu S. G. Faruque[5], Mercedes Pascual[6,7]

1 Center for Ocean-Land-Atmosphere Studies, Fairfax, Virginia, United States of America, **2** Institut Català de Ciències del Clima (IC3), Barcelona, Catalunya, Spain, **3** Institució Catalana de Recerca i Estudis Avançats, Barcelona, Catalunya, Spain, **4** University of North Carolina Chapel Hill, Chapel Hill, North Carolina, United States of America, **5** International Centre for Diarrheal Disease Research, Dhaka, Bangladesh, **6** Department of Ecology and Evolutionary Biology University of Michigan, Ann Arbor, Michigan, United States of America, **7** Howard Hughes Medical Institute, Chevy Chase, Maryland, United States of America

Abstract

Background: Comparative studies of the associations between different infectious diseases and climate variability, such as the El Niño-Southern Oscillation, are lacking. Diarrheal illnesses, particularly cholera and shigellosis, provide an important opportunity to apply a comparative approach. Cholera and shigellosis have significant global mortality and morbidity burden, pronounced differences in transmission pathways and pathogen ecologies, and there is an established climate link with cholera. In particular, the specific ecology of *Vibrio cholerae* is often invoked to explain the sensitivity of that disease to climate.

Methods and Findings: The extensive surveillance data of the International Center for Diarrheal Disease Research, Bangladesh are used here to revisit the known associations between cholera and climate, and to address their similarity to previously unexplored patterns for shigellosis. Monthly case data for both the city of Dhaka and a rural area known as Matlab are analyzed with respect to their association with El Niño and flooding. Linear correlations are examined between flooding and cumulative cases, as well as for flooding and El Niño. Rank-correlation maps are also computed between disease cases in the post-monsoon epidemic season and sea surface temperatures in the Pacific. Similar climate associations are found for both diseases and both locations. Increased cases follow increased monsoon flooding and increased sea surface temperatures in the preceding winter corresponding to an El Niño event.

Conclusions: The similarity in association patterns suggests a systemic breakdown in population health with changing environmental conditions, in which climate variability acts primarily through increasing the exposure risk of the human population. We discuss these results in the context of the on-going debate on the relative importance of the environmental reservoir vs. secondary transmission, as well as the implications for the use of El Niño as an early indicator of flooding and enteric disease risk.

Editor: Wei-Chun Chin, University of California, Merced, United States of America

Funding: This work was funded by the United States National Oceanic and Atmospheric Administration grant # F020704. The authors further acknowledge the support of core donors that provide unrestricted support to the International Centre for Diarrheal Disease Research, Bangladesh (icddr,b) for its operations and research. Current donors providing unrestricted support include the Australian International Development Agency, the government of the People's Republic of Bangladesh, the Canadian International Development Agency, the Swedish International Development Cooperative Agency, and the Department for International Development, United Kingdom. The authors gratefully acknowledge these donors for their support and commitment to icddr,b's research efforts. M. Pascual is an investigator of the Howard Hughes Medical Institute. The funders had no role in study design, data collection and analysis, decision to publish, or preparation of the manuscript.

Competing Interests: The authors have declared that no competing interests exist.

* Email: bcash@gmu.edu

Introduction

Comparative studies of associations between climate variability and human health across different infectious diseases are largely lacking. Potential climate influences are typically addressed only for specific infections and locations for which sufficiently long retrospective records exist. Such comparison studies, however, are instrumental in identifying systemic breakdowns in human health at the population level that do not depend on specific pathogen ecologies or epidemiology. Similarities in responses to climate forcing instead signal common mechanisms and, in so doing, identify key pathways of action for intervention. In addition, associations between disease risk and slowly varying features of the climate system allow for the possibility of developing early warning systems for disease risk in the affected areas.

Diarrheal illnesses provide one important disease class for the application of a comparative approach. Cholera, arguably the paradigmatic water-borne diarrheal disease, is caused by the bacteria *Vibrio cholerae* and has been responsible for numerous pandemics throughout history, including the current era [1]. Infection generally results from ingesting water contaminated with the bacteria, and left untreated leads to mortality rates as high as 50% [2]. Global mortality rates for cholera are estimated at ~3% [3]. Mortality for shigellosis, another widely spread diarrheal illness that is caused by bacteria of the *Shigella* genus can reach 5–15% for some strains in areas with poor medical care [4–5]. The infectious dose for shigellosis is also substantially lower than for cholera and the disease is responsible for significant mortality and morbidity in the developing world [6]. Given their global mortality and morbidity burden, the potentially pronounced differences in transmission pathways and pathogen ecologies, and the existing evidence for a role of climate forcing on cholera, cholera and shigellosis represent excellent candidates for a comparative study on their associations with climate.

Endemic cholera has been prominent in studies on the influence of climate variability on diarrheal diseases. In particular, the El Niño-Southern Oscillation (ENSO), widely recognized as one of the most significant modes of interannual climate variability, has been shown to affect the severity of seasonal outbreaks in Bangladesh [7–12]. Favorable conditions for increased cholera risk in the fall have been shown to be associated with positive ENSO (El Niño) events in the preceding winter, thus establishing ENSO as a potential early-warning indicator for Bangladesh cholera outbreaks. At the local level increased rainfall and associated flooding have also been shown to increase fall cholera cases, and represent the means by which the remote influence of ENSO in transmitted to Bangladesh [11], [13].

The particular attention paid to cholera is due in no small part to the extended record of cases available for Bangladesh, advances on the microbial ecology of *Vibrio cholerae*, and the recognition that the pathogen survives outside the human host in aquatic environments such as estuaries and brackish water [14–16]. Climate conditions favoring the population growth or survival of the pathogen would exacerbate transmission through environmental aquatic reservoirs. This paradigm has led to an emphasis on mechanisms that are pathogen specific in mediating the effect of climate variability. An alternative, although not necessarily exclusive view, is one in which the vulnerability of the human host plays a key role and at seasonal and interannual time scales is modified by anomalous climate conditions such as extreme floods [17–19].

The relationship between water-borne bacterial diseases in Bangladesh and the monsoon rains is of particular interest, given that Bangladesh lies at the confluence of three major rivers (Ganges/Padma, Brahmaputra, Megna) in an extensive estuarine region that is considered the hearth of cholera. Bangladesh is also a low-lying country that experiences some of the highest rainfall totals in the Indian monsoon region and is inundated to a greater or lesser degree on an annual basis. While a certain degree of flooding is necessary to maintain the fertility of the delta system and associated agriculture, major flooding events have resulted in serious loss of life and destruction of infrastructure throughout Bangladesh's history [20]. Given the evidence linking flooding and post-monsoon cholera outbreaks [17–18], [22–24], it is of particular interest to consider what role the severity of annual flooding might play for shigellosis in that same region and season, particularly in the context of potential remote forcing by ENSO.

The extensive surveillance program of the International Center for Diarrheal Diseases Research, Bangladesh (icddr,b) makes it possible for us to revisit here the known associations between cholera and climate variability, and to specifically inquire about the possibility of similar but unknown patterns for shigellosis. In the results presented below, we show that there are indeed similar associations between cholera and shigellosis cases in Bangladesh and flooding, as well as for cholera and shigellosis cases and sea surface temperatures in the tropical Pacific. These similar associations have significant implications for the mechanisms behind the influence of climate on enteric disease outbreaks in Bangladesh, as well as for the use of ENSO as an early warning indicator of outbreak risk.

We indeed find a strong similarity of association patterns for post-monsoon outbreaks, whose implications for the mechanisms behind the influence of climate forcing we discuss.

Data and Methodology

Ethics Statement

The Diarrheal Disease Surveillance System (DDSS) of icddr,b is a routine ongoing activity of the Dhaka and Matlab Hospital, which has been approved by the Research Review Committee (RRC) and Ethical Review Committee (ERC) of icddr,b. At the time of enrollment, verbal consent was taken from the adult patients and caregivers or guardians in case of the children patients, with the information to be stored in the hospital database and used for conducting research. This verbal consent was documented by keeping a check mark in the questionnaire, which was again shown to the adult patients or the parents/guardians of children patients. Patients or parents/guardians were assured about the non-disclosure of information collected from them, and were also informed about the use of data for improving patient care activities as well as scientific research and publication without disclosing the name or identity of the patients. ERC was satisfied with the voluntary participation, maintenance of the rights of the participants and confidential handling of personal information by the hospital physicians and has approved this consent procedure.

Data

Flood Affected Area (FAA), expressed as the percentage of the total area of Bangladesh inundated, was obtained from the annual reports of the Bangladesh Flood Forecasting and Warning Center (FFWC; http://www.ffwc.gov.bd). Values range from 0.2% in 1994 to a remarkable 68% during the severe flooding of 1998. Although FAA is only available as annual values, flooding in Bangladesh is dominated by the rainy season (June-September; JJAS). The reported FAA for each year was taken to be representative of this period.

The NINO34 index is a standard and widely used measure of the strength and state of ENSO, the dominant mode of climate variability on interannual timescales. Values were provided by the National Oceanic and Atmospheric Administration (NOAA) Climate Prediction Center. NINO34 is defined as the area-averaged sea surface temperature (SST) over the region (5°S-5°N, 120°W-170°W) and is presented here as 3-month running mean anomalies calculated relative to the 1971-2000 base period. Gridded SST values used to calculate the rank correlation maps (see below) were taken from the Hadley Centre Sea Ice and Sea Surface Temperature (HadISST) v1.1 data set [25].

The disease data analyzed in this work was taken from two surveillance programs overseen by the icddr,b. In one program, based in icddr,b's Dhaka Hospital, stool specimens from every 25th patient were tested for cholera and shigellosis from 1979–1995, and from every 50th patient from 1996 onwards. The second surveillance program is located in Matlab, Bangladesh, in a rural area approximately 57 km southeast of the capital of Dhaka. In contrast to the Dhaka hospital, patients attended to at the Matlab hospital are mostly those presenting symptoms of severe diarrheal illness. Stool specimens of all diarrhea patients from the Health and Demographic Surveillance System (HDSS) area were tested for shigellosis and cholera. In both locations cases were separated by causative species and strain, and in the analysis presented here we focus exclusively on cases due to the dominant form of the each disease for our period of study, which is 1983–2010. For cholera this was this El Tor biotype, which replaced the former Classical biotype in the past decades and is now the dominant strain both in Bangladesh and around the world. For shigellosis *S. flexneri* represent the dominant form of the disease in Bangladesh.

Time series of the monthly cases (Fig. 1a) and the magnitude of the fall peak (Fig. 1b) for the two diseases in both Matlab and Dhaka show that, in addition to significant interannual variability for both diseases and locations, cholera cases exceed those of shigellosis and that there is a clear downward trend in Dhaka shigellosis cases for this period.

Methodology

Our focus in this work is on interannual variations in disease outbreaks, as opposed to longer-term trends, and as such all data was detrended prior to analysis. As a check on the sensitivity of our results to the removal of the long-term trends we first analyzed data detrended using a simple linear regression. We then repeated the analysis using data detrended via Singular Spectrum Analaysis (SSA), which allows for a more flexible and nonlinear definition of the trend [26]. Our results were not sensitive to the choice of detrending technique (See File S1) and as such results reported here are based on the simpler linear method.

To quantify the magnitude and geographical extent of the link between the occurrence of water borne disease cases and potential environmental drivers, such as SST, we calculate Spearman rank-correlations between reported cases, flooding, and SST (see also [11], [27]). We employed rank-correlation, rather than the more common Pearson's correlation, because it is a non-parametric method more suitable for use with the non-normally distributed flooding and disease data. The rank-correlation, ρ, is calculated as

$$\rho = \frac{n^3 - \frac{D_1 + D_2}{2} - 6\sum_{i=1}^{n} d_i^2}{\sqrt{(n^3 - D_1)(n^3 - D_2)}} \quad (1)$$

in the case where the data includes ties [28], where n is the number of months, d_i is the difference in rank for each month, and D_1 and D_2 are the sum of the cubes of the sizes of the ties in the first and second samples, respectively, where the size of a tie is defined as the number of months with the same value. For $n>20$ we can test for the significance of the above quantity using the transformed, normally distributed variable

$$\omega = (\rho + \frac{6}{n(n^2-1)})\sqrt{n-1} \quad (2)$$

Results and Discussion

Time series of monthly cases (Fig. 1a) and the magnitude of the fall peak (Fig. 1b) of cholera and shigellosis in Matlab and Dhaka show that, in addition to the significant interannual variability for both diseases and locations, there is a downward trend in Dhaka shigellosis cases for this period that is significant at the 95% level (as determined by SSA; see File S1 for details). The significance of the trend is further emphasized by the fact that only for Dhaka shigellosis do results made using the detrended and raw case data differ.

As noted in the Introduction, previous studies have identified a clear statistical association, as well as a physical link, between post-monsoon cholera cases in Matlab and ENSO events in the preceding winter. Building on this previous work (e.g., [11–12]), we calculate the rank correlation between shigellosis cases during the 'fall peak' (August-December; ASOND) and SST at every grid point for the preceding boreal winter (December-February; DJF). Calculating the correlation for each grid point, rather than for a single index defined for a limited and predetermined region, allows for a fuller description of the association between disease outbreaks and global SST. Calculating correlation maps for multiple diseases and locations allows for a richer comparison of their associations with SST as well.

The correlation map for ASOND cholera in Matlab and DJF SST (Fig. 2a) produces a pattern that closely resembles the one for Matlab shigellosis (Fig. 2b), particularly through the tropical regions. This visual similarity is confirmed by the very high pattern correlation of 0.88 between the two maps. While there are minor differences between the patterns for cholera and shigellosis in the Indian Ocean, the diagnosed relationship with the tropical Pacific is nearly identical. Moreover, the maps also closely resemble the pattern of SST anomalies that mark the mature phase of a warm ENSO event, and both series are significantly correlated with the NINO34 index (0.42 for cholera, 0.55 for shigellosis; both $p<0.05$). This apparent association with El Niño was explored previously for Matlab cholera [11], in which experiments with a general circulation model confirmed the physical significance of the correlation pattern and its correspondence to ENSO. This analysis was essential in establishing that the patterns identified by the rank-correlation analysis do indeed represent ENSO, and do not resemble the ENSO pattern merely by chance. The close resemblance between the correlation patterns for cholera and shigellosis strongly implies that shigellosis is responding in a similar manner to the remote forcing from ENSO.

Applying this same correlation map analysis to Dhaka cholera (Fig. 3a) and shigellosis (Fig. 3b) cases, we again find strong similarities in the association patterns for the two diseases. While the Dhaka cholera map closely resembles the two Matlab maps, the highest correlations values are shifted towards the central Pacific for shigellosis. This shift results in a lower correlation between the two Dhaka patterns (0.72) than we find for Matlab, and a lower value of the correlation with the NINO34 index (0.54 for cholera, 0.21 for shigellosis; cholera correlation $p<<0.01$, shigellosis correlation not significant).

The fact that Dhaka shigellosis shows a statistically significant correlation with SST across a broad section of the tropical Pacific, while at the same time showing a relatively low correlation with the NINO34 index, highlights the advantages of analyzing correlation patterns rather than focusing on single indices. This shift in the region of significant correlations between Dhaka shigellosis and SST also suggests a closer association with the central, rather than eastern, Pacific component of ENSO. Thus, despite the dramatic differences in ecology between the two pathogens and the environments of the two study sites, we find a clear association between post-monsoon cases and ENSO in the preceding winter for both diseases and locations.

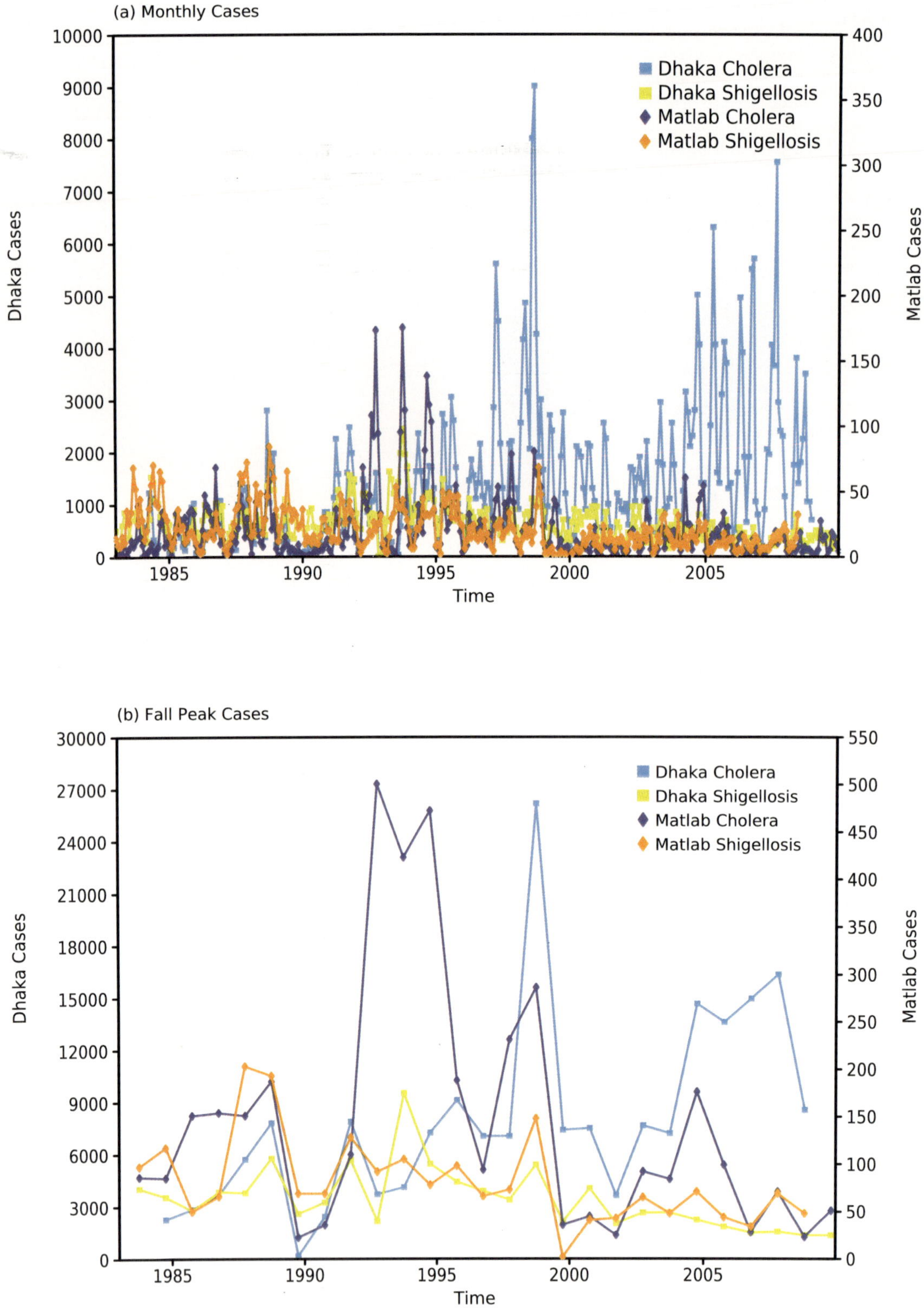

Figure 1. Time series of (a) monthly *S. flexneri* shigellosis and *V. cholerae* El Tor cholera cases and (b) cases during the fall peak (August-December; ASOND) from 1983–2009 for Dhaka and Matlab.

Earlier work (e.g., [11–12]) advanced the theory that enhanced local rainfall and subsequent flooding is the mediating factor between tropical SST anomalies and cholera cases in Bangladesh. Enhanced local rainfall linked to remote SST anomalies has also been associated with increased malaria cases in northwest India [27]. Consistent with this mechanism, we find strong positive

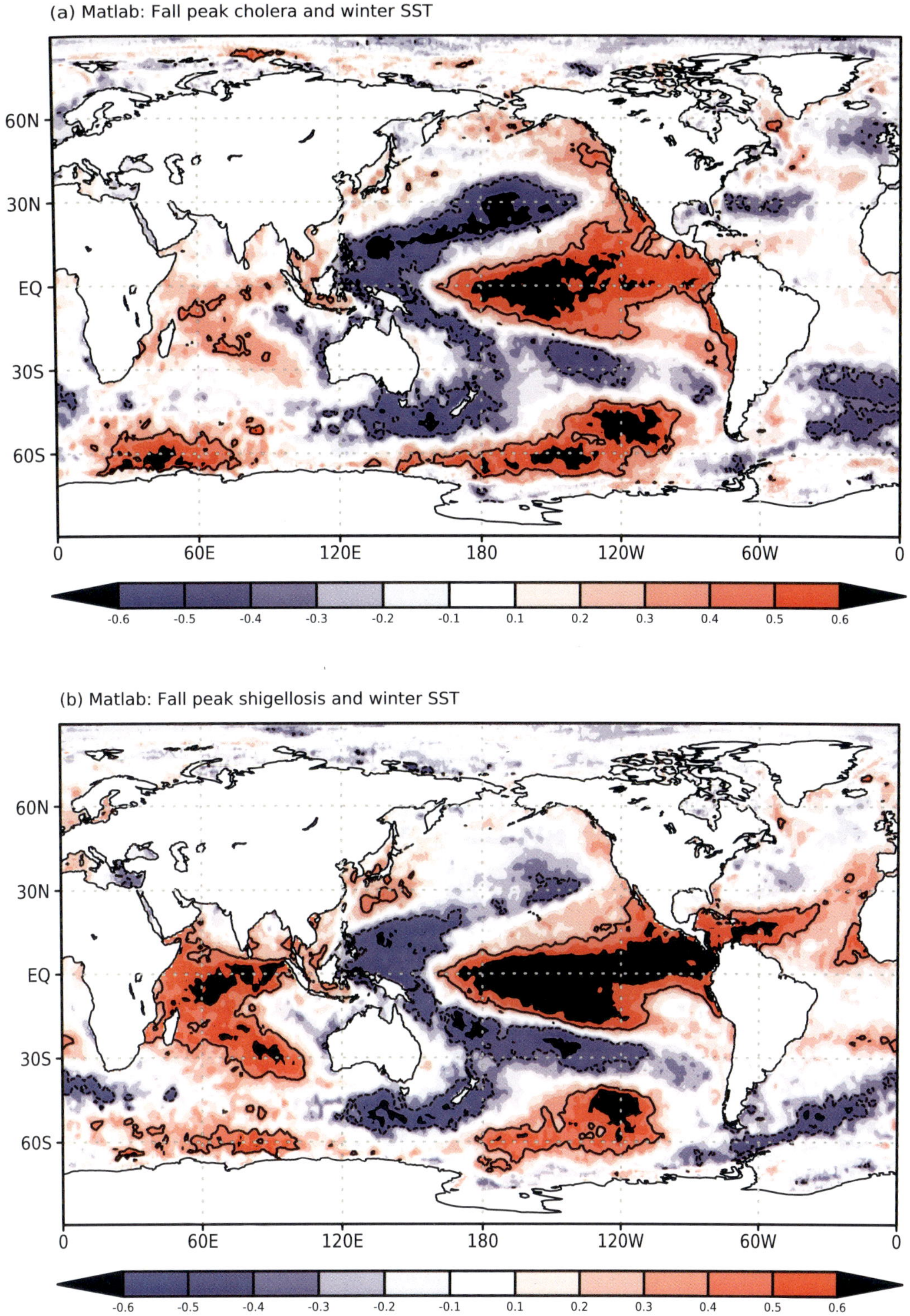

Figure 2. Rank-correlation maps for Matlab (a) fall peak (August-December; ASOND) El Tor cholera and (b) ASOND *S. flexneri* shigellosis cases and preceding December-February sea surface temperature (SST). Maps are correlated at a value of 0.88 for the subregion (35S, 35N).

associations between FAA and both cholera (Fig. 4) and shigellosis (Fig. 5) cases in both locations. The relationship is particularly clear for the Dhaka fall peak in cholera cases (Fig. 4a), with no notable outliers and a rank correlation coefficient of 0.74 ($p \ll 0.01$). In contrast, for the Matlab data the period from 1992–1994 stands out sharply as an outlier, with 2–3 times the number of cases compared to other years with similar FAA. If this period is excluded the rank correlation coefficient with FAA is 0.54 (p<

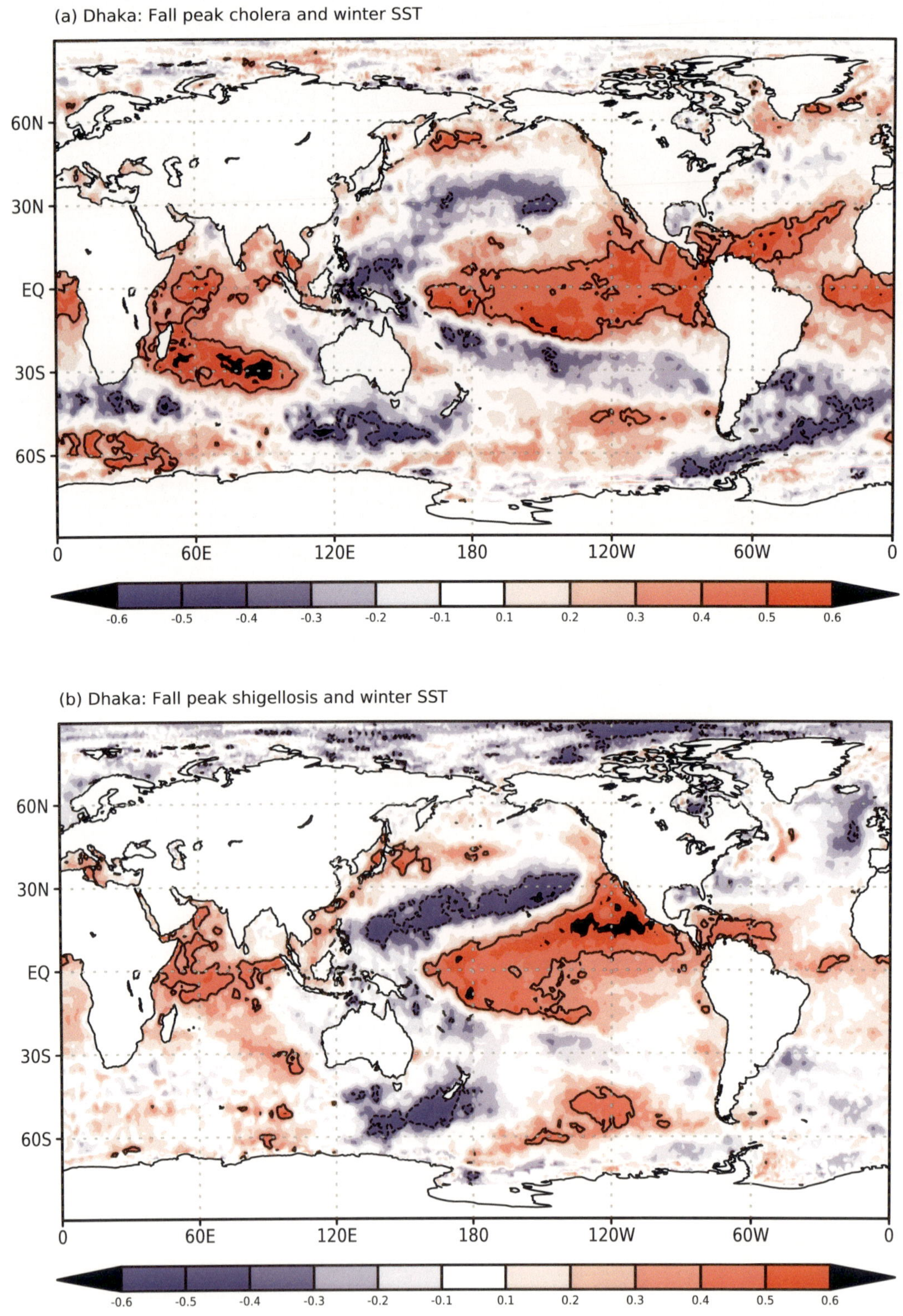

Figure 3. Rank-correlation maps for Dhaka (a) fall peak (August-December; ASOND) El Tor cholera and (b) ASOND *S. flexneri* shigellosis cases and preceding December-February sea surface temperature (SST). Maps are correlated at a value of 0.72 for the subregion (35S, 35N).

0.01; correlation is negligible if 1992–1994 are included). We do not find similar elevated values for this period in Dhaka. In addition, while 2007 was a year of heavy flooding and increased cholera prevalence in Dhaka, cases are relatively low in the Matlab record.

It is not known whether the inconsistencies in the cholera records for the two locations reflect sampling differences between

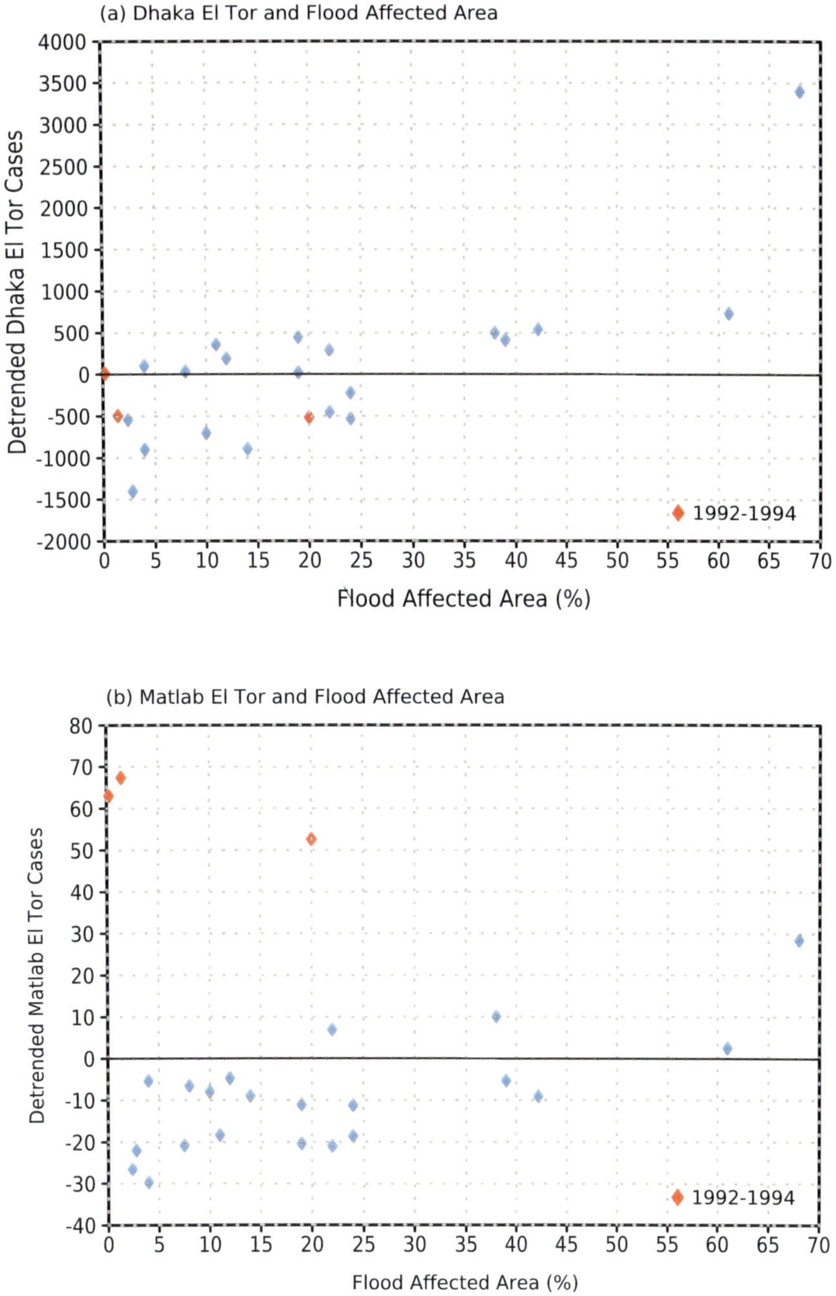

Figure 4. (a) Flood Affected Area (FAA) and linearly detrended fall peak (August-December; ASOND) Matlab El Tor cholera cases. Rank correlation of 0.56 when 1992–1994 removed. (b) FAA and linearly detrended ASOND Dhaka El Tor cholera incidence. Rank correlation of 0.74.

the large, urban environment of Dhaka and the smaller, more rural environment of Matlab, or if they reflect a degree of localization in outbreaks. One difference in the sampling methodology is that in Matlab only patients who come from the Health and Demographic Surveillance System (HDSS) area are included in the study, while in Dhaka any patient who arrives at the hospital is included. It should also be noted that 1992–1994 is the period in which 0139 Bengal emerged in Bangladesh, and this may be related to the unusual values from Matlab.

For shigellosis there is somewhat greater scatter at lower levels of FAA (Fig. 5) than for cholera, perhaps reflecting the fact that shigellosis requires a much smaller infectious dose than cholera [6]. Overall the correlation with FAA is comparable to that of cholera (0.74 and 0.50 for Matlab and Dhaka, respectively, $p << 0.01$). Interestingly, the 1992–1994 period is unremarkable for shigellosis in Matlab but is a partial outlier for Dhaka (note that correlation between Dhaka shigellosis and NINO34 increases from 0.21 to 0.41 if these years are removed), further suggesting that enteric disease in Bangladesh during these three years merits additional investigation.

The above analysis establishes that the annual flood affected area provides a clear predictor for the number of diarrheal disease cases in Bangladesh during the fall peak. However, it does so at very short leads. The fall peak (ASOND) overlaps with the end of

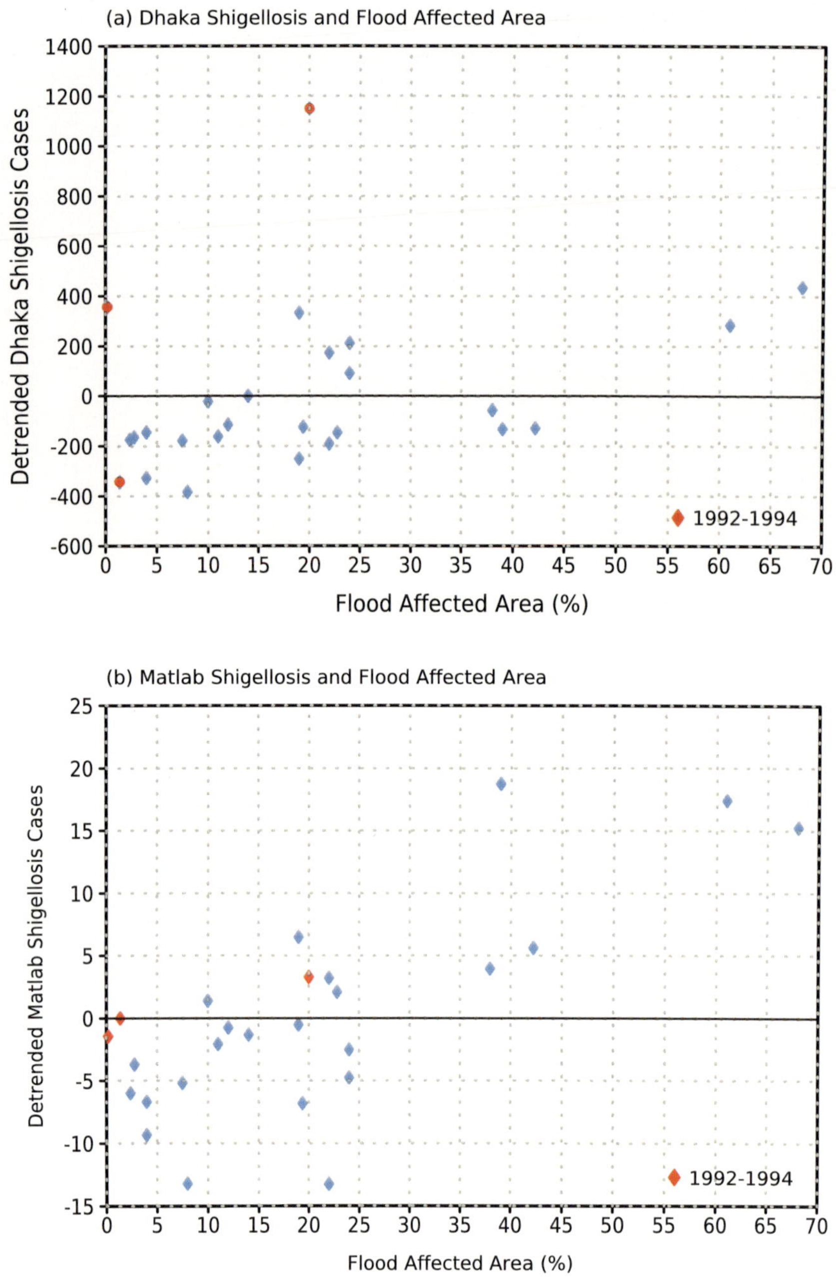

Figure 5. (a) Flood Affected Area (FAA) and linearly detrended fall peak (August-December; ASOND) Matlab *S. flexneri* shigellosis cases. Rank correlation of 0.74. (b) FAA and linearly detrended ASOND Dhaka *S. flexneri* shigellosis incidence. Rank correlation of 0.50.

the monsoon period (JJAS), providing only limited advanced warning for public health officials. In order to increase the lead-time of risk forecasts, we further explore the link between disease cases and ENSO (Figs. 2 and 3) in light of the association between disease cases and flooding (Figs. 4 and 5). Years with FAA below 30% are not strongly associated with the value of the NINO34 index (Fig. 6) for any of the three preceding seasons considered (December-January-February, DJF; March-April-May, MAM; June-July-August, JJA). FAA values above 30%, however, are not seen following negative DJF NINO34 values (Fig. 6a). For MAM (Fig. 6b) and JJA (Fig. 6c), these more severe floods can be associated with either positive or negative values of the NINO34 index. Hence, ENSO indices for the spring and summer seasons cannot be used to discriminate between strong and weak flooding years and thus high and low risk disease seasons.

Summary and Conclusions

Cholera and shigellosis are two prominent diarrheal illnesses that together are responsible for significant mortality and morbidity throughout the developing world, including Bangladesh. The causative organisms, *V. cholerae* and *S. flexneri*, differ significantly in their ecology, transmission pathways, and infectious doses, among other features. Despite these differences, our analysis of case data taken from two separate surveillance sites in Bangladesh demonstrates that interannual variations in the severity of the fall outbreaks of both diseases are closely and

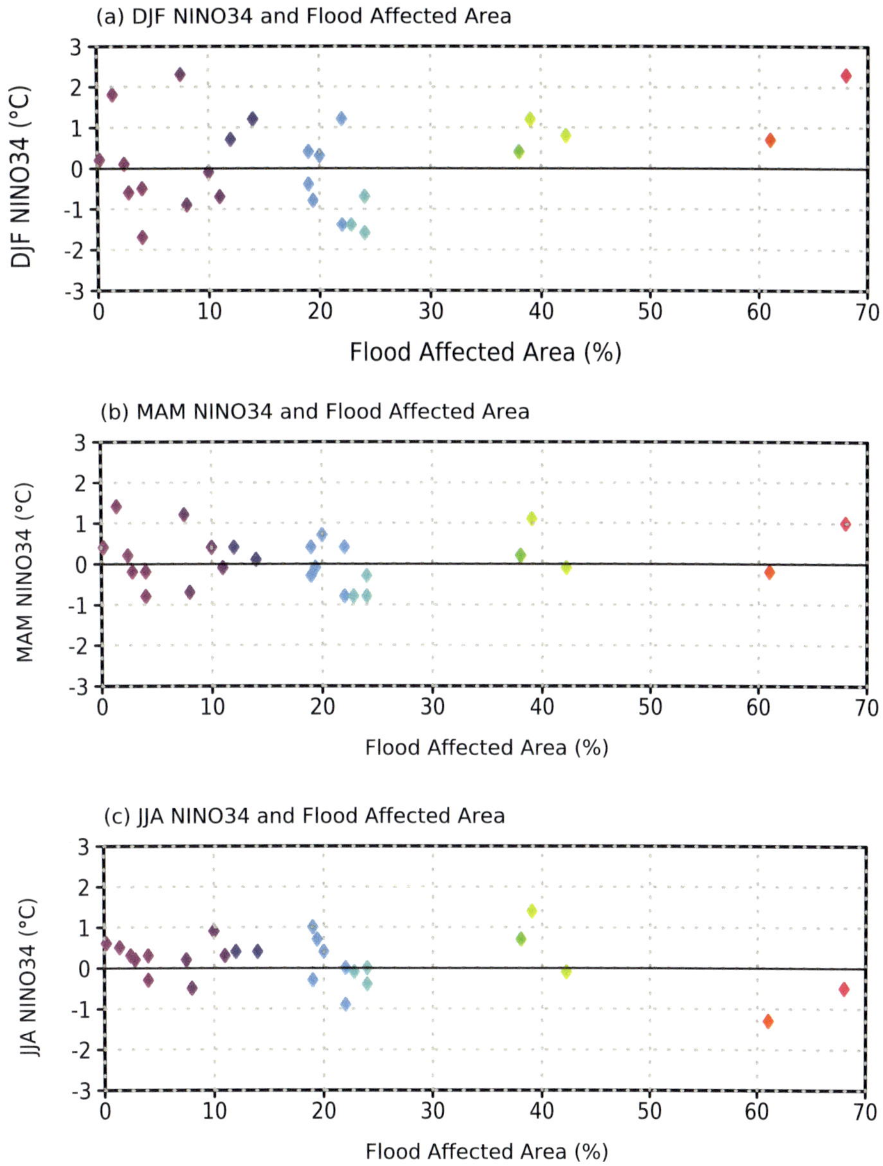

Figure 6. Flood Affected Area (FAA) versus (a) December-February (DJF) NINO34 index, (b) March-May (MAM) NINO34 index, and (c) June-August (JJA) NINO34 index.

similarly associated with the areal extent of the annual monsoon floods. Of potentially greater significance, particularly from the perspective of risk forecasting, we also find that both the monsoon floods and post-monsoon disease outbreaks are significantly correlated with ENSO activity in the preceding winter.

This association between winter ENSO and Bangladesh flooding is consistent with previous work [29], which identified a linear relationship between flooding and DJF NINO34 values. However, that study did not address the asymmetry between positive and negative ENSO events, or the variations in flooding between positive events. Recent work [30] suggests that the lag of two seasons between ENSO during DJF and the summer monsoon flooding is related to the excitation of a coupled air-sea mode of variability in the Indian Ocean region, which allows the impact of DJF ENSO anomalies to persist into summer. It is interesting to note that the magnitude of the flooding is not strongly correlated with the magnitude of the index, indicating that more than just ENSO is playing a role.

The striking similarity in the association between cholera and shigella and climate variability, despite the significant differences in the ecology of the two pathogens, strongly suggests that the two diseases share a similar transmission pathway in the post-monsoon period. Flooding inevitably increases the potential for exposure to contaminated water, an increase in risk likely to be exacerbated by the attendant overcrowding and breakdown in sanitary infrastructure. Flooding also, inevitably, subjects individuals to heightened stress, which is known to affect immune response and increases susceptibility to infectious disease [31]. While the relationship between flooding and El Tor cases in Bangladesh has been noted before (e.g., [13], [22–23], as has as an increase in shigellosis for the large flooding events or 1988, 1998 and 2004 [17], this general association between flooding, cholera, and shigellosis has not been explored previously.

The association between flooding and shigellosis, in conjunction with the association between flooding and cholera is of particular interest because it demonstrates that the association between post-monsoon cholera cases and flooding is not unique. Rather it suggests that it is the general increase in exposure risk of the human population that follows flooding, rather than the specific ecology of any one pathogen, which underlies the impact of climate variability on diarrheal disease in Bangladesh. In particular our analysis demonstrates that a long-lived environmental reservoir connected to primary transmission, which is known to exist for cholera but not for shigellosis, is not a necessary condition for flooding to drive post-monsoon disease cases in. It instead suggests that climate variability acts by modulating secondary transmission, where the latter can involve different pathways, through water or food or person to person contact, and is characterized by a dependency on previous levels of infection in the population [16].

Our findings have focused on the post-monsoon season in part because of the established role of ENSO during the preceding winter on cholera during this part of the year, through the pathway of increased precipitation and flooding. It is worth mentioning however that the disease exhibits an additional, pre-monsoon, peak and the overall seasonal pattern is known to vary regionally, in particular with respect to the relative importance of the two seasons [22], [24]. Comparisons with other diarrheal diseases at this regional level would be informative. Similarly, comparison of spatio-temporal patterns within a large urban environment such as Dhaka would further elucidate similarities and differences in epidemiology, especially given the reported heterogeneity within the city itself in the response to ENSO [18].

Linking cholera and shigellosis to flooding provides a physical mechanism for environmental influence on the interannual variability of the two diseases; linking flooding to ENSO provides a potential mechanism for forecasting risk. Our analysis shows that the most severe flooding events in Bangladesh follow warm winter conditions in the central and eastern tropical Pacific; none follow cold conditions. This relationship allows for an initial prediction of flooding and disease risk to be made as early as the end of the boreal winter; the risk of severe flooding and associated disease outbreaks should be substantially reduced when ENSO is in a negative state. Understanding why severe flooding follows warm winter Pacific SST in only a subset of years, as well as why the relationship is not linear with the magnitude of the SST anomalies is critical to improving the accuracy of disease risk forecasts, and is the subject of ongoing research. Likewise, expanding comparative analysis to include other water-borne and vector-borne infections should further refine our understanding of the fundamental processes underlying the connections between climate variability and disease outbreaks.

Author Contributions

Conceived and designed the experiments: BAC MP. Performed the experiments: BAC. Analyzed the data: BAC XR ME MY AF MP. Contributed reagents/materials/analysis tools: BAC XR ME MY AF MP. Contributed to the writing of the manuscript: BAC XR ME MY AF MP.

References

1. Kohn GC (1995) Encyclopedia of plague and pestilence. New York: Wordsworth Reference, 408 pp.
2. Cook GC (1996) Management of cholera: the vital role of rehydration. In: Cholera and the Ecology of *Vibrio Cholerae*, (B. S. Drasar and B. D. Forrest, Eds) Suffolk: Chapman and Hall, 54–94.
3. Ali M, Lopez AL, You YA, Kim YE, Sah B, et al. (2012) The global burden of cholera. Bull World Health Organ 90: 209–218, doi:10.2471/BLT.11.093427
4. Rahaman MM, Khan MM, Aziz KMS, Islam MS, Kibriya AK (1975) An outbreak of dysentery caused by *Shigella dysenteriae* type 1 on a Coral Island in the Bay of Bengal. The Journal of Infectious Diseases 132: 15–19.
5. Kotloff KL, Winickoff JP, Ivanoff B, Clemens JD, Swerdlow DL, et al. (1999) Global burden of *Shigella* infections: implications for vaccine development and implementation of control strategies. Bull World Health Organ, 77: 651–666.
6. Emch M, Ali Md, Yunus Md (2008) Risk areas and neighborhood-level risk factors for *Shigella dysenteriae 1* and *Shigella flexneri*. Health & Place 14: 96–105.
7. Pascual M, Rodó X, Ellner SP, Colwell RR, Bouma MJ (2000) Cholera dynamics and El Niño-Southern Oscillation. Science 8: 1766–1769.
8. Pascual M, Bouma MJ, Dobson AP (2002) Cholera and climate: revisiting the quantitative evidence. Microbes Infect 4: 237–245.
9. Rodó X, Pascual M, Fuchs G, Faruque ASG (2002) ENSO and cholera: A nonstationary link related to climate change? PNAS 99: 12901–12906.
10. Koelle K, Pascual M (2004) Disentangling extrinsic from intrinsic factors in disease dynamics: A nonlinear time series approach with an application to cholera. American Naturalist 163: 901–913.
11. Cash BA, Rodó X, Kinter III JL (2008) Links between tropical Pacific SST and cholera incidence in Bangladesh: Role of the eastern and central tropical Pacific. J Climate 21: 4647–4663.
12. Cash BA, Rodó X, Kinter III JL, Yunus Md (2010) Disentangling the impact of ENSO and Indian Ocean variability on the regional climate of Bangladesh: Implications for cholera risk. J Climate 23: 2817–2831.
13. Koelle K, Rodó X, Pascual M, Yunus Md, Mostafa G (2005) Refractory periods and climate forcing in cholera dynamics. Nature 436: 696–700.
14. Colwell RR (1996) Global climate and infectious disease: The cholera paradigm. Science 274: 2025–2031.
15. Lipp EK, Huq A, Colwell RR (2002) Effects of global climate on infectious disease: the cholera model. Clinical Microbiology Reviews 15: 757–770.
16. Codeço CT, Coelho FC (2006) Trends in Cholera Epidemiology. PLoS Med 3: e42; doi:10.1371/journal.pmed.0030042 [Online 31 January 2006].
17. Schwartz BS, Harris JB, Khan AI, Larocque RC, Sack DA, et al. (2006) Diarrheal epidemics in dhaka, bangladesh, during three consecutive floods: 1988, 1998, and 2004. Am J Trop Med Hyg 74: 1067–1073.
18. Reiner RC Jr, King AA, Emch M, Yunus Md, Faruque ASG, Pascual M (2012) Highly localized sensitivity to climate forcing drives endemic cholera in a megacity. PNAS 109: 2033–2036.
19. Rinaldo A, Bertuzzo E, Mari L, Righetto L, Blokesch M, et al. (2012) Reassessment of the 2010–2011 Haiti cholera outbreak and rainfall-driven multiseason projections. PNAS 109: 6602–6607, doi:10.1073/pnas.1203333109.
20. Hossain Md S (2009) Annual flood report 2009. 76 pp, Bangladesh Flood Warning and Forecast Center, Dhaka, Bangladesh.
21. Koelle K, Pascual M, Yunus Md (2005) Pathogen adaptation to seasonal forcing and climate change. Pro. Royal Soc, B 272: 971–977.
22. Akanda AS, Jutla AS, Islam S (2009) Dual peak cholera transmission in Bengal Delta: A hydroclimatological explanation. Geophys Res Lett 36: L19401.
23. Akanda AS, Jutla AS, Alam M, de Magny GC, Siddique AK, et al. (2011) Hydroclimatic influences on seasonal and spatial cholera transmission cycles: Implications for public health intervention in the Bengal Delta. Water Resour. Res 47: doi:10.1029/2010WR009914 [Online 10 May 2011].
24. Bertuzzo E, Mari L, Righetto L, Gatto M, Casagrandi R (2012) Hydroclimatology of dual-peak annual cholera incidence: Insights from a spatially explicit model. Geophys Res Lett 39: doi:10.1029/2011GL050723 [Online 10 March 2012].
25. Rayner NA, et al. (2003) Global analyses of sea surface temperature, sea ice, and night marine air temperature since the late nineteenth century. J Geophys Res 108: doi:10.1029/2002JD002670 [Online 17 July 2003].
26. Ghil M., et al. (2002) Advanced spectral methods for climatic time series. Reviews of Geophysics 40: 1.1–1.41.
27. Cash BA, Rodó X, Ballester J, Bouma MJ, Baeza A, et al. (2013) Malaria epidemics and the influence of the tropical South Atlantic on the Indian monsoon. Nature Climate Change 3: 502–507.
28. Kraft CH, van Eden C (1968) *A nonparametric introduction to statistics*. The Macmillan Company.
29. Chowdhury MR, Ward MN (2007) Seasonal flooding in Bangladesh – variability and predictability. Hydro Proc 21: 335–347.
30. Kosaka Y, Xie S-P, Lau N-C, Vecchi G (2013) Origin of seasonal predictability for summer climate over the Northwestern Pacific. PNAS 110: 7574–7579.
31. Marsland AL, Bachen AH, Cohen S, Rabin B, Manuck SB (2002) Stress, immune reactivity and susceptibility to infectious disease. Physiology and Behavior 711–716.

The Periplasmic Enzyme, AnsB, of *Shigella flexneri* Modulates Bacterial Adherence to Host Epithelial Cells

Divya T. George[1], Ulrike Mathesius[2], Carolyn A. Behm[1], Naresh K. Verma[1]*

1 Division of Biomedical Science and Biochemistry, Research School of Biology, The Australian National University, Canberra, Australia, **2** Division of Plant Science, Research School of Biology, The Australian National University, Canberra, Australia

Abstract

S. flexneri strains, most frequently linked with endemic outbreaks of shigellosis, invade the colonic and rectal epithelium of their host and cause severe tissue damage. Here we have attempted to elucidate the contribution of the periplasmic enzyme, L-asparaginase (AnsB) to the pathogenesis of *S. flexneri*. Using a reverse genetic approach we found that *ansB* mutants showed reduced adherence to epithelial cells *in vitro* and attenuation in two *in vivo* models of shigellosis, the *Caenorhabditis elegans* and the murine pulmonary model. To investigate how AnsB affects bacterial adherence, we compared the proteomes of the *ansB* mutant with its wild type parental strain using two dimensional differential in-gel electrophoresis and identified the outer membrane protein, OmpA as up-regulated in *ansB* mutant cells. Bacterial OmpA, is a prominent outer membrane protein whose activity has been found to be required for bacterial pathogenesis. Overexpression of OmpA in wild type *S. flexneri* serotype 3b resulted in decreasing the adherence of this virulent strain, suggesting that the up-regulation of OmpA in *ansB* mutants contributes to the reduced adherence of this mutant strain. The data presented here is the first report that links the metabolic enzyme AnsB to *S. flexneri* pathogenesis.

Editor: Rajeev Misra, Arizona State University, United States of America

Funding: The authors have no support or funding to report.

Competing Interests: The authors have declared that no competing interests exist.

* E-mail: Naresh.Verma@anu.edu.au

Introduction

Shigellosis, more commonly known as bacillary dysentery, is a diarrhoeal infirmity ensuing from an acute inflammatory reaction in the gastrointestinal (GI) tract caused by the enteric bacterium *Shigella*. There are four recognized species of the genus *Shigella*, namely *S. flexneri*, *S. dysenteriae*, *S. boydii*, and *S. sonnei* [1]. Of the four species, *S. flexneri* strains are most frequently linked with endemic outbreaks of shigellosis in the developing world. *S. flexneri* invades the colonic and rectal epithelium of its host and causes severe tissue damage, which manifests in a spectrum of clinical symptoms ranging from watery diarrhea to severe dysentery characterized by fever, abdominal cramping and bloody mucoid stool [2]. Most cases of shigellosis are self-limiting, however in certain individuals, especially malnourished infants, untreated disease can result in several complications which can be fatal [3].

Although a lot has been unraveled about the various steps involved in the pathogenesis of *S. flexneri*, a complete picture of the bacterial genes that are expressed exclusively during infection of host cells has not been elucidated. A clear understanding of bacterial genes expressed at various host-pathogen interfaces can pave the way to the identification of potential attenuation targets and vaccine candidate antigens. In an attempt to identify immunogenic proteins expressed during infection, Jennison and colleagues [4] used 2-dimensional gel electrophoresis (2-DE) followed by immunoblotting with sera from convalescent shigellosis patients, to screen the soluble and membrane protein profiles of *S. flexneri* 2457T. In their study, the chromosomally encoded, metabolic, periplasmic enzyme, L-asparaginase (AnsB) was identified to be immunogenic. This protein is of interest as AnsB has been found to be antigenic in a number of other enteric bacterial species [5–8], and has not been characterized in *S. flexneri*, thereby making it a potential attenuation target for vaccine development.

The *E. coli* L-asparaginase (AnsB) protein, which shares 99.1% amino acid identity with *S. flexneri* AnsB, is an enzyme that converts asparagine to aspartate and ammonia. AnsB has high affinity for L-asparagine and the expression of *ansB* is induced by anaerobiosis and positively regulated by the cyclic AMP receptor protein (CRP) and the product of the *fnr* gene [9].

In this study, a reverse genetic approach was used to characterize AnsB in *S. flexneri* and determine if this enzyme is required for bacterial pathogenesis. Recombineering, a lambda red-mediated PCR-based approach [10], was used to knockout the *ansB* gene from a virulent, wild type serotype 3b strain of *S. flexneri*. The effect of *ansB* mutation on bacterial physiology and virulence was analyzed using *in vitro* growth studies, cell culture assays and two *in vivo* models of shigellosis, namely the murine pulmonary model and the *C. elegans* infection model, a new potential animal model of shigellosis [11]. The results of this study indicate that the activity of AnsB is required during the initial stages of bacterial pathogenesis, as *in vitro* bacterial adherence assays clearly showed that *ansB* mutants had decreased adherence to host cells. To gain further insight into how AnsB affects bacterial adherence, we screened the proteomes of the *ansB* mutant and wild type *S. flexneri* strains and found that mutant cells up-regulate the expression of the prominent outer membrane protein, OmpA. These findings highlight the importance of AnsB in the pathogenesis of *S. flexneri*, paving the way to designing new therapeutic or vaccine strategies.

Materials and Methods

All mice experiments were performed under the protocol approved by the Australian National University Experimentation Ethics Committee.

Bacterial strains and growth conditions

All *S. flexneri* strains used were derivatives of the highly virulent *S. flexneri* 3b strain, SFL1520, obtained from the International Centre for Diarrhoeal Diseases Research Bangladesh (ICDDRB). Bacterial cultures were grown routinely in Luria Bertani (LB) broth or on LB agar plates. Where appropriate, antibiotic selection was with ampicillin (100 µg/mL) and/or kanamycin (50 µg/mL). For growth studies under nutrient stress, Minimal Essential media (MM) was used. *E. coli* strains were grown and maintained at 37°C, while *S. flexneri* cultures were grown at 30°C to maintain the virulence plasmid.

Recombinant DNA methods

Restriction endonucleases (New England Biolabs), alkaline phosphatase (Fermentas) and T4 DNA ligase (Promega) were used in accordance with the manufacturer's specifications. Plasmids were maintained in the *E. coli* strain JM109 [12] and isolated using the alkaline lysis method [13] or the QIAprep Spin MiniPrep kit (Qiagen). All primers were synthesized by Sigma-Aldrich. All sequencing was performed at the Biomolecular Resource Facility, Australian National University. PCR was carried out using the high fidelity *PfuUltraII* polymerase (Stratagene) for cloning and sequencing or *iTaq* (Scientifix) for screening.

Construction of mutant strains

Recombineering was used to generate knockouts in SFL1520. A linear knockout template consisting of the *kanamycin* resistance gene flanked by ~1000 bp regions showing homology to the upstream and downstream regions of each of the target genes was generated using PCR. Electrocompetent cells of the wild-type SFL1520, transformed with either of the helper plasmids pKD46 or pKM208 [10], were prepared. Freshly prepared electrocompetent cells were transformed with 1–2 µg of each purified knockout template. Transformed cells were recovered in Super Optimal Broth with Catabolite repression (SOC) [14] for 4 hours to allow for homologous recombination. Recovered cells were plated on LB agar containing 50 µg/mL kanamycin and incubated at 30°C for up to 3 days. Resulting colonies were routinely restreaked onto fresh LB agar plates containing 50 µg/mL kanamycin to eliminate false positives. Colonies were then screened for successful gene disruption by colony PCR and sequencing, after which the presence of the virulence plasmid in both mutant strains was confirmed using PCR to amplify two virulence plasmid indicator genes, *apyI* and *virG*. These genes were chosen as they lie on opposite sides of the 220 kb virulence plasmid.

Growth studies

Overnight cultures of strains were diluted 1:20 in LB as well as MM and sampled at 30 minute intervals. Growth studies were carried out at 30°C and 37°C under aerobic conditions.

SDS PAGE and Western Blot

The secretion of type 3 effector proteins was induced using congo red (final concentration 10 mM) for 30 minutes. Bacterial cells were harvested by centrifugation and the supernatants were passed through 0.45 µm filters to eliminate cellular debris. Secretory proteins were precipitated using 25% trichloroacetic acid (TCA) in acetone. Protein precipitates were washed twice using acetone and pellets were allowed to dry completely, after which they were resuspended in solubilization buffer (9 M urea, 4% CHAPS, 1% DTT, 1% ampholytes, 35 mM tris base). Protein concentration was estimated using the BCA kit (Pierce) according to the manufacturer's instructions and 20 µg of proteins in the supernatant samples were loaded onto 12% (v/v) SDS-PAGE gels for Western blots. The gels were stained with Coomassie Brilliant blue R250 to ensure equal loading of samples. Once samples were equalized the separated proteins were transferred onto Hybond-P PVDF membranes (Millipore) and blocked in 5% skimmed milk in Phosphate Buffered Saline (PBS) at 4°C overnight. Following blocking, the membranes were washed thrice in PBS containing 0.05% (v/v) Tween-20 (PBST) (Sigma). Membranes were then incubated with the primary antibodies (Anti-IpaB and Anti-IpaD antisera generated in-house in mice) for 2 hours. Unbound antibodies were washed off using three washes with PBST as outlined above, following which the membranes were incubated with the secondary antibodies (Anti-mouse IgG; Sigma) for 1 hour. Membranes were washed thrice as done previously. The binding of antibodies was then detected by chemiluminescence using SuperSignal West Pico Chemiluminescent Substrate (Pierce) as described by the manufacturer. Chemiluminescence was then detected using the Fisher Biotec chemiluminescence system.

Reverse transcription polymerase chain reaction (RT-PCR) and Quantitative Real-time Reverse transcription polymerase chain reaction (qRT-PCR)

For both RT-PCR and qRT-PCR, RNA was isolated using Trizol reagent (Invitorgen) according to the manufacturer's instructions. Briefly, overnight cultures of *S. flexneri* strains, (SFL1520, SFL2283 or SFL2443) were diluted 1:50 and grown to log phase at 37°C. 1×10^9 CFU were harvested and treated with 1 mL Trizol reagent followed by incubation at room temperature for 5 minutes. Samples were treated with 200 µl chloroform to separate RNA from DNA and proteins. RNA in the aqueous phase was washed with chloroform and precipitated using 2 volumes of isopropanol. RNA pellets were collected by centrifugation and washed using 1 mL freshly prepared 75% ethanol. RNA pellets were air-dried after ethanol wash and suspended in 50 µl of nuclease-free water. The isolated RNA was cleaned up using the Qiagen RNeasy Kit; this step was performed to remove any residual DNA and organic salts. Isolated RNA was treated with Turbo DNase (Ambion) to minimise any contaminating genomic DNA. cDNA was made from 200 ng of RNA using Superscript II (Invitrogen) according to the manufacturer's instructions. qRT-PCR was performed on the cDNA samples using the power SYBR Green RT-PCR kit (Applied Biosystems) according to the manufacturer's instructions except that primers were used at a final concentration of 0.4 µM and the final reaction volume was reduced to 10 µl. Expression of *hisG* was used as a control to normalize the expression of all genes studied. All Real-Time RT-PCRs were performed in triplicate with a no reverse transcriptase (NRT) and a no template control (NTC) set up for each run. Reactions were run in a Rotor-Gene Q Real-Time cycler (Qiagen).

Measurement of asparaginase activity

Asparaginase activity of SFL1520 and SFL2283 was measured using the ammonia assay kit (Sigma) with log phase culture supernatants, according to the manufacturer's instructions. Bacterial cells expressing L-asparaginase would break down asparagine with the release of ammonia, thus increased ammonia levels correlate with increased hydrolysis of asparagine. Briefly, fresh log phase cells were harvested and washed once in PBS, and 3×10^8 colony forming units (CFU) of bacteria was resuspended in 1 ml PBS with 5 mM asparagine. Aliquots were taken after 30, 60, 90 and 180 minutes of incubation at 37°C and centrifuged to collect bacterial cells. The ammonia concentration in the cell-free supernatants was measured using the ammonia assay kit, according to the manufacturer's guidelines.

In vitro adherence assay

BHK cells in 6-well plates were infected with 4×10^8 CFU of each bacterial strain. Bacterial cells were allowed to infect the monolayer for 90 minutes at 37°C, 5% CO_2. Unbound bacterial cells were washed off the BHK monolayer using PBS, after which the mammalian cells were lysed using 0.05% (v/v) Triton-X in PBS. Appropriate dilutions of the cell lysates were plated on LB agar plates carrying the appropriate antibiotics to determine the number of adherent bacterial cells.

Coverslip adherence assay

The coverslip adherence assay was performed based on the protocol developed by Cravioto *et al*, [15]. Briefly, overnight cultures of all *S. flexneri* strains grown at 30°C were diluted and grown to log phase at 37°C ($OD_{600}=0.6$–0.8). 4×10^8 CFU of each strain was used to infect a confluent layer of BHK cells grown on coverslips placed within wells of 6-well culture plates. The plates were incubated for 90 minutes at 37°C to allow for infection. The coverslips were then washed thrice in PBS to remove any unbound bacterial cells. Samples were fixed using fresh 70% (v/v) methanol and stained for 30 minutes using 10% (v/v) Giemsa stain. Excess stain was washed off. Coverslips were mounted on glass slides and examined using an oil immersion lens.

C. elegans strains and growth conditions

The *C. elegans* wild type N2 strain [16] was used in this study. Nematodes were maintained at 22°C on modified nematode growth medium (NGM) agar medium seeded with *E. coli* OP50 [16]. A synchronous population of *C. elegans* was established by isolating eggs from adult worms through bleaching [17]. After hatching, L1 worms were transferred to NGM agar plates seeded with *E. coli* OP50 and allowed to grow at 22°C until they reached the L4 stage.

C. elegans bacterial accumulation

All bacterial strains used for the accumulation assay were grown overnight at 37°C on NG agar medium to stimulate expression of virulence plasmid-encoded genes [11]. Plates were cooled to room temperature before they were inoculated with 50–100 nematodes (L4s). The worms were allowed incubated at 22°C for 24 hours after which 10 worms were picked and washed thoroughly using sterile S-basal with 1 mM sodium azide. Worms were then treated with 200 mg/mL gentamycin for 3 hours to remove surface-bound bacterial cells, after which they were washed thoroughly to remove any residual antibiotic. Washed worms were suspended in S-basal +0.1% Triton-X and lysed by mechanical disruption using glass beads as described by [18]. Appropriate dilutions of the lysates were plated onto LB agar with the appropriate antibiotics, to obtain gut bacterial counts. In order to visualize bacterial accumulation within nematode guts, worms were fed *S. flexneri* strains tagged with GFP^+. Following 24 hours of infection, bacterial fluorescence was observed using the EVOS digital inverted microscope (AMG) and quantified using the Infinite M1000 Pro (Tecan).

C. elegans survival assays

Overnight cultures of *S. flexneri* strains maintained at 30°C were diluted 1: 50 in LB media and grown to log phase at 37°C. A synchronized population of L4 stage *C. elegans* worms was treated with 200 µg/mL gentamycin for 3 hours, after which they were washed thoroughly with S-basal to remove any residual antibiotic. Approximately 20 washed L4s were transferred into each well of a 24-well plate containing 100 µL of the appropriate log-phase bacterial culture to be tested. The volume of solution in each well was adjusted to 500 µL with S-basal and plates were incubated at 22°C. The number of live worms in each well was scored every 12 hours and the percentage survival was calculated. Worms that showed no pharyngeal pumping and remained immobile on tapping the plate were considered dead. A minimum of three replicates for each test strain was set up per trial.

Mouse pulmonary model of shigellosis

6–8 week old female Balb/c mice weighing approximately 20–25 g (Animal Resource Centre, WA) were inoculated intranasally with a sub-lethal dose (2×10^7 CFU/10 µL) of either the pathogenic wild type SFL1520 strain or SFL2283 (Δ*ansB*). The mice were lightly anesthetized with isoflurane prior to inoculation. 20 mice were euthanized 24 hours post infection and their lungs were extracted and homogenized in PBS with 0.05% Triton-X. Appropriate dilutions of the homogenates were plated on LB agar with antibiotics, where appropriate, to obtain the live counts of intracellular bacteria per lung.

Isolation of total bacterial protein for two-dimensional gel electrophoresis

Overnight cultures of SFL1520 (wild type parent) and SFL2283 (Δ*ansB*) grown in LB at 30°C were diluted 1/100 and grown to log phase at 37°C. Bacterial cells were collected and washed thrice using cell wash solution (10 mM Tris pH 8.0, 5 mM magnesium acetate). Bacterial pellets were resuspended in 500 µl of cell lysis buffer containing 7 M urea, 2 M thiourea, 30 mM tris-base, 4%(w/v) CHAPS and Complete Protease Inhibitor (Roche) and incubated on ice for 10 minutes. Subsequently, the suspensions were sonicated 10 times for 15 s with 30 s intervals, on ice. Cellular debris was sedimented by centrifugation. Supernatants were treated with 10 volumes of ice-cold acetone and incubated at −20°C overnight to precipitate proteins. The protein pellets were washed thrice using ice-cold acetone, following which they were dried. Acetone-free proteins were solubilized in 200 µl of cell lysis buffer and pH was adjusted to 8.5. For 2-dimensional (2-D) gel electrophoresis, total protein from wild type and *ansB* mutant strains were isolated in triplicate over three independent experiments. Protein concentration was determined using the BCA kit (Pierce) and 500 µg of each protein sample was labeled with fluorescent dyes Cy3 or Cy5 (GE Healthcare); an internal standard, consisting of a mixture of 250 µg of each sample, was labeled with Cy2. Samples were labeled with the CyDye DIGE Fluors (minimal dyes) for Ettan DIGE kit (GE Healthcare), according to the manufacturer's instructions, with minor modifications as described by Mathesius *et al*, 2001. Briefly, 500 µg of each protein sample was labeled with 400 pmol amine reactive cyanine freshly dissolved in anhydrous dimethyl formamide. CyDye labeling was carried out on ice and in the dark for 30 minutes. Each reaction was terminated using 10 nmol lysine to eliminate any unbound dye. Labeled samples were treated with DTT (20 mg/ml) and Bio-ampholytes (50 µl/ml). To identify differences in the proteomes of SFL1520 and SFL2283, 500 µg of total protein from the wild type parent (SFL1520) labeled with

Cy3 or Cy5 was combined with 500 μg of oppositely labeled proteins from the Δ*ansB* mutant strain. Each wild type-mutant pair was then mixed with 500 μg of the combined protein preparations of all protein samples that were labeled with Cy2 as an internal control.

2-D electrophoresis

2-D electrophoresis was performed in darkness to maintain the stability of the Cy dyes. Immobiline pH 3–10 NL Drystrips (24 cm, GE Healthcare) were used for the first dimension isoelectric focusing (IEF). The strips were rehydrated overnight in rehydration solution containing, 8 M urea, 0.5% (w/v) CHAPS, 0.2% (w/v) DTT, 0.52% (w/v) bio-ampholytes and 0.6% (w/v) bromophenol blue. Wild type-mutant pairs with internal controls were loaded onto rehydrated Immobiline strips and IEF was carried out in a Multiphor II electrophoresis system (GE Healthcare) at 20°C for a total of 35,000 volt hours [19].

For separation of proteins across the second dimension, self-cast 12.5% SDS-PAGE gels were cast using the EttanDALTsix system (GE Healthcare). The gels were cast using low fluorescence glass plates, which are compatible with visualizing the CyDyes. Focused first dimension strips were equilibrated as described by [19] and placed on the second dimension gels. SDS-PAGE was carried out at 10°C in SDS running buffer (25 mM Tris, pH 8.0, 192 mM glycine and 0.1% SDS) at 600 V, 10 mA, and 2.5 W per gel for the first hour; 600 V, 40 mA, and 13 W per gel until the bromophenol blue front reached the bottom of the gel.

Gel imaging and image analysis

After the second dimension electrophoresis, DIGE-labeled proteins were visualized using a Typhoon Trio laser scanner (GE Healthcare). Gels were scanned with the specific excitation wavelengths of Cy3 (532-nm laser and a 580-nm band pass 30 emission filter), Cy5 (633-nm laser and a 670-nm band pass 30 emission filter) and Cy2 (488-nm laser and a 580-nm band pass 40 emission filter). Spot detection and analysis was carried out using DeCyder Version 5 (GE Healthcare) software followed by careful manual confirmation and rematching of matching errors. Statistics and identification of differentially expressed spots were carried out in the DeCyder DIA and BVA modules (one-way ANOVA).

In-gel trypsin digestion of protein spots and mass spectrometry

After analysis of gel images, identified spots of interest were excised from the 2D-DIGE gels using an Ettan spot picker (GE Healthcare). The spot picker was calibrated and tested several times prior to spot excision. In-gel trypsin digest was carried out as described by Mathesius *et al*, 2001 with a few modifications. Briefly, excised protein spots were washed four times in acetonitrile: 50 mM ammonium bicarbonate (50:50, v/v). Spots were then dried in 100% acetonitrile for 30 minutes following which they were air-dried to eliminate all acetonitrile. Gel pieces were then rehydrated with a trypsin solution (20 units; Promega) and incubated for 2 hours at 4°C followed by overnight incubation at 37°C. Peptides were then extracted from the gel pieces using an extraction buffer consisting of acetonitrile: water: trifluroacetuic acid (TFA) (50%:50%:1%, v/v) followed by gentle sonication in a sonic water bath for 40 minutes. This extraction step was performed twice using a reduced volume of extraction buffer and 20 minutes sonication. Peptides were collected and dried completely to remove all traces of TFA. Dried peptides were resuspended in 20 μl of acetonitrile:water:formic acid (10%:89.9%:0.1%, v/v) of which 6 μl were loaded onto the mass spectrometer. The peptides were identified at the Mass Spectrometry Facility, The Australian National University, on an Agilent 6530 Q-TOF LC/MS (Santa Clara, CA, USA) with a ChipCube ion source interface (Agilent Technologies, Inc., Palo Alto, CA) containing a liquid chromatographic chip (ProtID-Chip-150(II), separation: 150 mm×75 μm, enrichment: 4 mm 40 nL, packed with 5 μm Zorbax 300SB-C18 particles) The LC separation system included a binary capillary pump operated at a flow rate of 4 μL/min, used for loading the samples, and a nanoflow gradient pump using a linear gradient from 8 to 38% mobile phase B in 47 min at a flow rate of 300 nL/min. The column was then washed with 90% mobile phase B for 5 min. Mobile phase A 0.1% formic acid and mobile phase B was 90% acetonitrile/water containing 0.1% formic acid.

The spray from the chip was subjected to positive polarity electrospray ionisation (ESI) using the following settings: gas flow rate 4 L/min, gas temperature 300°C, capillary voltage 1900 V, fragmentor 175 V, skimmer 65 V and octopole RF peak 750 V. The instrument was run in extended dynamic range mode with data dependent acquisition switching between MS (m/z 100–1700 at 3 spectra/s) and MS/MS (m/z 50–1700 at 3 spectra/s), measuring the collision induced dissociation (CID) fragment spectra of the three most intense precursor ions with charge states 2, 3 and ≥3 with a 15 s dynamic exclusion time, within a cycle time of 1.4 s. The collision energy was automatically set by the Agilent MassHunter Acquisition software (slope 3, offset 2). The m/z values of all ions present in the mass spectra were corrected against two reference ions (purine, $[MH]^+$ m/z 112.985587 and 1H, 1H, 3H tetra(fluoropropoxy)phosphazine, $[MH]^+$ m/z 922.0097). Data was acquired and analysed with Agilent Technologies MassHunter software (version B.4.0).

Proteins were identified through Peptide Mass Fingerprinting using MASCOT (Matrix Science). One missed cleavage per peptide was allowed and a mass tolerance between 0.3 and 0.1 Da was used in all searches. Carbamidomethylation was set as a fixed modification and oxidation (M) as a variable. We searched the Ludwig database under taxonomy *Shigella flexneri* on the MASCOT database at the Australian Proteomic Computation Facility (APCF).

Results

Insertional inactivation of *ansB* in the wild type *S. flexneri* serotype 3b strain

The *ansB* gene was successfully disrupted in wild type *S. flexneri* serotype 3b (SFL1520) using recombineering to produce *ΔansB* (SFL2283). Excessive handling and manipulation of *S. flexneri* strains often results in the loss of the virulence plasmid, therefore the presence of the virulence plasmid in *S. flexneri* serotype 3b (SFL1520) and *ΔansB* (SFL2283) was confirmed by PCR before every virulence assay performed in this study as described in the methods.

S. flexneri virulence-plasmid encoded invasion protein antigens (Ipa) are important components of the type three secretion needle complex, required for virulence. In order to determine whether *ΔansB* (SFL2283) efficiently expressed and secreted virulence-plasmid encoded proteins, we investigated the expression and secretory levels of IpaB and IpaD, two key components of the type three secretory apparatus, using western immunoblots. Western immunoblots showed no differences in the expression and secretion of IpaB and IpaD in *ΔansB* (SFL2283) and the wild type serotype 3b strains (SFL1520) (Figure S1), thus suggesting that expression and secretion of key virulence plasmid-encoded proteins remain unaffected by the *ansB* mutation.

Prior to carrying out any physiological studies, we confirmed that the *ansB* gene was expressed in wild type serotype 3b (SFL1520) when grown *in vitro* under nutrient rich and starved conditions, using reverse transcriptase PCR (RT-PCR) (data not shown). AnsB is an identified L-asparaginase in *E. coli*; to determine if this function was conserved in *S. flexneri*, we used an ammonia assay to measure levels of ammonia released when bacterial cells were treated with asparagine. Ammonia assays showed that wild type *S. flexneri* serotype 3b (carrying intact *ansB*) released significantly more ammonia than the Δ*ansB* strain (Figure 1). These results suggest that AnsB in *S. flexneri* functions as an L-asparaginase.

The activity of AnsB is not essential for bacterial growth *in vitro*

Once we established that the *ansB* gene was expressed and functional in *S. flexneri* serotype 3b when grown *in vitro*, we carried out *in vitro* growth studies to determine whether the metabolic activity of AnsB was required for bacterial growth. No mutation-related growth retardation was observed when strains were grown under nutrient rich (LB media) conditions at both 37°C and 30°C (Figure S2.A). To determine if *ansB* expression was required for growth under stress conditions, growth studies were carried out under reduced nutrient conditions using minimal essential salts media (MM) (Figure S2.B). No significant ($p>0.05$, unpaired t-test) growth retardation was exhibited by the *ansB* mutant strain, suggesting that, although this metabolic gene is expressed, its activity is not vital for bacterial growth *in vitro*.

AnsB activity is required for *S. flexneri* adherence to baby hamster kidney (BHK) cells

in vitro adherence assays were performed to investigate whether the activity of AnsB contributed to bacterial adherence to epithelial cells. The Δ*ansB* (SFL2283) strain showed a significant drop in the number of adherent bacteria when compared with the wild type parental strain (SFL1520) (Figure 2.A). This decrease in adherence was restored upon complementation of the *ansB* mutation in SFL2309 (SFL2283 + plasmid expressing *ansB*).

In order to visualize the differences in adherence patterns of the mutant and wild type strains, a coverslip adherence assay was performed. Giemsa staining of infected BHK monolayers also showed a decrease in the number of adherent bacteria in monolayers infected with Δ*ansB* (SFL2283) (Figure 2.C) compared with wild type *S. flexneri* 3b (SFL1520) (Figure 2.B) and the ansB complemented strain SFL2309 (Figure 2.D). The number of adherent bacteria per BHK cell was determined in order to validate the microscopic findings. Δ*ansB* (SFL2283) cells showed a significant drop in the number of adherent bacterial cells when compared with SFL1520 and SFL2309 (Figure 2.E).

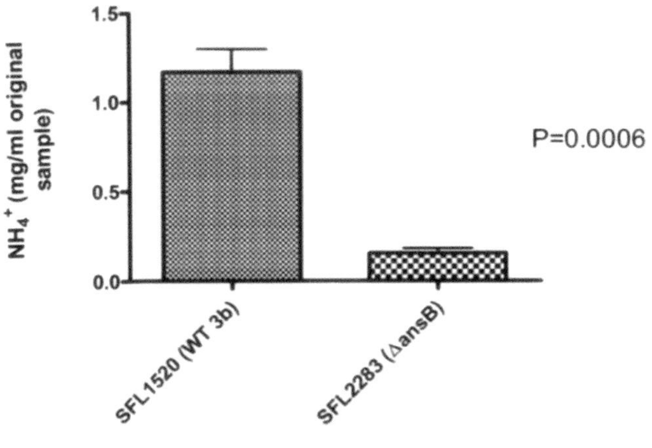

Figure 1. AnsB in *S. flexneri* hydrolyses asparagine. *S. flexneri* parental strain SFL1520 or isogenic mutant Δ*ansB* (SFL2283) at 3×10^8 colony forming units (CFU) per ml were incubated in phosphate buffered saline (PBS) with 5 mM asparagine. Ammonia production was measured after 60 minutes incubation at 37°C. Hydrolysis of asparagine was measured by quantifying ammonia production. There is a significant drop in the levels of released ammonia by *ansB* mutant cells ($p = 0.0006$, unpaired t-test). Error bars represent the standard error of means obtained from three independent experimental measurements.

AnsB activity is required for *S. flexneri*-mediated killing and bacterial accumulation in the intestinal lumen of *C. elegans*

To determine if the reduced adherence observed *in vitro* in the Δ*ansB* (SFL2283) strain had an effect on bacterial virulence; preliminary *in vivo* studies were carried out in *C. elegans*. Kesika and colleagues have previously reported that virulent *S. flexneri* serotype 2b kills *C. elegans* in liquid culture [18]. We performed liquid killing assays to compare the killing rates of Δ*ansB* (SFL2283) and wild type *S. flexneri* serotype 3b. *C. elegans* fed wild type *S. flexneri* 3b (SFL1520) died much faster (with 50% killing (TD_{50}) = 42±1 h) than worms maintained on Δ*ansB* (SFL2283) (<50% killing in 48 h) (Figure 3.A).

Burton E.A. *et al* [11] have demonstrated that virulent *S. flexneri* strains accumulate in the intestinal lumen and kill *C. elegans*, while avirulent *S. flexneri* strains are digested by the nematodes. To determine whether the survival of nematodes fed the Δ*ansB* strain correlated with low intraluminal bacterial numbers, *C. elegans* bacterial accumulation assays were performed. Results of bacterial accumulation assays correlate with nematode killing, as the wild type *S. flexneri* 3b strain (SFL1520) accumulated within the gut of the worms, while Δ*ansB* (SFL2283) cells were digested by the nematodes (Figure 3.B). Complementation of the *ansB* mutation restored the intestinal accumulation phenotype of the wild type strain.

In order to visualize bacterial accumulation, nematodes were fed GFP^+ tagged *S. flexneri* strains. Consistent with the bacterial accumulation assays, worms fed wild type *S. flexneri* 3b (SFL1520) showed accumulation of GFP^+ tagged bacterial cells within their intestinal lumen (Figure 3.C), while those fed the Δ*ansB* (SFL2283) strain failed to show GFP^+ accumulation (Figure 3.D). GFP^+ accumulation assays could not be carried out using the complemented strain as the plasmid expressing GFP^+ was not compatible with the plasmid used for the complementation of *ansB* mutation.

The enhanced survival of nematodes fed Δ*ansB* (SFL2283) and digestion of wild type *S. flexneri* 3b following mutation of *ansB* suggests that this metabolic enzyme is required for bacterial virulence.

AnsB activity is required for *S. flexneri* infection in the murine pulmonary model of shigellosis

Since preliminary *in vivo* studies in *C. elegans* indicated that the *ansB* mutant showed reduced virulence, the virulence of this strain was also assessed using the murine pulmonary model, an established animal model of shigellosis [21–23]. Virulent strains of *S. flexneri*, when inoculated intranasally, colonize the lungs of infected mice and cause pneumonia. The lung counts obtained from mice inoculated with the Δ*ansB* strain 24 hours post infection were significantly lower than the wild type strain ($p = 0.0035$,

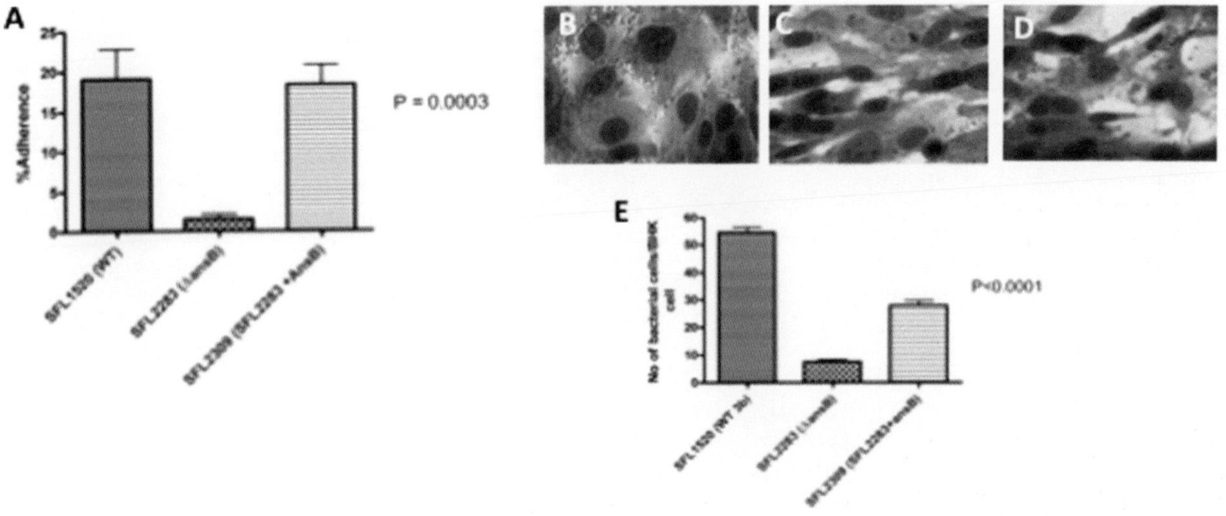

Figure 2. AnsB activity required for *S. flexneri* adherence to baby hamster kidney (BHK) cells. Results of *in vitro* adherence assays for wild type *S. flexneri* serotype 3b (SFL1520), Δ*ansB* (SFL2283) and complemented strain SFL2309 (SFL2283 + *ansB*). **A:** Bacterial adherence to baby hamster kidney cells plotted as percentage adherence, a ratio of the number of adherent and intracellular bacteria to the total number of bacterial cells in the infecting inoculum (y-axis). SFL2283 cells are significantly less adherent that SFL1520 and SFL2309 ($p = 0.0003$, One Way ANOVA). Results are the means of three independent blind repeats with standard errors. **B–D:** Results of coverslip adherence assay performed to compare the adherence of *S. flexneri* 3b wild type strain (SFL1520-**B**), Δ*ansB* (SFL2283-**C**) and complement of Δ*ansB* (SFL2309-**D**). **E:** A graph depicting the number of adherent bacteria counted per BHK cell under 1000× magnification (y-axis). The adherence of SFL2283 is significantly lower than SFL1520 and SFL2309 ($p < 0.0001$, One Way ANOVA). Results are the mean of 10 cells across 10 fields with standard errors, counted at random in a blind experiment.

unpaired t tests) (Figure 4), further demonstrating that AnsB activity is required for the virulence of *S. flexneri*.

2-Dimensional gel electrophoresis identifies changes in the *S. flexneri* proteome caused by *ansB* mutations

To gain insight into why the Δ*ansB* strain shows reduced adherence to epithelial cells, we used two dimensional differential in-gel electrophoresis (DIGE) to compare the proteomes of Δ*ansB* (SFL2283) and wild type *S. flexneri* serotype 3b (SFL1520) strains. Our proteomic studies identified 17 differentially expressed proteins in Δ*ansB* (SFL2283). Using liquid chromatography mass spectrometry (LC-MS) we identified 6 (out of 17) proteins as up-regulated in the Δ*ansB* (SFL2283) strain (RplL, Udp, Mdh, OmpA, GroEL and DnaK) (Table S1). Quantitative real-time reverse transcription polymerase chain reaction (qRT-PCR) was performed to confirm the results obtained in the DIGE analysis (Figure 5). We analysed the transcript levels of proteins identified in the DIGE analysis, in three independent biological replicates, using the bacterial *hisG* gene as a control gene to normalize the expression of all genes tested. Similar to our DIGE analysis, the expression of *rplL*, *udp*, *ompA*, *groEL* and *dnaK* was up-regulated in the Δ*ansB* (SFL2283) strain. However, no significant differences in the transcript levels of *mdh* were observed (Figure 5).

Overexpression of the outer membrane protein OmpA in wild type *S. flexneri* serotype 3b decreases bacterial adherence to BHK cells and virulence in *C. elegans*

Since the *ansB* mutant exhibited decreased adherence and up-regulation of OmpA, a prominent outer membrane protein, we decided to determine whether the up-regulation of OmpA in Δ*ansB* was responsible for the observed virulence phenotypes. To investigate whether the up-regulation of OmpA had an effect on bacterial virulence, we overexpressed OmpA in wild type 3b (SFL1520) by introducing a plasmid carrying *ompA* into SFL1520, to generate SFL2443 (SFL1520 + *ompA*). qRT-PCR was used to confirm that there was an increase in *ompA* transcripts in SFL2443 compared with the wild type strain (Figure 6). SFL2443 was then used to perform cell culture adherence assays and *in vivo C. elegans* virulence assays in order to assess whether the decreased adherence shown by the *ansB* mutant strain was a result of the up-regulation of outer membrane protein, OmpA.

Adherence assays performed using SFL2443 (SFL1520 + *ompA*) clearly indicate that the overexpression of OmpA in wild type *S. flexneri* serotype 3b significantly decreased the adherence of wild type cells (Figure 7.A). Similarly, *in vivo* bacterial accumulation assays in *C. elegans* showed that the overexpression of OmpA in wild type 3b, reduced bacterial accumulation in the nematodes to levels similar to Δ*ansB* (SFL2283) (Figure 7.B). Results of both the BHK adherence assays and *C. elegans* bacterial accumulation assays suggest that the up-regulation of the outer membrane protein OmpA is responsible for the decreased virulence of the Δ*ansB* strain.

ansB regulates the expression of *ompA* in *S. flexneri*

Since DIGE analysis indicated that OmpA levels were elevated in *ansB* mutant cells and virulence studies showed that the up-regulation of OmpA in wild type cells lead to decreased bacterial adherence, we decided to determine if the presence of AnsB does in fact affect the expression of *ompA*. In order to determine whether the presence of *ansB* had an effect on the expression of *ompA* in *S. flexneri*, qRT-PCR was performed to compare the levels of *ompA* transcripts in the wild type 3b strain, *ansB* mutant and the *ansB* mutant strain complemented with a plasmid copy of *ansB*. Using this approach, we show that on complementation of the *ansB* mutation, the levels of *ompA* transcripts are restored to wild type levels (Figure 8). These results suggest that *ansB* does in fact play a role in the regulation of *ompA* expression.

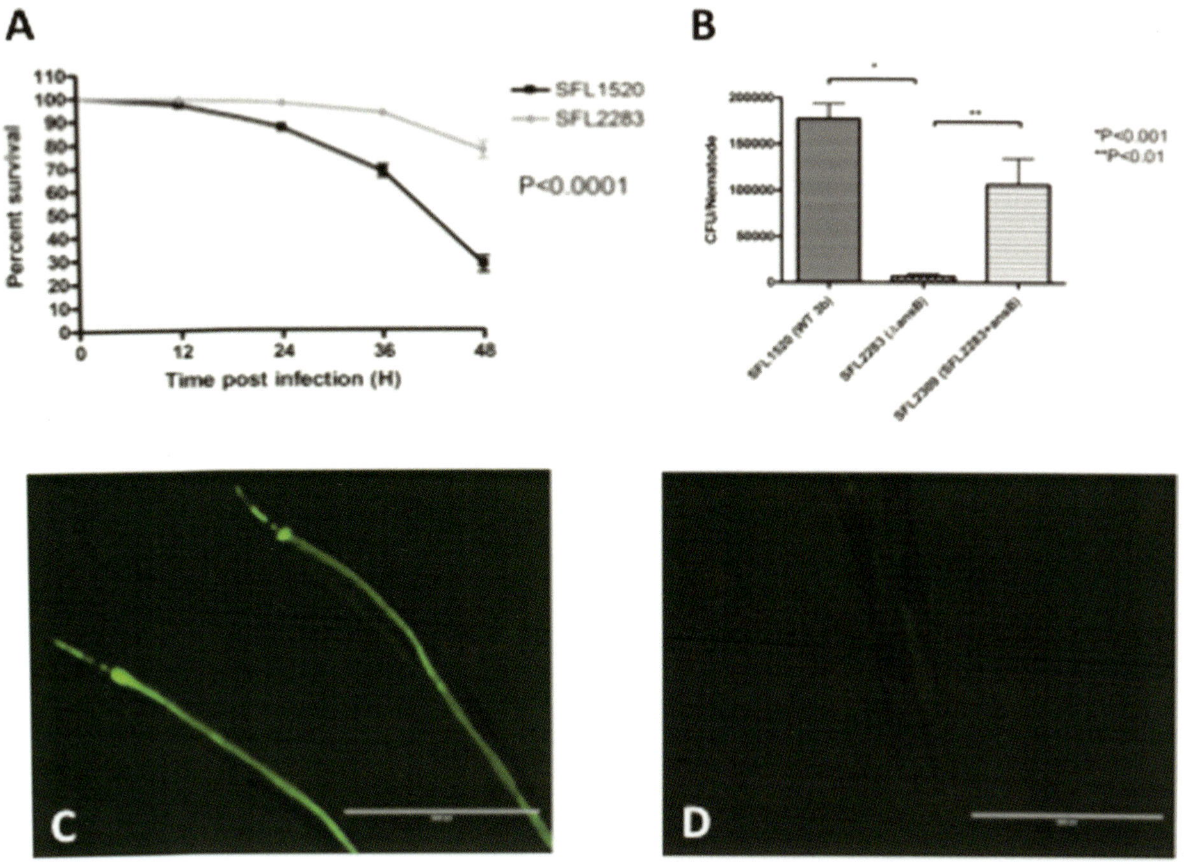

Figure 3. AnsB activity required for *S. flexneri*-mediated killing and bacterial accumulation in *C. elegans.* **A**: *S. flexneri*-mediated *C. elegans* liquid killing assays. 20 synchronized adult nematodes were treated with log phase cultures of *S. flexneri* 3b (SFL1520-black) or Δ*ansB* (SFL2283-grey) strains grown at 37°C to express virulence factors. Infected nematodes were monitored for 48 hours and survival was scored every 12 hours. Worms treated with the Δ*ansB* strain show a significant increase ($p<0.0001$, Logrank test) in survival rates compared to nematodes infected with wild type *S. flexneri* 3b. Error bars represent standard error of mean across at least 3 independent biological repeats. **B**: Bacterial accumulations assays; young adult hermaphrodite nematodes were fed SFL1520, SFL2283 or *ansB* complemented strain SFL2309 (SFL2283 + *ansB*) for 24 hours. 20 nematodes were picked and mechanically disrupted to release internalized bacteria. Diluted lysates were plated on LB agar plates carrying appropriate antibiotics, and colonies were scored in order to quantify *S. flexneri* cells associated with each nematode. There is a significant decrease in the accumulation of SFL2283 compared to SFL1520 and SFL2309 ($p<0.01$, One-way ANOVA). Error bars represent standard error of mean across 3 independent biological repeats. Young adult hermaphrodite nematodes infected as above with GFP^{+}- tagged SFL1520 (**C**) and SFL2283 (**D**). Wild type *S. flexneri* 3b accumulates in the nematode gut lumen and Δ*ansB* (SFL2283) strain fails to accumulate in the worm gut lumen. Scale bar = 400 μm.

Discussion

Here we characterize AnsB, a metabolic enzyme identified to be immunogenic in *S. flexneri* [4] and found that the activity of this enzyme is required for the virulence of *S. flexneri*. Using *in vitro* bacterial adherence assays and two *in vivo* models of shigellosis, we found a marked decrease in the adherence and virulence of the *ansB* mutant strain (SFL2283), clearly suggesting that AnsB is involved in the initial stages of *S. flexneri* pathogenesis.

The L-asparaginase activity of AnsB has previously been found to enhance bacterial colonization of mammalian cells by increased hydrolysis of asparagine in the case of *Campylobacter jejuni* [24–26] and *Helicobacter pylori* [6,27]. However, the role of this enzyme in *S. flexneri* virulence has not been elucidated. The results of ammonia release assays suggest that AnsB in *S. flexneri* functions as an L-asparaginase, as is the case in *E. coli* [9] and *Salmonella enterica* [28]. This reaction features in several metabolic pathways, including nitrogen, cyanoamino acid, alanine and aspartate metabolism [29].

The involvement of L-asparaginase activity in several metabolic pathways suggests that mutating *ansB* could lead to metabolic impairments, which in turn could decrease overall bacterial fitness. However, our *in vitro* growth studies found no differences in the growth rates of mutant and wild type cells, which suggests that although *ansB* is expressed and functional in wild type *S. flexneri* cells grown *in vitro*, its activity is not required for bacterial growth *in vitro* under nutrient rich or nutrient stressed conditions (Figure S2). The results of our growth studies are not surprising as AnsB in *E. coli*, is essential for growth under low oxygen, poor carbon source conditions by providing an alternative electron acceptor. Therefore although this gene is expressed in *S. flexneri* cells grown aerobically, the activity of this enzyme may only be critical under anaerobiosis [30]. Therefore further growth studies need to be performed under anaerobic conditions in order to determine whether *ansB* mutant cells show reduced bacterial fitness.

Successful establishment of bacterial infection requires adherence to host tissue. Members of the family *Enterobacteriaceae* use a plethora of strategies to adhere to host tissues, ranging from the use of pili to the secretion of highly specialized adhesion molecules

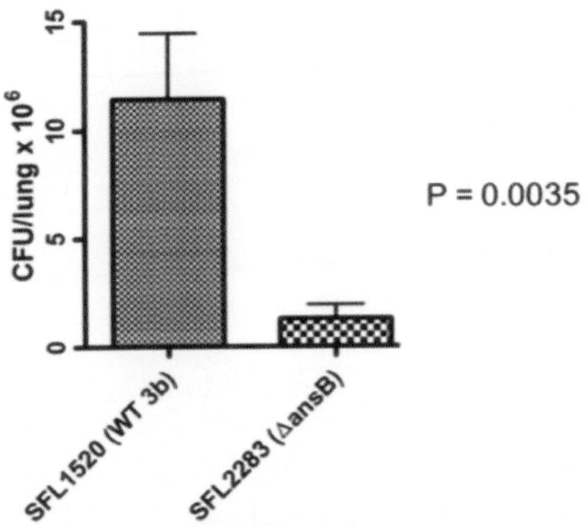

Figure 4. AnsB activity required for *S. flexneri* infection in the murine pulmonary model of shigellosis. Lung counts of mice inoculated intranasally with a sub-lethal dose (2×10^7 CFU) of *S. flexneri* 3b (SFL1520) and Δ*ansB* (SFL2283). 20 mice per strain were euthanized 24 hours post-inoculation, and their lungs were isolated and homogenized. Dilutions of the homogenates were plated to determine the number of intracellular bacterial cells 24 hours post inoculation. Results represent the mean values of lung counts obtained from 20 mice infected with each strain in a blind experiment with standard errors (error bars). There is a significant decrease in the lung counts of mice infected with the *ansB* mutant strain compared to mice infected with the wild type strain ($p = 0.0035$, unpaired t-test).

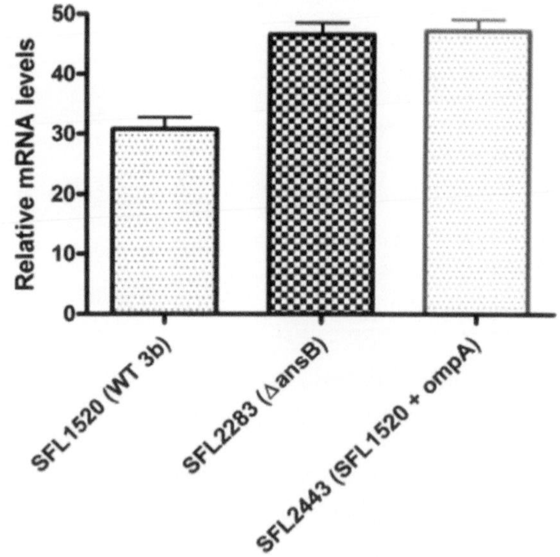

Figure 6. qRT-PCR analysis confirms the up-regulation of *ompA* in SFL2443 (wild type + *ompA*). qRT-PCR was used to compare the mRNA transcript levels of *ompA* in SFL1520 (wild type *S. flexneri* serotype 3b), SFL2283 (Δ*ansB*) and SFL2443 (SFL1520 + a plasmid carrying *ompA* to account for the up-regulation of OmpA seen in the Δ*ansB* mutant). Results represent the means of three biological repeats, each measured in triplicate and normalized to the control gene *hisG*. Error bars indicate the standard errors of the means. OmpA mRNA levels in SFL2443 are significantly higher than SFL1520 ($p<0.001$, unpaired t-test) and similar to the up-regulated levels seen in SFL2283 ($p>0.05$, unpaired t-test).

[31]. The molecular mechanisms used by *S. flexneri* to adhere to host cells are relatively unknown. Previous studies have shown that the bacterial Type III secretory Ipa proteins, especially IpaB, facilitate adherence to mammalian tissue [32–34]. In this study, western immunoblots confirmed that IpaB levels in Δ*ansB* and wild type cells are comparable (Figure S1.B), which suggests that there may be an IpaB-independent mechanism involved in *S. flexneri* adhesion to host cells.

DIGE analysis was performed to identify changes in the *S. flexneri* proteome in response to mutating *ansB*. Comparative analysis of proteomes of the *ans*B mutant and wild type *S. flexneri* strains showed that this mutation exerts pleiotropic effects on the expression of several *S. flexneri* proteins (Table S1), including proteins involved in stress responses (DnaK and GroEL), translation (RplL), metabolism (Udp and Mdh) and an outer membrane protein (OmpA). OmpA is a prominent outer membrane protein found in Gram negative bacteria, required to maintain the structural integrity of cellular outer membranes [35,36] and the role of this protein in Gram negative bacterial pathogenesis has been extensively studied [37–39]. Furthermore, studies in *E. coli* [40] and enterohemorrhagic *E. coli* (EHEC)

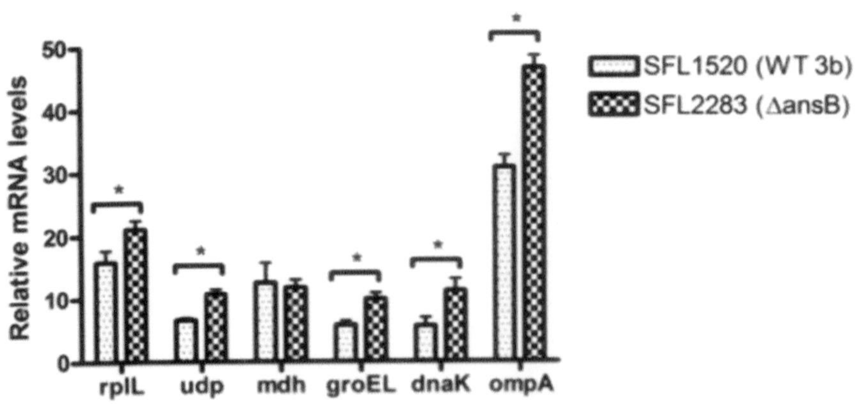

Figure 5. Reverse transcription quantitative PCR (qRT-PCR) analysis to confirm two dimensional differential in-gel electrophoresis (DIGE) analysis. Transcript levels of proteins identified by DIGE analysis, *rplL*, *udp*, *mdh*, *groEL*, *dnaK* and *ompA*, were measured in Δ*ansB* (SFL2283) and wild type *S. flexneri* serotype 3b (SFL1520) and expressed as a ratio of the *ansB* mutation-induced levels and the basal wild type levels. Data represent the means of three independent biological repeats, each replicate measured in triplicate and normalized to the control gene *hisG*. Asterisks indicate statistically significant differences calculated using unpaired Student's t-test ($p<0.05$).

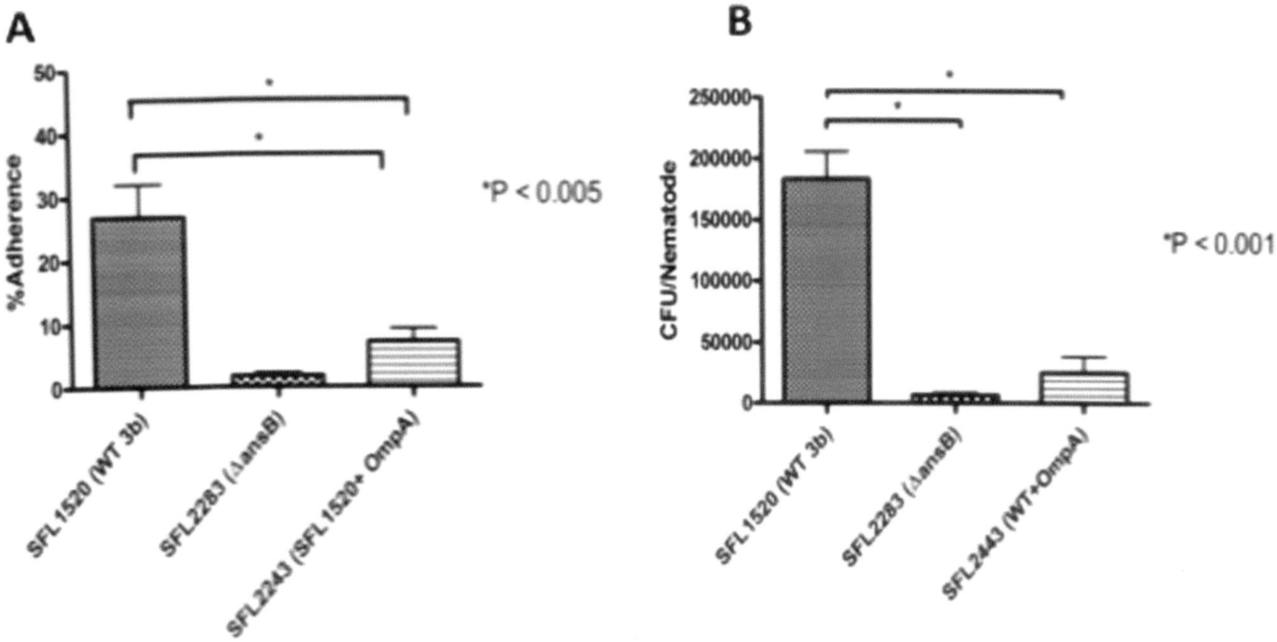

Figure 7. Overexpression of OmpA decreases *S. flexneri* adherence *in vitro* and virulence in *C. elegans*. A: Results of *in vitro* adherence assays for SFL2443 (SFL1520 + a plasmid expressing *ompA* to account for the up-regulating of OmpA seen in the Δ*ansB* mutant), wild type *S. flexneri* 3b (SFL1520), and Δ*ansB* (SFL2283) strains plotted as percentage adherence, a ratio of the number of adherent and intracellular bacteria to the total number of bacterial cells in the infecting inoculum (y-axis). The adherence of SFL1520 is significantly decreased as a result of the overexpression of OmpA in, SFL2443 ($p<0.005$, unpaired t-test). Results are the means of three independent blind repeats with standard errors (error bars).**B:** Results of *in vivo C. elegans* bacterial accumulation assays for SFL2443, SFL1520, SFL2283 strains. The accumulation of SFL1520 is significantly higher than SFL2443 ($p<0.001$, unpaired t-test). Results are the means of three independent blind repeats with standard errors (error bars).

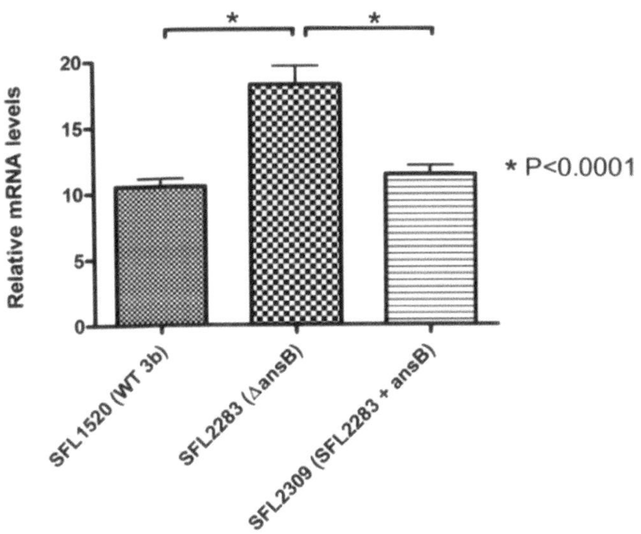

Figure 8. qRT-PCR analysis confirms that the presence of *ansB* regulates the expression of *ompA* in *S. flexneri*. qRT-PCR was used to compare the mRNA transcript levels of *ompA* in SFL1520 (wild type *S. flexneri* serotype 3b), SFL2283 (Δ*ansB*) and SFL2309 (SFL2283 + a plasmid carrying *ansB* to complement the *ansB* mutation). Results represent the means of three biological repeats each measured in triplicate and normalized to the control gene *hisG*. Error bars indicate the standard errors of the means. A significant increase in *ompA* expression is observed in SFL2285 ($p<0.0001$) when compared with SFL1520 and SFL2309. No significant differences were observed in the expression of *ompA* between the wild type parental strain (SFL1520) and the *ansB* complement (SFL2309) ($p>0.05$, unpaired t-test), suggesting that complementation of the *ansB* mutation in SFL2309, restores the expression of this gene to wild type levels.

[41,42] have found that OmpA plays a key role in the initial stages of bacterial adhesion and invasion. In this study we show that AnsB is required for the adherence of *S. flexneri*, and *ansB* mutant cells up-regulate the expression of OmpA, therefore the effect of overexpressing OmpA in *S. flexneri* was investigated.

ansB mutants showed an up-regulation of OmpA, it is generally believed that the overexpression of membrane proteins affects the integrity of cell membranes and cell viability [43]. Therefore the overexpression of OmpA would affect cellular protein homeostasis, which in turn would have an effect on the overall integrity of the cellular envelope. Therefore to determine the effects of elevated OmpA levels on bacterial adherence, we overexpressed OmpA in the wild type strain and found that the overexpression of this outer membrane protein decreased both bacterial adherence to BHK cells and accumulation in *C. elegans* (Figure 7.A and B). These results suggest that the up-regulation of OmpA in *ansB* mutant cells could disrupt the bacterial cell envelope integrity and therefore may be one of the factors that contribute to the decreased adherence of these mutant cells.

qRT-PCR analysis of *ompA* expression in the *ansB* complement showed that complementation of the *ansB* mutation resulted in decreased *ompA* expression. This result suggests that the presence of *ansB* directly or indirectly affects *ompA* expression. The expression of OmpA has been known to be environmentally responsive. In *E. coli*, OmpA levels are elevated in response to nitrogen shortage, to facilitate an increased uptake of peptides to alleviate the nitrogen shortage [44,45]. One of the identified functions of AnsB is to provide nitrogen and carbon sources from the hydrolysis of exogenous asparagine [46]. Nitrogen depletion increases the expression of *ansB* in yeast [47,48], suggesting that AnsB plays a role in nitrogen metabolism. *ansB* mutant cells would thus have lower nitrogen levels compared with wild type cells;

therefore we propose that the expression of OmpA in these mutant cells may be increased to alleviate this nitrogen shortage.

The exact mechanism involved in the AnsB-mediated regulation of OmpA remains unclear at this stage nonetheless our finding provided clear evidence suggesting that the presence of AnsB is required for the adherence of *S. flexneri* and for regulating OmpA levels.

Conclusions

Here we have shown that the periplasmic enzyme, AnsB, is required for the virulence of *S. flexneri. in vitro* cell culture assays indicate that this enzyme is essential for bacterial adherence. Differential in-gel electrophoresis showed that *ansB* mutants exert pleiotropic effects on the expression of a number of *S. flexneri* genes, including a prominent bacterial outer membrane protein, OmpA that is known to be required for adherence to host cells. We also show that the up-regulation of OmpA, could be one of the factors responsible for the defective adherence of *ansB* mutant cells. This is the first report in *S. flexneri* where the function of AnsB has been found to extend beyond its canonical metabolic role. The requirement of AnsB for the virulence of *S. flexneri* makes this gene an attractive candidate for designing new therapeutic measures and preventive approaches to curb the spread of shigellosis.

Supporting Information

Figure S1 *ansB* mutation does not affect the expression and secretion of invasion protein antigens-IpaB and IpaD. Secreted proteins were isolated from the *S. flexneri* serotype 3b parental strain (SFL1520), *ΔansB* (SFL2283) and a *S. flexneri* strain cured of the virulence plasmid (SFL1223) [20] used as a negative control. Proteins were separated using SDS-PAGE, following which they were electroblotted onto PVDF membranes and probed with anti-IpaB (**A**) and anti-IpaD (**B**) primary antibodies. The levels of secreted IpaB (~62 kDa) and IpaD (~34 kDa) produced by all strains was visualized using a chemiluminescence reader. No differences were observed in the secretory levels of both IpaB and IpaD between the wild type and *ansB* mutant strains.

Figure S2 AnsB activity is not required for *S. flexneri* growth *in vitro*. The growth curves of wild type *S. flexneri* serotype 3b (SFL1520) (black) and Δ*ansB* strain (SFL2283) (grey), plotted as optical density readings at 600 nm (OD_{600}) (y-axis) versus time (x-axis). **A**: Growth in Luria-Bertani (LB) broth at 37°C (bold lines) and at 30°C (dashed lines). **B**: Growth in minimal essential salts media (MM) at 37°C (bold lines) and at 30°C (dashed lines). No significant difference in the growth patterns of SFL1520 and SFL2283 were detected under all four conditions examined ($p > 0.05$, unpaired t-test). Error bars represent standard error of means obtained from three independent biological repeats.

Table S1 Differentially expressed spots in the *ansB* mutant.

Author Contributions

Conceived and designed the experiments: DG NV. Performed the experiments: DG. Analyzed the data: DG NV UM CB. Contributed reagents/materials/analysis tools: DG NV UM CB. Wrote the paper: DG NV UM CB.

References

1. Strockbine NA, Maurelli AT (2005) In Bergey's Manual of Systematic Bacteriology; Brenner DJ, Krieg, NR, Staley, JT editor. N Y: Springer.
2. Jennison AV, Verma NK (2004) *Shigella flexneri* infection: pathogenesis and vaccine development. FEMS Microbiol Rev 28: 43–58.
3. van den Broek JM, Roy SK, Khan WA, Ara G, Chakraborty B, et al. (2005) Risk factors for mortality due to shigellosis: a case control study among severely malnourished children in Bangladesh. J Health Popul Nutr 23: 259–265.
4. Jennison AV, Raqib R, Verma NK (2006) Immunoproteome analysis of soluble and membrane proteins of *Shigella flexneri* 2457T. World J Gastroenterol 12: 6683–6688.
5. Cheung NKV, Chau IY, Coccia PF (1986) Antibody response to *Escherichia coli* L-asparaginase - prognostic significance and clinical utility of antibody measurement. Am J Pediatr Hematol Oncol 8: 99–104.
6. Leduc D, Gallaud J, Stingl K, de Reuse H (2010) Coupled amino acid deamidase transport systems essential for *Helicobacter pylori* colonization. Infect Immun 78: 2782–2792.
7. Zautner AE, Ohk C, Tareen AM, Lugert R, Gross U (2012) Epidemiological association of *Campylobacter jejuni* groups with pathogenicity-associated genetic markers. BMC Microbiol 12: 171.
8. Kullas AL, McClelland M, Yang HJ, Tam JW, Torres A, et al. (2012) L-asparaginase II produced by *Salmonella typhimurium* inhibits T cell responses and mediates virulence. Cell Host Microbe 12: 791–798.
9. Jennings MP, Beacham IR (1990) Analysis of the *Escherichia coli* gene encoding L-asparaginase-Ii, AnsB, and its regulation by cyclic-amp receptor and Fnr proteins. J Bacteriol 172: 1491–1498.
10. Datsenko KA, Wanner BL (2000) One-step inactivation of chromosomal genes in *Escherichia coli* K-12 using PCR products. Proc Natl Acad Sci U S A 97: 6640–6645.
11. Burton EA, Pendergast AM, Aballay M (2006) The *Caenorhabditis elegans* ABL-1 tyrosine kinase is required for *Shigella flexneri* pathogenesis. Appl Environ Microbiol 72: 5043–5051.
12. Yanisch-Perron C, Vieira J, Messing J (1985) Improved M13 phage cloning vectors and host strains: nucleotide sequences of the M13mp18 and pUC19 vectors. Gene 33: 103–119.
13. Sambrook J, Fritsch EF, Maniatis T (1989) Molecular cloning: a laboratory manual: Cold Spring Harbor, N.Y.: Cold Spring Harbor Laboratory Press.
14. Hanahan D (1983) Studies on transformation of *Escherichia coli* with plasmids. J Mol Biol 166: 557–580.
15. Cravioto A, Gross RJ, Scotland SM, Rowe B (1979) Adhesive factor found in strains of *Escherichia coli* belonging to the traditional infantile enteropathogenic serotypes. Curr Microbiol 3: 95–99.
16. Brenner S (1974) The genetics of *Caenorhabditis elegans*. Genetics 77: 71–94.
17. Wood WB (1988) The nematode *Caenorhabditis elegans*; William B. Wood UoC, Boulder editor. New York: Cold Spring Harbor Monograph Laboratory Press.
18. Kesika P, Karutha Pandian S, Balamurugan K (2011) Analysis of *Shigella flexneri*-mediated infections in model organism *Caenorhabditis elegans*. Scand J Infect Dis 43: 286–295.
19. Mathesius U (2001) Flavonoids induced in cells undergoing nodule organogenesis in white clover are regulators of auxin breakdown by peroxidase. J Exp Botany 52: 419–426.
20. Maurelli AT, Blackmon B, Curtiss R III (1984) Loss of pigmentation in *Shigella flexneri* 2a is correlated with loss of virulence and virulence-associated plasmid. Infect Immun 43: 397–401.
21. Voino-Yasenetsky MV, Voino-Yasenetskaya MK (1962) Experimental pneumonia caused by bacteria of the *Shigella* group. Acta Morphol Acad Sci Hung 11: 439–454.
22. Mallett CP, VanDeVerg L, Collins HH, Hale TL (1993) Evaluation of *Shigella* vaccine safety and efficacy in an intranasally challenged mouse model. Vaccine 11: 190–196.
23. van de Verg LL, Mallett CP, Collins HH, Larsen T, Hammack C, et al. (1995) Antibody and cytokine responses in a mouse pulmonary model of *Shigella flexneri* serotype 2a infection. Infect Immun 63: 1947–1954.
24. Zautner AE, Ohk C, Tareen AM, Lugert R, Gross U (2012) Epidemiological association of *Campylobacter jejuni* groups with pathogenicity-associated genetic markers. BMC Microbiol 12: 171.
25. Thompson SA, Gaynor EC (2008) *Campylobacter jejuni* host tissue tropism: a consequence of its low-carb lifestyle? Cell Host & Microbe 4: 409–410.
26. de Haan CP, Llarena AK, Revez J, Hanninen ML (2012) Association of *Campylobacter jejuni* metabolic traits with multilocus sequence types. Appl Environ Microbiol 78: 5550–5551.
27. Shibayama K, Takeuchi H, Wachino J, Mori S, Arakawa Y (2011) Biochemical and pathophysiological characterization of *Helicobacter pylori* asparaginase. Microbiol Immunol 55: 408–417.
28. Jennings MP, Scott SP, Beacham IR (1993) Regulation of the *ansB* gene of *Salmonella enterica*. Mol Microbiol 9: 165–172.

29. Yang J, Chen L, Yu J, Sun L, Jin Q (2006) ShiBASE: an integrated database for comparative genomics of *Shigella*. Nucl Acids Res 34: 398–401.
30. Srikhanta YN, Atack JM, Beacham IR, Jennings MP (2013) Distinct physiological roles of two L-asparaginase isozymes of *Escherichia coli*. Biochem Biophys Res Comm. 436: 362–365.
31. Pizarro-Cerda J, Cossart P (2006) Bacterial adhesion and entry into host cells. Cell 124: 715–727.
32. Watarai M, Funato S, Sasakawa C (1996) Interaction of Ipa proteins of *Shigella flexneri* with alpha5beta1 integrin promotes entry of the bacteria into mammalian cells. J Exp Med 183: 991–999.
33. Skoudy A, Mounier J, Aruffo A, Ohayon H, Gounon P, et al. (2000) CD44 binds to the *Shigella* IpaB protein and participates in bacterial invasion of epithelial cells. Cell Microbiol 2: 19–33.
34. Lafont F, Tran Van Nhieu G, Hanada K, Sansonetti P, van der Goot FG (2002) Initial steps of *Shigella* infection depend on the cholesterol/sphingolipid raft-mediated CD44-IpaB interaction. EMBO J 21: 4449–4457.
35. Rasmussen AA, Eriksen M, Gilany K, Udesen C, Franch T, et al. (2005) Regulation of ompA mRNA stability: the role of a small regulatory RNA in growth phase-dependent control. Mol Microbiol 58: 1421–1429.
36. Johansen J, Eriksen M, Kallipolitis B, Valentin-Hansen P (2008) Down-regulation of outer membrane proteins by noncoding RNAs: unraveling the cAMP-CRP- and sigmaE-dependent CyaR-ompX regulatory case. J Mol Biol 383: 1–9.
37. Krishnan S, Prasadarao NV (2012) Outer membrane protein A and OprF: versatile roles in Gram-negative bacterial infections. FEBS J 279: 919–931.
38. Smith SG, Mahon V, Lambert MA, Fagan RP (2007) A molecular Swiss army knife: OmpA structure, function and expression. FEMS Microbiol Lett 273: 1–11.
39. Confer AW, Ayalew S (2013) The OmpA family of proteins: roles in bacterial pathogenesis and immunity. Vet Microbiol 163: 207–222.
40. Shin S, Lu G, Cai M, Kim KS (2005) *Escherichia coli* outer membrane protein A adheres to human brain microvascular endothelial cells. Biochem Biophys Res Commun 330: 1199–1204.
41. Torres AG, Kaper JB (2003) Multiple elements controlling adherence of enterohemorrhagic *Escherichia coli* O157:H7 to HeLa cells. Infect Immun 71: 4985–4995.
42. Torres AG, Li Y, Tutt CB, Xin L, Eaves-Pyles T, et al. (2006) Outer membrane protein A of *Escherichia coli* O157:H7 stimulates dendritic cell activation. Infect Immun 74: 2676–2685.
43. Wagner S, Bader ML, Drew D, de Gier JW (2006) Rationalizing membrane protein overexpression. Trends Biotechnol 24: 364–371.
44. Baev MV, Baev D, Radek AJ, Campbell JW (2006) Growth of *Escherichia coli* MG1655 on LB medium: determining metabolic strategy with transcriptional microarrays. Appl Microbiol Biotechnol 71: 323–328.
45. Payne JW, Smith MW (1994) Peptide transport by Micro-organisms. Adv Microbiol Physiol 36:1–80.
46. Jennings MP, Beacham IR (1993) Co-dependent positive regulation of the *ansB* promoter of *Escherichia coli* by CRP and the FNR protein: a molecular analysis. Mol Microbiol 9: 155–164.
47. Dunlop PC, Roon RJ (1975) L-Asparaginase of *Saccharomyces cerevisiae*: an extracellular Enzyme. J Bacteriol 122: 1017–1024.
48. Pauling KD, Jones GE (1980) Asparaginase II of Saccharomyces cerevisiae: inactivation during the transition to stationary phase. Biochim Biophys Acta 616: 271–282.

15

Viral Gastroenteritis Associated with Genogroup II Norovirus among U.S. Military Personnel in Turkey, 2009

Salwa F. Ahmed[1]*, John D. Klena[1], Manal Mostafa[1], Jessica Dogantemur[2], Tracy Middleton[2], James Hanson[2], Peter J. Sebeny[1]

1 United States Naval Medical Research Unit No.3, Cairo, Egypt, **2** Incirlik Air Base, Incirlik, Turkey

Abstract

The present study demonstrates that multiple NoV genotypes belonging to genogroup II contributed to an acute gastroenteritis outbreak at a US military facility in Turkey that was associated with significant negative operational impact. Norovirus (NoV) is an important pathogen associated with acute gastroenteritis among military populations. We describe the genotypes of NoV outbreak occurred at a United States military facility in Turkey. Stool samples were collected from 37 out of 97 patients presenting to the clinic on base with acute gastroenteritis and evaluated for bacterial and viral pathogens. NoV genogroup II (GII) was identified by RT-PCR in 43% (16/37) stool samples. Phylogenetic analysis of a 260 base pair fragment of the NoV capsid gene from ten stool samples indicated the circulation of multiple and rare genotypes of GII NoV during the outbreak. We detected four GII.8 isolates, three GII.15, two GII.9 and a sole GII.10 NoV. Viral sequences could be grouped into four clusters, three of which have not been previously reported in Turkey. The fact that current NoV outbreak was caused by rare genotypes highlights the importance of norovirus strain typing. While NoV genogroup II is recognized as causative agent of outbreak, circulation of current genotypes has been rarely observed in large number of outbreaks.

Editor: Dhanasekaran Vijaykrishna, Duke-NUS Gradute Medical School, Singapore

Funding: This work was supported by the Military Infectious Disease Research Program (MIDRP) proposal D0105_09_N3 - The Epidemiology and Management of Diarrhea Among Deployed US Forces to CENTCOM and EUCOM theaters of operation. The funders had no role in study design, data collection and analysis, decision to publish, or preparation of the manuscript.

Competing Interests: The authors have declared that no competing interests exist.

* E-mail: salwa.fouad.eg@med.navy.mil

Introduction

Human noroviruses (NoV) are the most common cause of outbreaks of acute gastroenteritis, worldwide [1]. Annually, NoV have been estimated to be implicated in 21 million cases of acute gastroenteritis in the United States [2], and is the most common cause of diarrhea in adults [3]. One in fourteen people will have a norovirus infection each year, and most people will have suffered several NoV infections within their lifetime [2]. Worldwide, it has been estimated that over 218,000 of pediatric deaths that are attributed to gastrointestinal disease each year from a total of 1.6 million can be directly attributed to NoV illness [3]. Most children will have at least one NoV infection within the first 5 years of life [4]. Sporadic NoV infection has been reported as second to rotavirus as an enteric pathogen associated with gastroenteritis among children [5].

Norovirus is recognized as a major cause of gastroenteritis outbreaks in military populations [6], and other semi-closed or closed institutions such as hospitals, elder care homes, cruise ships, and nurseries [7]. Norovirus strains were a major cause of outbreaks and sporadic cases of gastroenteritis among US ground troops during the Persian Gulf War in 1991, where NoV infection was in one report the most common cause of disability [6] as well as coalition forces in Gulf War II and the Afghanistan campaign beginning in 2002 [8,9,10,11]. As many as 73% of enteric viral gastroenteritis cases among British troops deployed from 2002–2007 were associated with NoV [9]. In 2002, a NoV outbreak among British forces deployed to Afghanistan forced medical evacuations to European hospitals because of severe dehydration and other complications, resulting in closure of the field hospital, leaving the remaining military contingent without full medical services until the outbreak could be characterized [8]. Studies from an array of military units continue to demonstrate that NoV outbreaks have the capacity to impede force readiness and have even caused the stand down of the entire air wing of a battle group [12].

Norovirus belong to the family *Caliciviridae* and have a single-stranded, positive-sense RNA genome that is genetically highly variable, with five known genogroups [1], three (GI, GII, GIV) of which are associated with human disease [1]. The GII NoV are most commonly associated with human disease, with 19 known genotypes [13]; strains of genotype GII.4 in particular are recognized as a dominant circulating strain. Between 1995 and 2006, genotype GII.4 caused at least four pandemic seasons during which novel GII.4 variants rapidly emerged and displaced previously circulating strains [14]. Because of the dramatic increase in GII.4 NoV outbreaks in the past several years, much of the attention with respect to NoV control has focused on strains of this genotype. However, other NoV strains are always circulating, causing local and regional outbreaks [15].

In May 2009, a significant increase in acute gastroenteritis (AGE) cases was noted in the American health clinic at Incirlik Air Base (IAB) in Adana, Turkey. This increased rate of AGE led to discussions with local Turkish military public health authorities, which confirmed that the Turkish military community and the residents of Adana were also experiencing an anecdotal increase in AGE illnesses [16]. An epidemiologic investigation was launched to attempt to identify the cause and possible source of this AGE outbreak at IAB.

Materials and Methods

Clinical and Epidemiologic Methods

The current investigation describes a gastrointestinal outbreak which occurred on a US military base in Turkey. The main objective was to identify the etiological agent(s) responsible for the outbreak as a public health response to formulate containment strategy and provide data that would support an appropriate intervention control strategy. The project was conducted as an activity not involving human research, therefore IRB review was not required. Participants voluntarily agreed to provide stool samples and complete the questionnaire information.

IAB is located in the village of Incirlik, about six miles from the city of Adana in southeastern Turkey. It is a Turkish military complex, composed of both Turkish and American personnel. The American component has approximately 1250 active duty personnel and 1300 civilians and dependents. The vast majority of U.S. military and their dependents live and work on the base, but travel within and outside Turkey is common for base personnel and their families.

Due to a rapid increased report of AGE in the local community and anecdotal cases reported among US personnel at IAB in May, 2009, a clinic case-based investigation was performed. The goal of this investigation was to identify whether an outbreak was underway and if so, to determine the scope of the outbreak, the etiologic agent and its source, in order to mitigate risk and minimize impact as necessary. Patients presenting with diarrhea were requested to fill in a brief self-completed survey starting on 18 May, 2009. The survey collected demographic information, clinical signs and symptoms, and risk factors. Patients were asked to voluntarily submit a diarrheal stool sample for laboratory analysis. The case-based investigation ended on 18 June, 2009 as gastroenteritis cases dropped to a frequency typical for summer.

To identify the frequency of patients presenting with AGE just prior to the beginning of the presumed outbreak and continuing over time (from May 17–June 27, 2009), data from the clinic's electronic medical record was utilized by public health officials. This was done through identification of cases with a disease non-battle injury (DNI) code of 'gastrointestinal, infectious' which encompasses AGE, to characterize the likely onset and duration of the outbreak.

Microbiological Analysis

Stool samples were collected in clean stool hats and transferred into a sample cup and stored at 4°C until initial testing. An aliquot of each sample was tested locally using an ELISA for NoV (IDEIA Oxoid (Ely) Ltd, Denmark House, Angel Drove, UK). An additional aliquot of each specimen was also tested by EIA for *Cryptosporidium parvum*, *Entamoeba histolytica*, and *Giardia lamblia* (Techlab Inc., Blacksburg, VA, USA). The remaining sample was stored in Cary-Blair transport medium until transferred to the enteric disease research laboratory at US Naval Medical Research Unit No.3, Cairo, Egypt. In Cairo, standard bacterial culture investigation was performed to detect *Campylobacter* spp., *Salmonella* spp., *Shigella* spp., and *Vibrio* spp. Bacterial isolates were identified and confirmed using standard biochemical methods, and antibiotic sensitivity was determined via disk-diffusion (Becton Dickinson, Cockeysville, MD, USA), and/or E-tests (AB- Biodisk, Sölna, Sweden) as guided by the Clinical Laboratory Standards Institute (CLSI) [17]. EIA was also performed to test for astrovirus, rotavirus, adenovirus, and repeated for NoV (IDEIA, Oxoid, UK) according to the manufacturer's instructions. DNA was extracted from *Escherichia coli*-like colonies grown on MacConkey-lactose medium and subsequently tested for the enterotoxin genes *eltB* and *estA* [18].

RNA Extraction, RT-PCR and cDNA Sequencing

Viral RNA was extracted from 140 μl of a 10% fecal suspension in vertrel/water solution using a QIAamp Viral RNA Mini Kit (QIAGEN, Valencia, CA, USA) according to the manufacturer's protocol. Identification of NoV was performed by RT-PCR as previously described [19]. Genogroup II NoV was identified using primers targeting GII-specific regions in the 5′ capsid gene as described [20]. PCR amplicons from NoV-positive specimens were sequenced using the ABI Prism Big Dye Terminator cycle sequencing kit and an ABI Prism 3100 DNA sequence (Applied Biosystems, Foster City, CA, USA). Sequences were aligned against NoV capsid sequences obtained from Genbank using BioEdit software, version 5.1. Phylogenetic analysis was carried out using MEGA 5.0 [21] and a dendrogram was constructed using the neighbor-joining method with genetic distance modeled using the Kimura 2-parameter model [22]. Statistical confidence for the phylogenetic branches was assessed by bootstrap analysis (2,000 replicates) [23]. The tree is drawn to scale, with branch lengths in the same units as those of the evolutionary distances used to infer the phylogenetic tree [24].

Results

From the electronic medical record review from 18 May to 19 Jun 2009, 187 patients presented to the IAB clinic with AGE. The peak incidence of AGE cases was during the week of 31 May–06 June with a total of 71 patients seeking medical care at the clinic (Figure 1), with the outbreak occurring from 26 May to 15 June, 2009. Of the 187, 82 patients completed the case survey, 79% reported diarrhea, 46% reported vomiting, and 29% reported fever (Table 1). The median number of days between symptom onset and clinic visit was 2 days (interquartile range 1, 5). During the 7 days prior to symptoms, 73% of respondents reported travelling off base, 56% reported eating off base, and 24% reported using an outdoor pool.

Stool samples were collected from 37 patients; only 22 of these patients completed the survey questionnaire. Of the 22 stool samples collected along with a completed survey form, 9 were positive for NoV and we could identify their clinical characteristics. Of the NoV positive cases, 44% (4/9) suffered from nausea, 78% (7/9) had watery diarrhea and 67% (6/9) experienced vomiting. No significant difference was noticed between cases positive for NoV as opposed to negative cases in regard to consumption of bottled water, eating and travelling off base, pool usage and presence of a family member with a similar symptom.

Norovirus genogroup II was detected in 43% (16/37) stool samples by RT-PCR. Three of the 16 NoV positive cases were identified with a second enteropathogen: *C. jejuni*, *C. parvum*, or ETEC whereas enteropathogens were recovered from 59% (22/37) of remaining cases (Table 2). With regards to identification of other sole-pathogen infections, 5% (2/37) were positive for *Salmonella* group B, 3% (1/37) were positive for ETEC; 3% (1/37) were positive for *Cryptosporidium*, and 5% (2/37) were positive by EIA for rotavirus; 41% (15/37) of the samples were negative for all pathogens tested (Table 2).

Figure 1. Distribution of AGE cases from 18 May – 23 June 2009 evaluated in the clinic identified from AHLTA* (A), and associated stool sample testing results for NoV (B).

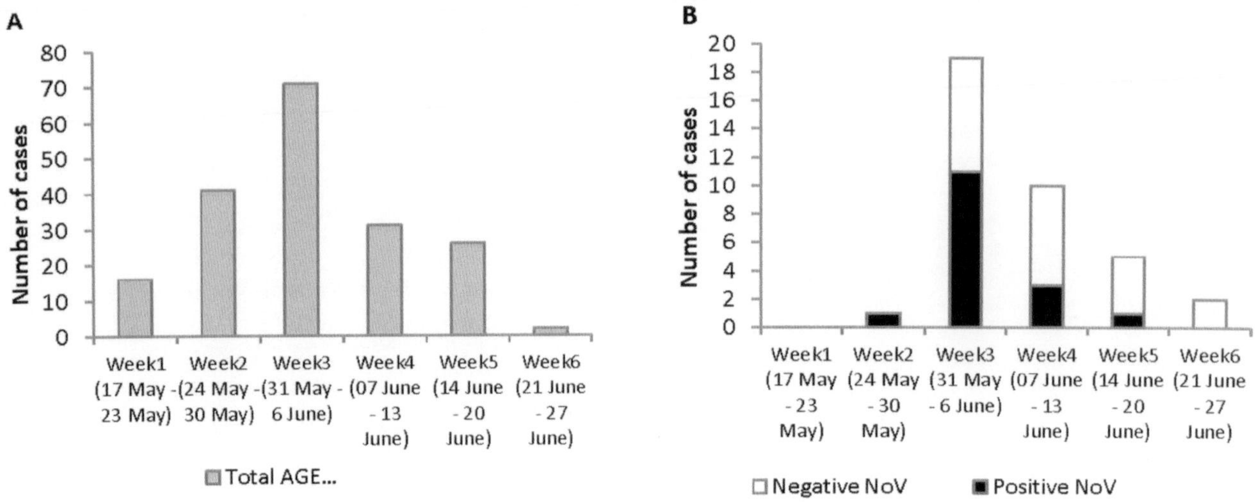

* AHLTA: Armed Forces Health Longitudinal Technology Application database, a United States Department of Defense - electronic medical record encompassing all branches of the armed services.

Figure 1. Distribution of AGE cases from 18 May –23 June 2009 evaluated in the clinic identified from AHLTA* (A), and associated stool sample testing results for NoV (B).

We were able to amplify a fragment of the gene encoding NoV capsid protein from 10 of the 16 NoV-positive stool samples; a phylogenetic analysis based on sequence comparison of these products indicated that multiple and rare genotypes of GII NoV were circulating during the outbreak (Figure 2). Four indistinguishable strains (Group I; accession number: JF895615, JF89616, JF973385, JF895613) could be typed as GII.8. A second group of two strains (Group II; accession number: JF895614, JF973386) could be typed as GII.9 and had 99% nucleotide sequence similarity with prototype strain Idaho Falls (accession number AY054299). A third group included one strain that could be typed as GII.10 (Group III; accession number JF895609). Yet another three strains belonged to genotype II.15 (Group IV; accession number: JF895612, JF895610, JF8956111) which had 98–99% nucleotide sequence similarity with other GII.15 strains in the GenBank database.

Table 1. Characteristics and activities of gastroenteritis cases reported by case-based surveillance survey responders.

Characteristics	Total; n = 82
Age: Median (IQR)	27(23–35)
Gender: Male, n (%)	51(62)
Symptoms, n (%)	
Watery diarrhea	65(79)
Nausea	52(63)
Vomiting	38(46)
Fever	24(29)
Headache	42(51)
Chills	31(38)
Stomach and/or abdominal pain	63(77)
Base facilities, n (%)	
Consumption of vegetables, fruits, meat, milk off base	46(56)
Consumption of bottled water	56(68)
Travel off base	60(73)
Self-report of an ill family member	22(27)
Outdoor Pool	20(24)

Discussion

This report summarizes the results of an AGE outbreak investigation at a US military facility in Turkey that was associated with significant negative operational impact, degrading mission readiness with nearly 20% of the American population in a one month period affected. Initiation of a clinic case-based investiga-

Table 2. Distribution of pathogens identified from stool samples (n = 37).

Pathogen detected (Method)	Sole, n (%)	Mixed, n (%)
Cryptosporidium (EIA)	1(3)	1(3)
ETEC (PCR)	2(5)	1(3)
Norovirus (PCR)	13(35)	3(8)
Rotavirus (EIA)	2(6)	0(0)
Campylobacter (culture)	0(0)	1(3)
Salmonella (culture)	2(5)	0(0)

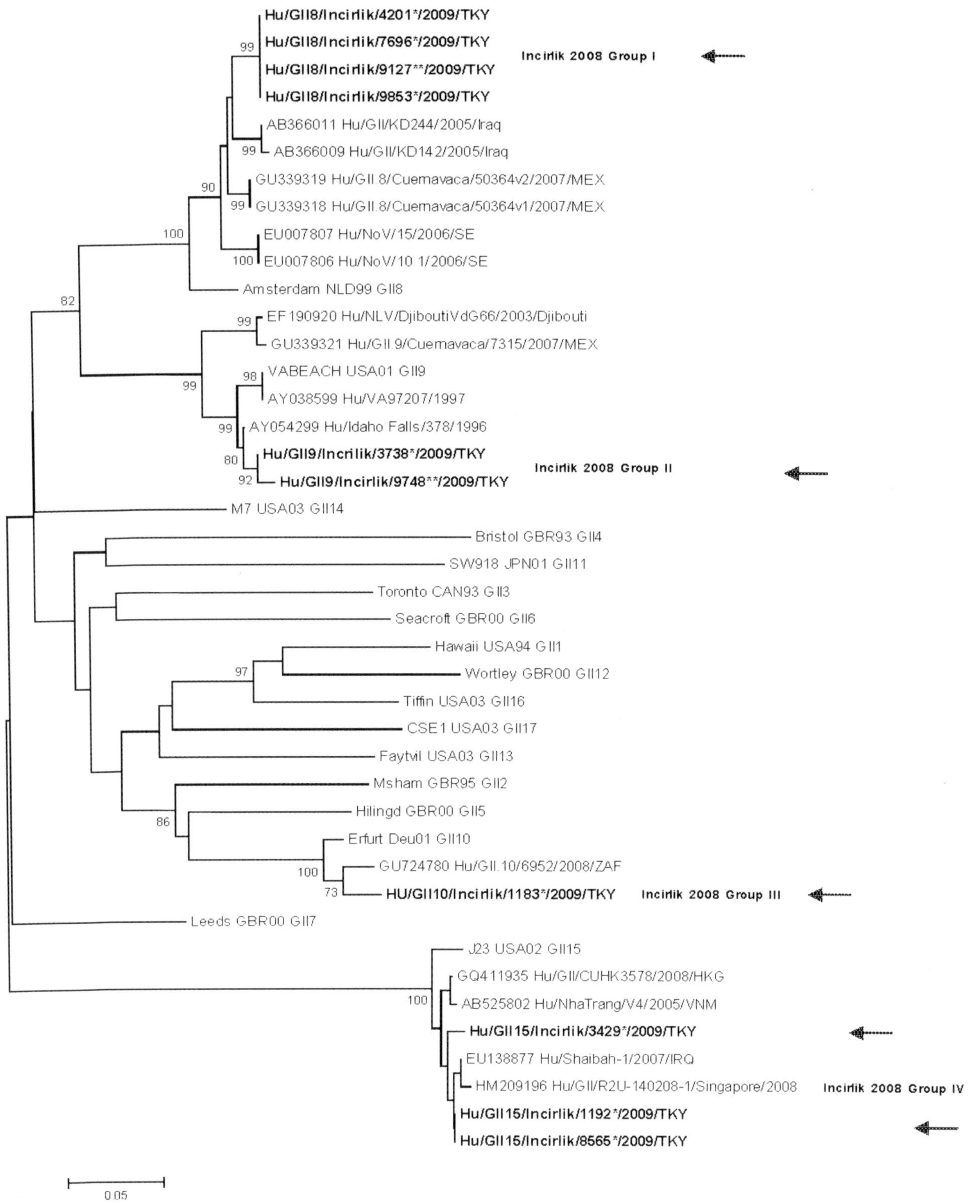

Figure 2. Phylogenetic analysis based on the partial capsid gene of NoV isolates from Turkey.

Figure 2. The evolutionary history was inferred using the Neighbor-Joining method. The optimal tree with the sum of branch length = 2.38 is shown. The percentage of replicate trees in which the associated taxa clustered together in the bootstrap test (2000 replicates) are shown next to the branches. Boot strap values below 70% were considered insignificant and are not shown. The tree is drawn to scale, with branch lengths in the same units as those of the evolutionary distances used to infer the phylogenetic tree. The evolutionary distances were computed using the Kimura 2-parameter method and are in the units of the number of base substitutions per site. The analysis involved 42 nucleotide sequences. Codon positions included were 1st+2nd+3rd+Noncoding. All positions containing gaps and missing data were eliminated. There were a total of 260 positions in the final dataset. Bold sequences represent strains from current study.

tion yielded 37 stool samples in which NoV was detected in 43% (16/37) of the samples with 81% (13/16) of the positive NoV samples identified without a copathogen.

DNA sequencing data demonstrated that several relatively rare genotypes of NoV contributed to this outbreak. Among the 16 NoV positive samples identified, 4 different genotypes were identified. Two of the NoV strains (Shaibah-like, and KD244-like) were previously reported in Iraq and only from deployed troops, while the other two genotypes were reported in South Africa and in the US [25,26]. In Turkey little systematic data on circulating NoV genotypes exist. However, GIIb/GII.4 strains have been frequently identified in Turkish children with gastroenteritis; strains belonging to this genotype have been found in Europe and mainly in children [27]. Our phylogenetic analysis, although based only on partial sequences from the capsid gene, showed unique strains not previously reported in Turkey. The capsid region of the NoV genome demonstrates great genetic diversity with 20% amino acid differences across capsid sequences [28]. The gene encoding the capsid region is widely used for classification of NoV and provides a reliable marker for genotyping NoV [29]. Homologous recombination, in particular at the junction between ORF1 and ORF2, but also within ORF2 contributes significantly to this high degree of variation [30]. Full capsid sequencing analyses is the gold standard for genotyping of NoV strains, however, for clinical samples with low copy numbers, amplifying and sequence analysis of partial capsid sequences is more practical and is only slightly less discriminatory than full capsid sequencing [31]. In addition, full capsid sequencing has been used to distinguish differences between closely related GII.4 variants [32]; this genotype was not the predominant NoV in our study and partial capsid sequencing sufficiently demonstrated viral relationships.

Previous reports from British troops deployed to Iraq indicated that two NoV strains were responsible for cases of gastroenteritis. Similar mixed NoV outbreaks have been previously observed and are often attributed to systematic failure of cooking/cleaning/drinking water supplies [33]. One limitation of this investigation was that the survey was not used to capture data from a control group (persons without recent AGE); thus we were unable to perform a risk factor analysis. Another limitation was the lack of of environmental samples that could be tested for NoV in order to track the source of outbreak.

To our knowledge a formal outbreak investigation in the Turkish population was never performed. With the reported lack of sensitivity of commercial norovirus EIAs [34], it is important to use molecular diagnostics such as real-time RT-PCR for detection of NoV [35,36]. Norovirus strain typing of samples collected during outbreaks of AGE in the military is infrequently done. However, with NoV being the most important cause of foodborne illness in the US [2], a full epidemiologic investigation of AGE illness in the military including strain typing of stool samples may be able to limit the magnitude of the outbreak, link unrelated cases to a single contaminated food or water source, and better identify future risks of NoV illness in the military. As a part of the efforts to reduce the risk of outbreaks of NoV gastroenteritis, the US Department of Defense research community is working with US Centers for Disease Control and Prevention to join the electronic NoV outbreak surveillance network CaliciNet [36]. This NoV surveillance network provides centralized reporting of causative NoV strains in the US, epidemiologic information such as likely transmission route, and viral typing information. By combining this existing information new observations, such as seasonality of outbreaks or patterns of emergence of new variants or frequency of food- and waterborne exposure, can be more broadly studied.

NoVs are an important cause of both outbreaks and sporadic disease among military service members. Although usually self-limited, NoV has been associated with significant operational impact. The global significance of the emergence of NoV in recent years as well as its association with military operations, and its divergent molecular epidemiology highlight the need to perform surveillance of circulating NoV infections to characterize and detect evolving strains. This is particularly important now that efforts are underway to develop a NoV vaccine.

Acknowledgments

We are grateful to Col Johnson and Lt Col Green for their support with the outbreak investigation. We would also like to thank MSgt Christopher Duffy, TSgt Angelita Pfeiffer, SSgt Tiffany (Woods) Mitchell and SSgt Christa (Lewis) Premo for their technical assistance in the laboratory at IAB. The laboratory support of Ms.Mireille Kamel is gratefully acknowledged.

We are indebted to Dr J.Vinjé for his review and critique of this manuscript.

Author's disclaimer. The views expressed in this article are those of the author and do not necessarily reflect the official policy or the opinions of the Department of the Navy, Centers for Disease Control and Prevention.

Author Contributions

Conceived and designed the experiments: SFA JDK. Analyzed the data: SFA JDK MM. Wrote the paper: SFA JDK JD. Coordinated outbreak response, epidemiological data and fecal sample collection: TM. Coordinated Incirlik laboratory support: JH. Provided oversight of data analysis, reporting, and manuscript revision: PJS.

References

1. Patel MM, Hall AJ, Vinje J, Parashar UD (2009) Norovirus: a comprehensive review. J Clin Virol 44: 1–8.
2. Scallan E, Hoekstra RM, Angulo FJ, Tauxe RV, Widdowson M-A, et al. (2011) Foodborne illness acquired in the United States–major pathogens. Emerg Infect Dis17: 7–15.
3. Koo HL, Ajami N, Atmar RL, DuPont HL (2010) Noroviruses: The leading cause of gastroenteritis worldwide. Discov. Med10: 61–70.
4. Lopman B, Armstrong B, Atchison C, Gray JJ (2009) Host, weather and virological factors drive norovirus epidemiology: time-series analysis of laboratory surveillance data in England and Wales. PLoS One 4: e6671.
5. Patel MM, Widdowson MA, Glass RI, Akazawa K, Vinjé J, et al. (2008) Parashar UD. Systematic literature review of role of noroviruses in sporadic gastroenteritis. Emerg Infect Dis 14: 1224–31.
6. McCarthy M, Estes MK, Hyams KC (2000) Norwalk-like virus infection in military forces: epidemic potential, sporadic disease, and the future direction of prevention and control efforts. Systematic literature review of role of Noroviruses in sporadic gastroenteritis. J Infect is181: S387–91.
7. Gallimore CI, Richards AF, Gray JJ (2003) Molecular diversity of noroviruses associated with outbreaks on cruise ships: comparison with strains circulating within the UK. Commun Dis Public Health. 6(4): 285–93.

8. Centers for Disease Control and Prevention (CDC) (2002) Outbreak of acute gastroenteritis associated with Norwalk-like viruses among British military personnel Afghanistan, May 2002 MMWR Morb Mortal Wkly Rep 51: 477–9.
9. Bailey MS, Gallimore CI, Lines LD, Green AD, Lopman BA, et al. (2008) Viral gastroenteritis outbreaks in deployed British troops during 2002–7. J R Army Med Corps 154: 156–9.
10. Goodgame R (2007) Systematic literature review of role of noroviruses in sporadic gastroenteritis. Curr Infect Dis Rep 9: 102–9.
11. Thornton SA, Sherman SS, Farkas T, Zhong W, Torres P, et al. (2005) Gastroenteritis in US Marines during Operation Iraqi Freedom. Clin Infect Dis 40: 519–25.
12. Matson DO (2005) Norovirus gastroenteritis in US marines in Iraq. Clin Infect Dis 40: 526–7.
13. Siebenga JJ, Vennema H, Zheng DP, Vinjé J, Lee BE, et al. (2009) Norovirus illness is a global problem: emergence and spread of Norovirus GII.4 variants, 2001–2007. J Infect Dis 200: 802–12.
14. Siebenga JJ, Vennema H, Renckens B, de Bruin E, van der Veer B, et al. (2007) Epochal evolution of GGII.4 Norovirus capsid proteins from 1995 to 2006. J Virol 9: 932–41.
15. Kroneman A, Verhoef L, Harris J, Vennema H, Duizer E, et al. (2008) Analysis of integrated virological and epidemiological reports of Norovirus outbreaks collected within the Foodborne viruses in Europe network from 1 Jul 2001 to 30 June 2006. J Clin Microbiol 46: 2959–65.
16. Real-World Spring 2009 Disease outbreak After Action report–Incirlik AB, Turkey.
17. CLSI (2009) Clinical Laboratory Standars Institute. Performance standards for antimicrobial susceptibility testing, 19 information supplement. M100-S19.9 (3). Wayne, Pennsylvania (USA).
18. Nada RA, Shaheen HI, Touni I, Fahmy D, Armstrong AW, et al. (2010) Design and validation of a multiplex polymerase chain reaction for the identification of enterotoxigenic Escherichia coli and associated colonization factor antigens. Diag Microbiol Infect Dis 67: 134–42.
19. Kojima S, Kageyama T, Fukushi S, Hoshino FB, Shinohara M, et al. (2002) Genogroup-specific PCR primers for detection of Norwalk-like viruses. Journal of Virological Methods 100: 107–114.
20. KageyamaT, Shinohara M, Uchida K, Fukushi S, Hoshino FB, et al. (2004) Coexistence of multiple genotypes, including newly identified genotypes, in outbreaks of gastroenteritis due to *Norovirus* in Japan. J Clin Microbiol 42: 2988–95.
21. Tamura K, Peterson D, Peterson N, Stecher G, Nei M, et al. (2011) MEGA5: Molecular evolutionary genetics analysis using maximum likelihood, evolutionary distance, and maximum parsimony methods. Mol Biol Evol 28: 2731–39.
22. Kimura M (1980) A simple method for estimating evolutionary rate of base substitutions through comparative studies of nucleotide sequences. J Mol Evol 16: 111–20.
23. Saitou N, Nei M (1987) The neighbor-joining method: A new method for reconstructing phylogenetic trees. Mol Biol Evol 4: 406–25.
24. Felsenstein J (1985) Confidence limits on phylogenies: An approach using the bootstrap. Evolution 39: 783–91.
25. Mans J, de Villiers JC, du Plessis NM, Avenant T, Taylor MB (2010) Emerging norovirus GII.4 2008 variant detected in hospitalised paediatric patients in South Africa. J Clin Virol. 49(4): 258–64.
26. Fankhauser RL, Noel JS, Monroe SS, Ando T, Glass RI (1998) Molecular epidemiology of "Norwalk-like viruses" in outbreaks of gastroenteritis in the United States. J Infect Dis. 178(6): 1571–8.
27. Altindis M, Bányai K, Kalayci R, Gulamber C, Koken R, et al. (2009) Frequency of norovirus in stool samples from hospitalized children due to acute gastroenteritis in Anatolia, Turkey, 2006–2007. Scand J Infect Dis 41: 685–8.
28. Vinjé J, Green J, Lewis DC, Gallimore CI, Brown DW, et al. (2000) Genetic polymorphism across regions of the three open reading frames of "Norwalk-like viruses". Arch Virol. 145(2): 223–41.
29. Gallimore CI, Iturriza-Gomara M, Xerry J, Adigwe J, Gray JJ (2007) Inter-seasonal diversity of norovirus genotypes: emergence and selection of virus variants. Arch Virol. 52(7): 1295–303.
30. Allen DJ, Gray JJ, Gallimore CI, Xerry J, Iturriza-Gómara M (2008) Analysis of amino acid variation in the P2 domain of the GII-4 norovirus VP1 protein reveals putative variant-specific epitopes. PLoS One. 23; 3(1): e1485.
31. Vinjé J, Hamidjaja RA, Sobsey MD (2004) Development and application of a capsid VP1 (region D) based reverse transcription PCR assay for genotyping of genogroup I and II noroviruses. J Virol Methods. 116(2): 109–17.
32. MMWR Recomm Rep (2011) Updated norovirus outbreak management and disease prevention guidelines. 60(RR-3): 1–18.
33. O'Reilly CE, Bowen AB, Perez NE, Sarisky JP, Shepherd CA, et al. (2007) A waterborne outbreak of gastroenteritis with multiple etiologies among resort island visitors and residents: Ohio, 2004. Clin Infect Dis 44: 506–12.
34. Costantini V, Grenz L, Fritzinger A, Lewis D, Biggs C, et al. (2010) Diagnostic accuracy and analytical sensitivity of IDEIA Norovirus assay for routine screening of human norovirus. J Clin Microbiol 48(8): 2770–8.
35. Mattison K, Grudeski E, Auk B, Charest H, Drews SJ, et al. (2009) Multicenter comparison of two norovirus ORF2-based genotyping protocols. J Clin Microbiol 47(12): 3927–32.
36. Everardo Vega, Jan Vinjé (2011) Novel GII.12 Norovirus Strain, United States, 2009–2010. Emerg Infect Dis 17(8): 1516–8.

16

Rapid and Sensitive Detection of *Plesiomonas shigelloides* by Loop-Mediated Isothermal Amplification of the *hugA* Gene

Shuang Meng, Jianguo Xu, Yanwen Xiong, Changyun Ye*

State Key Laboratory for Infectious Disease Prevention and Control, National Institute for Communicable Disease Control and Prevention, Chinese Center for Disease Control and Prevention, Changping, Beijing, People's Republic of China

Abstract

Plesiomonas shigelloides is one of the causative agents of human gastroenteritis, with increasing number of reports describing such infections in recent years. In this study, the *hugA* gene was chosen as the target to design loop-mediated isothermal amplification (LAMP) assays for the rapid, specific, and sensitive detection of *P. shigelloides*. The performance of the assay with reference plasmids and spiked human stools as samples was evaluated and compared with those of quantitative PCR (qPCR). No false-positive results were observed for the 32 non-*P. shigelloides* strains used to evaluate assay specificity. The limit of detection for *P. shigelloides* was approximately 20 copies per reaction in reference plasmids and 5×10^3 CFU per gram in spiked human stool, which were more sensitive than the results of qPCR. When applied in human stool samples spiked with 2 low levels of *P. shigelloides*, the LAMP assays achieved accurate detection after 6-h enrichment. In conclusion, the LAMP assay developed in this study is a valuable method for rapid, cost-effective, and simple detection of *P. shigelloides* in basic clinical and field laboratories in the rural areas of China.

Editor: Stefan Bereswill, Charité-University Medicine Berlin, Germany

Funding: This work was supported by the National Science and Technology Key Project on Major Infectious Diseases (2008ZX10004-001, 2009ZX10004-101, 2011ZX10004-001). The funders had no role in study design, data collection and analysis, decision to publish, or preparation of the manuscript.

Competing Interests: The authors have declared that no competing interests exist.

* E-mail: yechangyun@icdc.cn

Introduction

Plesiomonas shigelloides is a motile, oxidase-positive, facultatively anaerobic, gram-negative rod bacterium, which is presently classified in the family *Vibrionaceae* [1]. *P. shigelloides* has been isolated from a variety of environmental sources, primarily aquatic [2–4], and is distributed worldwide. Moreover, *P. shigelloides* has been associated with seafood-associated outbreaks [5]. *P. shigelloides* has been implicated as an agent of human gastroenteritis for many years, with an increasing number of reports describing such infections during the recent years [6]. This bacterium is also of considerable clinical importance as the etiological agent responsible for different types of opportunistic infections [7].

Although extra-intestinal infections such as septicemia, cellulitis, and meningitis caused by *P. shigelloides* are rarely reported, it has been associated with secondary infections in immunocompromised patients [8–10]. Salerno et al [12] also described an infection of *P. shigelloides* with a fatal outcome in a newborn. Since most laboratories concentrate on recovery of *Salmonella*, *Shigella*, *E. coli* and other classical enteropathogens, *P. shigelloides* may be overlooked during routine culture of stool samples. The lack of routine analysis for *P. shigelloides* in cases of gastroenteritis leads to only sporadic and occasional identification of this bacterium [11]. However, the greatest challenge to clinicians and epidemiologist is the lack of a rapid, early, and accurate diagnostic method for the detection of *P. shigelloides* as an emerging infectious disease in China.

Several methods such as culture studies and biochemical assays have been developed for detection and identification of *P. shigelloides*. Despite their effectiveness and accuracy, these assays are time consuming, usually requiring up to 5 days to complete. The isolation of *P. shigelloides* from clinical samples has often been unsuccessful owing to the fastidious nature of the organism and the low level of transient bacteremia associated with the disease process. Rapid, specific, and sensitive nucleic acid amplification tests (NAATs) such as standard and real-time PCR have been developed to detect *P. shigelloides* by targeting genes encoding for major virulence factors [5,13–14]. The major limitation to the widespread use of these assays is the fact that a sophisticated thermal cycler is an indispensable requirement of such tests, thereby limiting their wide applicability.

Recently, a novel NAAT technology termed loop-mediated isothermal amplification (LAMP) has attracted a great deal of attention as a rapid, accurate, and cost-effective method for detection of pathogens in clinical diagnostics [15,16]. LAMP employs 4–6 specially designed primers and a strand-displacing Bst DNA polymerase (isolated from *Bacillus stearothermophilus*) to amplify up to 10^9 target DNA copies under isothermal conditions (60°C–65°C) within an hour [15], making LAMP a potentially rapid and simple diagnostic tool for detection of *P. shigelloides* infection. In this study, we aimed to develop a rapid, sensitive, and highly specific LAMP assay to detect *P. shigelloides* and evaluate the assay performance with pathogen-simulated human stool.

Materials and Methods

Ethics statement

Feces samples were acquired with the written informed consent from a healthy donor. This study was reviewed and approved by the ethics committee of the National Institute for Communicable Disease Control and Prevention, China CDC, according to the medical research regulations of the Ministry of Health, China.

Bacterial strains and culture conditions

A total of 52 strains (20 *P. shigelloides* and 32 non-*P. shigelloides* strains, as described in Table 1) was used for specificity testing. The bacterial load of the strains used for specificity evaluation was 10^5 pg/μL, which is high enough to avoid the false-negative amplification. Strain ATCC 51903 was used for the assay optimization , sensitivity evaluation, and simulating human stool samples. *P. shigelloides* and *Enterobacteriaceae* were cultured at 37°C overnight on brain heart infusion agar (BHI; BD Diagnostic Systems, Sparks, MD, USA). Non-*Enterobacteriaceae* strains were grown on blood agar, except for *Vibrio* strains, for which trypticase soy agar (TSA) supplemented with 2% NaCl was used. *Campylobacter* strains were grown under microaerophilic conditions (85% N_2, 10% CO_2, and 5% O_2).

LAMP primers and reaction conditions

A set of 6 primers targeted toward the *hugA* gene of the species *P. shigelloides* were designed using PrimerExplorer V4 software (Eiken Chemical Co. Ltd., Tokyo, Japan) based on the conserved sequences determined by the alignment of the *hugA* gene sequences obtained from GenBank. The primers shown in Table 2 were synthesized by Sangon Biotech (Shanghai, China). The primer sequences and their positions in the expression site of the *hugA* gene are shown in Fig. 1. All LAMP reactions were performed with the Loopamp Kit (Eiken Chemical Co. Ltd., Tokyo, Japan) in a 25-μL mixture containing 1.6 μM FIP and BIP primers (each), 0.8 μM LF and LB primers (each), 0.2 μM F3 and B3 primers (each), 20 mM Tris-HCl (pH 8.8), 10 mM KCl, 8 mM $MgSO_4$, 10 mM $(NH4)_2SO_4$, 0.1% Tween 20, 0.8 M betaine, 1.4 mM deoxynucleoside triphosphates (dNTPs; each), and 1 μL of Bst DNA polymerase (8 U/μL). The reaction mixture was incubated in a real-time turbidimeter LA320 (Teramecs, Tokyo, Japan) at 65°C for 60 min, followed by 80°C for 5 min to terminate the reaction. Positive and negative samples were distinguished from one another by a turbidity cutoff value of 0.1. After amplification, the LAMP products were detected by electrophoresis on 2% agarose gels with ethidium bromide staining or were determined by visual inspection after adding 1 μL of 1,000× SYBR green I.

Reference plasmid

To determine the sensitivity of the LAMP assay, a recombinant plasmid containing the target sequence of the *hugA* gene from the *P. shigelloides* strain (ATCC 51903) was constructed as follows: 1) A pair of primers was designed to span the sequences between the F3 and B3 primers; forward primer hugA-F (5′-GCGGTCTCCGGTTTCAAAT-3′) and reverse primer hugA-R (5′-GTTACCGGGTCTGCGTTATG-3′); 2) the PCR products (259 bp) were cloned into the pEASY-T1 vector using the pEASY-T1 Cloning Kit (Transgen, Beijing, China); 3) the recombinant plasmid was quantified with a NanoPhotometer (Implen, Munich, Germany) and was serially diluted (to concentrations of 1×10^6, 10^5, 10^4, 10^3, 10^2, 10^1, and 10^0 copies/μL) in order to evaluate the limit of detection and the reproducibility of the LAMP assay.

Table 1. Strains used in this study.

Latin name	Strain	Strains number
Plesiomonas shigelloides	ATCC51903	1
	Isolated strains	19
Enteropathogenic E. coli	Isolated strain	1
Enterotoxigenic E. coli	Isolated strain	1
Enteroinvasive E. coli	Isolated strain	1
Enterohemorrhagic E. coli	EDL933	1
Enteroaggregative E. coli	Isolated strain	1
Salmonella enteric	ATCC14028	1
Shigella flexneri	Isolated strain	1
Shigella sonnei	ATCC25931	1
Salmonella typhi	H98125	1
Klebsiella pneumoniae	ATCC700603	1
Proteus vulgaris	Isolated strain	1
Aeromonas veronii	1.2205	1
Clostridium perfringens	Isolated strain	1
Enterobacter cloacae	Isolated strain	1
Serratia marcescens	Isolated strain	1
Vibrio parahaemolyticus	ATCC17802	1
Staphylococcus aureus	ATCC6538	1
Streptococcus pneumoniae	Isolated strain	1
Streptococcus pyogenes	Isolated strain	1
Streptococcus sanguis	Isolated strain	1
Streptococcus salivarius	Isolated strain	1
Streptococcus bovis	Isolated strain	1
Enterococcus faecalis	ATCC35667	1
Yersinia enterocolitica	ATCC23715	1
Pseudomonas aeruginosa	ATCC15442	1
Aeromonas hydrophila	ATCC7966	1
Listeria monocytogenes	54003	2
Enterobacter sakazakii	ATCC51329	1
Campylobacter jejuni	ATCC33291	1
Vibrio minicus	Isolated strain	1
Vibrio vulnificus	Isolated strain	1
Vibrio fluvialis	Isolated strain	1

Evaluation of the sensitivity, specificity, and reproducibility of the LAMP assay

To compare the sensitivities of the LAMP assay and quantitative PCR (qPCR), the serially diluted reference plasmids (at concentrations of 1×10^6, 10^5, 10^4, 10^3, 10^2, 10^1, and 10^0 copies/μL) containing the target DNA were used to define the limit of detection. The qPCR assay was performed with the primers and probe in Table 2. qPCR amplification was performed in a 20-μL reaction volume containing 0.25 μM primer (each), 0.18 μM probe, 1× Premix (Takara Bio, Inc., Otsu, Japan) Ex Taq^{TM}, and 2 μL of DNA template. The assays were conducted using the PCR settings of pre-denaturation at 95°C for 30 s, 40 cycles of denaturation at 94°C for 5 s, and extension at 60°C for 34 s in an ABI PRISM system (Applied Biosystems, Carlsbad, CA, US). Fluorescence readings were acquired using the 6-carboxyfluorescein (FAM) channel.

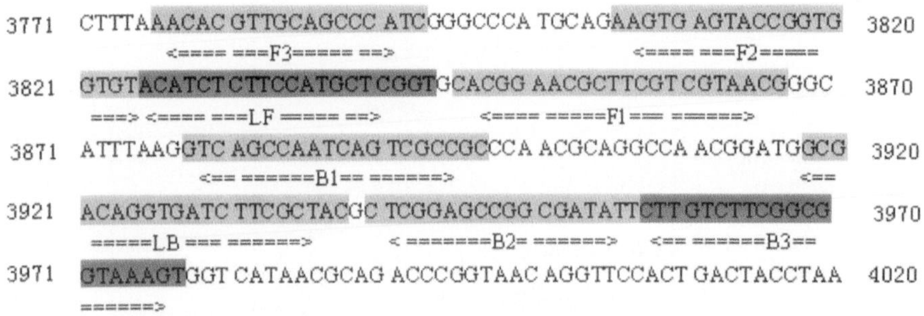

Figure 1. Names and locations of target sequences used as primers for the expression site of *hugA* LAMP.

Genomic DNA of the 32 non-*P. shigelloides* strains were detected by LAMP to determine the specificity of the *hugA* LAMP assay. All detection assays were performed in triplicate.

A set of 3 reference plasmids with varying concentrations (10^6, 10^4, and 10^2 copies/μL) was amplified in two ways (10 times on 1 day and once on each of 10 days) to evaluate the reproducibility of the LAMP assay. The intra-assay coefficient of variation (CVi) and inter-assay coefficient of variation (CVo) were analyzed at the time of peak precipitation, as measured by turbidity on a real-time turbidimeter. Statistical analyses were conducted using SAS software version 9.1.

LAMP application in simulated human stools

Human stool specimens were obtained from a healthy donor and immediately processed. We have screened the human stool specimens by culture assay and PCR, no *P. shigelloides* strain was detected and no positive amplification of *P. shigelloides* DNA was observed. To determine the detection limit of LAMP in human stool, serial 10-fold dilutions of a mid-log-phase culture of *P. shigelloides* grown in BHI were prepared in phosphate-buffered saline (PBS) and quantified using the standard plating method, resulting in spiking levels between 5×10^7 and 5×10^1 CFU/g stool. Aliquots (0.2 g) of the stools were removed for DNA extraction with a QIAamp DNA stool mini kit (QIAGEN, Venlo, Netherlands). This experiment was independently repeated 3 times, and the supernatants (2 μL) were used for both LAMP and qPCR. In addition, the capability of the LAMP assay to detect low levels of *P. shigelloides* in human stool was evaluated. For this application, simulated human stool samples were spiked with *P. shigelloides* cultures at 2 levels: 1 to 2 and 10 to 20 CFU/0.5 g. The samples were homogenized with buffered peptone water (BPW; BD Diagnostic Systems) supplemented with 50 μg/mL ampicillin (Sigma-Aldrich, St. Louis, MO, USA), followed by incubation at 37°C for up to 10 h. Aliquots (1 mL) of the enrichment broth were removed at 4, 6, 8, and 10 h, and processed similarly by QIAamp DNA stool mini kit (QIAGEN). Two microliters of the sample DNA extracts were subjected to both LAMP and qPCR assays, which were repeated twice for each sample.

Results

Specificity of the LAMP assay

The specificity of the LAMP assay targeting *hugA* gene was tested with 52 bacterial strains (Table 1). Positive amplifications were observed in 20 *P. shigelloides* strains within a 60-min incubation period. By contrast, 32 non-*P. shigelloides* strains were not amplified after a 60-min incubation period. This result indicates that no false-positive amplifications were observed with these heterologous species in the LAMP assay.

Sensitivity of LAMP assay

The limit of detection of LAMP (Fig. 2A) and qPCR for the *hugA* gene were 20 and 200 copies/reaction, respectively. This result indicates that the LAMP assay is more sensitive than qPCR for detecting *P. shigelloides* DNA. The LAMP products could also be detected by electrophoresis (Fig. 2C) and visual inspection after adding 1 μL of 1,000× SYBR green I (Fig. 2D).

Table 2. LAMP and qPCR primers used in this study to detect *P. shigelloides*.

Assay type	Primer/Probe name	Sequence (5′-3′)	Position
hugA-LAMP	F3	AACACGTTGCAGCCCATC	3776–3973
	B3	ACTTTACCGCCGAAGACAAG	3958–3977
	FIP	CGTTACGACGAAGCGTTCCGTGAAGTGAGTACCGGTGGTGT	3846–3867, 3806–3824
	BIP	GTCAGCCAATCAGTCGCCGCAATATCGCCGGCTCCGAG	3878–3897, 3940–3957
	LF	ACCGAGCATGGAAGAGATGT	3825–3844
	LB	GCGACAGGTGATCTTCGCTAC	3918–3938
hugA-qPCR	F	GGAATATCGGCCTGTACAT	4022–4040
	R	TATGGCGGCGATATTTA	4121–4137
	Probe	FAM-CCCCAGACTTTGCTGCGACCATCGG-BHQ-1	4046–4070

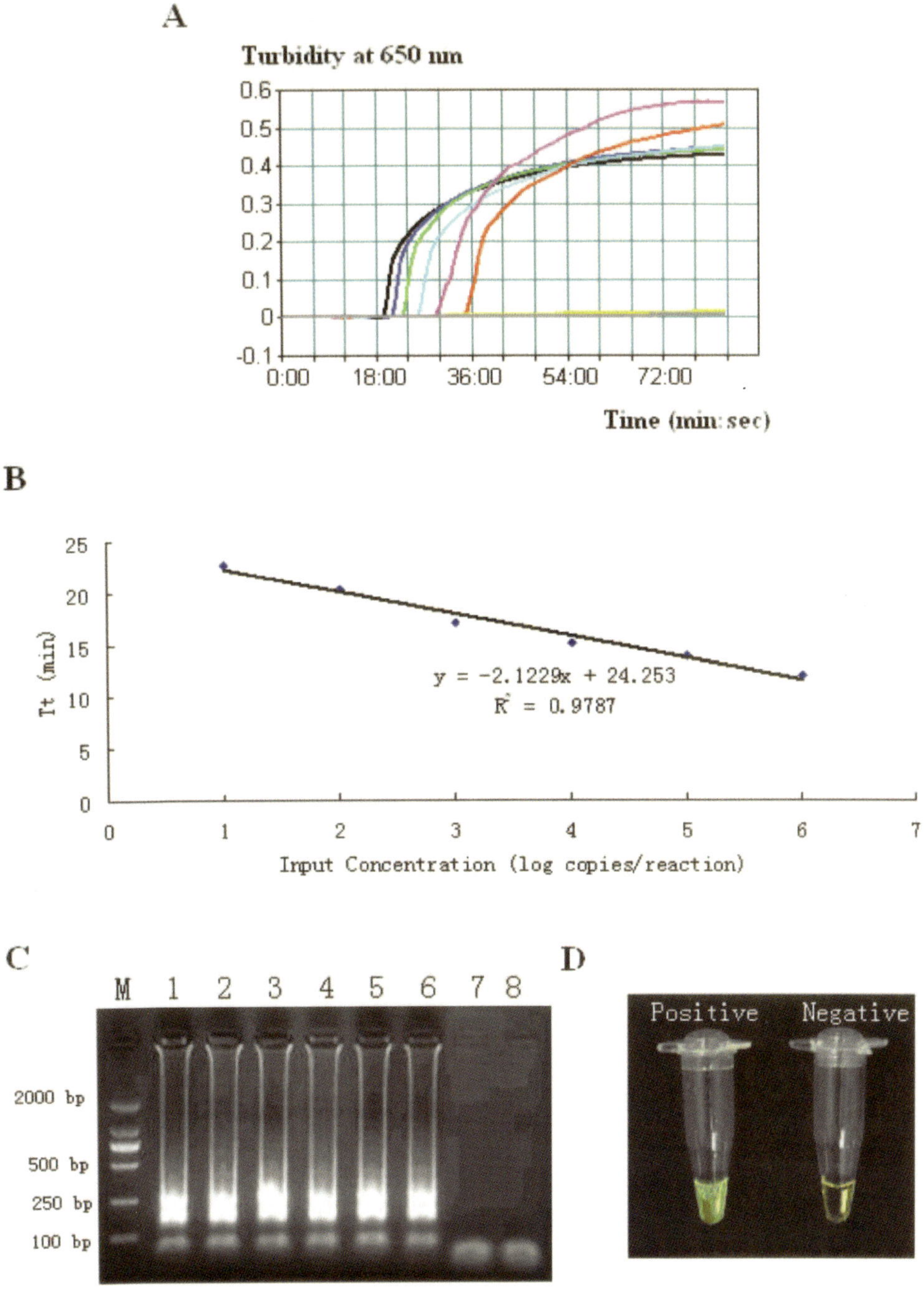

Figure 2. Real-time sensitivity and detection limit of *hugA*-LAMP. (A) Real-time sensitivity of *hugA*-LAMP as monitored by the measurement of turbidity (optimal density at 650 nm). A turbidity of >0.1 was considered to be positive for *hugA*-LAMP. The detection limit was 20 copies/reaction. (B) The relation between the threshold time (Tt) of each sample and the log copies/reaction. The standard curve was drawn on the basis of 3 independent repeats and the linear relationship R^2=0.9787. (C) Sensitivities of electrophoretic analysis of *hugA*-LAMP amplified products. Lane M: DL2000 marker; lane 1: 2×10^6 copies/reaction; lane 2: 2×10^5 copies/reaction; lane 3: 2×10^4 copies/reaction; lane 4: 2×10^3 copies/reaction; lane 5: 2×10^2 copies/reaction; lane 6: 2×10^1 copies/reaction; lane 7: 2×10^0 copies/reaction; lane 8: no template. (D) SYBR green I fluorescent dye-mediated monitoring of *hugA*-LAMP assay amplification. The original orange color of the SYBR Green I changed to green in case of positive amplification, whereas the original orange color was retained for a negative control with no amplification.

Reproducibility of LAMP assay

The CVi was assessed by testing 3 reference plasmids with varying concentrations (10^6, 10^4, and 10^2 copies/μL), 10 times in a single run, whereas the CVo was assessed by testing the same plasmids 10 times in 10 separate runs. The CVi ranged from 1.21% to 1.54%, while the CVo ranged from 2.17% to 3.23%.

Evaluation of LAMP assay in simulated human stool

The detection limit of LAMP in simulated human stool was also examined. The LAMP assays detected the presence of *P. shigelloides* strains down to as little as 5×10^3 CFU/g. By comparison, the qPCR assays had a detection limit of 5×10^4 CFU/g for *hugA* gene in simulated human stool samples (data not shown). Table 3

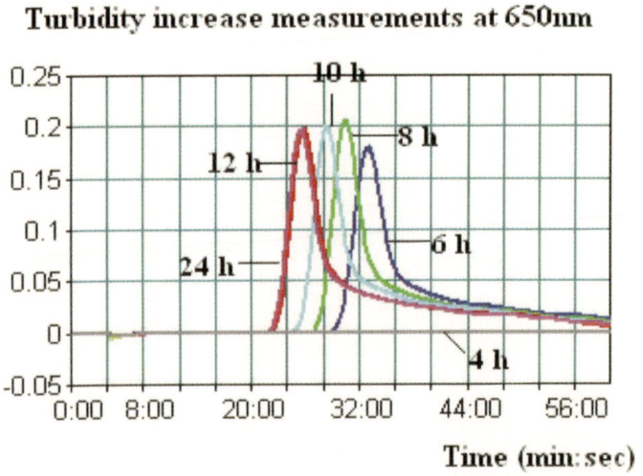

Figure 3. A typical LAMP amplification graph generated when testing human stool samples spiked with the low level of P. shigelloides strain after various enrichment periods (4, 6, 8, 10, 12, and 24 h). In this graph, the human stool sample was spiked with 1.3 CFU of Strain ATCC 51903.

summarizes LAMP and qPCR results in human stool samples spiked with 2 low levels (1 to 2 and 10 to 20 CFU/0.5 g) of *P. shigelloides* strains after various enrichment periods. A typical LAMP judgment graph generated for human stool enrichment samples is shown in Fig. 3. Regardless of spiking levels, none of the 4-h-enrichment samples tested positive for *P. shigelloides* by either LAMP or qPCR. We observed positive results with LAMP at 6 h with significantly higher threshold time (Tt) values, while for samples enriched for 8, 10, 12, and 24 h, lower and stable Tt values were observed. A similar trend of detection was observed for qPCR (Table 3). In addition, qPCR results were presented by cycles, which were approximately 1 min/cycle. Therefore, an additional 20–40 min of amplification time was needed for qPCR when testing the same enrichment sample.

Discussion

Some reports have suggested that *P. shigelloides* may cause enteric diseases in normal hosts [5,17]. Moreover, septicemia, cellulitis, meningitis, and cholecystitis due to *P. shigelloides* have also been documented among immunocompromised patients or patients with other underlying conditions [8–10]. The mortality rate associated with *Plesiomonas*-induced septicemia is high [18]. Individuals with serious infections are faced with the lack of a rapid and sensitive diagnostic method and inappropriate antimicrobial therapy, and therefore, they, often, cannot receive timely treatment, leading to diseases and fatal outcomes.

It is well known that the bacteriological methods available for the isolation and identification of *P. shigelloides* are tedious and lengthy. Modified PCR techniques such as nested PCR and real-time PCR are complicated and require a high-precision thermal cycler, and therefore, they are not adapted to diagnosing *P. shigelloides* in basic clinical and field laboratories in rural areas. In contrast, the LAMP assay reported in this study is advantageous because of the following 3 features: rapid reaction, simple operation, and easy detection. The LAMP assay does not require sophisticated and expensive equipment, maintaining a constant temperature of 60°C–65°C for 1 h is sufficient for the reaction [16]. These features demonstrate that the LAMP assay is suitable for the detection of *P. shigelloides* in basic clinical and field laboratories in rural areas.

Although the pathogenesis of *P. shigelloides*-associated gastroenteritis has not yet been elucidated, a number of potential virulence factors have been described [19,20]. Acquisition of iron is known to be involved in the virulence of a variety of bacterial pathogens [21,22]. Heme is the most abundant source of iron in the body, and many pathogenic bacteria possess heme transport systems. The *hugA* gene, one of the characterized genes encoded in the heme iron utilization system of *P. shigelloides*, encodes an outer membrane receptor that is required for heme iron utilization.

In this study, all *hugA* gene sequences of *P. shigelloides* recorded in the GeneBank were aligned, and the LAMP primers were designed on the basis of the conserved regions. We tested 32 non-*P. shigelloides* strains to evaluate the specificity of the *hugA* LAMP assay for the bacteria, with the results showing that the specificity of the LAMP assay was 100%.

To the best of our knowledge, this is the first study applying the novel LAMP technology for the detection of *P. shigelloides* in human stool. Previously, spiked samples were usually enriched overnight without characterizing the effects of different enrichment times on the detection outcomes [23,24]. In this study, *P. shigelloides* strain ATCC 51903 was used in experiments with simulated human stool samples, with the LAMP assays having a detection limit of 5×10^3 CFU/g stool. Positive detection occurred after a 6-h period of enrichment, and consistently thereafter, for the human stool samples spiked with 2 low levels (1 to 2 and 10 to 20 CFU/0.5 g) of ATCC 51903. We observed that the LAMP assay performed better than qPCR with respect to detection limit and assay speed in spiked human stool. In general, molecular level-based detection methods such as PCR and LAMP are subjected to a variety of inhibitors present in clinical samples. Some researchers have reported that the Bst polymerase in LAMP is less sensitive to the presence of inhibitors than the Taq polymerase used in classic PCR [25,26]. Our results showed that the LAMP assay is more accurate and sensitive than qPCR methods using simulated human stool samples, and proved markedly faster than qPCR by at least 20 min, thereby significantly shortening the total assay time.

In conclusion, the LAMP assay was successfully validated in this study for rapidity, sensitivity, specificity, and robustness; thus, this assay may serve as an effective means for screening *P. shigelloides* in

Table 3. Comparison of LAMP and qPCR assays in human stool samples spiked with low levels of *P. shigelloides*.

Cell level (no. of CFU/ 0.5 g)	LAMP Tt (min) after enrichment						qPCR CT (cycles) after enrichment					
	4 h	**6 h**	**8 h**	**10 h**	**12 h**	**24 h**	**4 h**	**6 h**	**8 h**	**10 h**	**12 h**	**24 h**
1–2	Not available	30.3	27.1	25.2	22.7	22.4	Not available	36.5	33.2	30.8	29.6	29.1
10–20	Not available	28.5	25.3	23.8	21.5	21.3	Not available	33.7	29.1	27.7	26.3	25.8

clinical samples. We proved that the LAMP assay demonstrated superior performance to qPCR in simulated human stool samples, and may facilitate rapid and reliable diagnosis of *P. shigelloides* infections in basic clinical and field laboratories in rural areas.

Author Contributions

Conceived and designed the experiments: SM CY JX. Performed the experiments: SM. Analyzed the data: SM YX. Contributed reagents/materials/analysis tools: SM YX. Wrote the paper: SM CY.

References

1. Garrity GM, Bell JA, Lilburn TG (2003) Taxonomic outline of the procaryotes. Bergey's Manual of Systematic Bacteriology, 2nd edn. Release 4.0 Available: http://141.150.157.80/bergeysoutline/main.htm.
2. Krovacek K, Eriksson LM, González-Rey C (2000) Isolation, biochemical and serological characterisation of *Plesiomonas shigelloides* from freshwater in Northern Europe. Comp Immunol Microbiol Infect Dis 23:45–51.
3. Reinhardt JF, George WL (1985) *Plesiomonas shigelloides*-associated diarrhea. JAMA 253:3294–3295.
4. Escobar JC, Bhavnani D, Trueba G (2012) *Plesiomonas shigelloides* infection, Ecuador, 2004–2008. Emerg Infect Dis 18:322–324.
5. González-Rey C, Svenson SB, Bravo L (2000) Specific detection of *Plesiomonas shigelloides* isolated from aquatic environments, animals and human diarrhoeal cases by PCR based on 23S rRNA gene. FEMS Immunol Med Microbiol 29:107–113.
6. Wouafo M, Pouillot R, Kwetche PF (2006) An acute foodborne outbreak due to *Plesiomonas shigelloides* in Yaounde, Cameroon. Foodborne Pathog Dis 3:209–211.
7. Miller WA, Miller MA, Gardner IA (2006) *Salmonella* spp., *Vibrio* spp., *Clostridium perfringens*, and *Plesiomonas shigelloides* in marine and freshwater invertebrates from coastal California ecosystems. Microb Ecol 52:198–206.
8. Schneider F, Lang N, Reibke R (2009) *Plesiomonas shigelloides* pneumonia. Med Mal Infect 39:397–400.
9. Ozdemir O, Sari S, Terzioglu S (2010) *Plesiomonas shigelloides* sepsis and meningoencephalitis in a surviving neonate. J Microbiol Immunol Infect 43:344–346.
10. Auxiliadora-Martins M, Bellissimo-Rodrigues F, Viana JM (2010) Septic shock caused by *Plesiomonas shigelloides* in a patient with sickle beta-zero thalassemia. Heart Lung 39:335–339.
11. Chan SS, Ng KC, Lyon DJ (2003) Acute bacterial gastroenteritis: a study of adult patients with positive stool cultures treated in the emergency department. Emerg Med J 20:335–338.
12. Salerno A, Čižnár I, Krovacek K (2010) Phenotypic characterization and putative virulence factors of human, animal and environmental isolates of *Plesiomonas shigelloides*. Folia Microbiol (Praha) 55:641–647.
13. Herrera FC, Santos JA, Otero A (2006) Occurrence of *Plesiomonas shigelloides* in displayed portions of saltwater fish determined by a PCR assay based on the hugA gene. Int J Food Microbiol 108:233–238.
14. Gu W, Levin RE (2006) Quantitative detection of *Plesiomonas shigelloides* in clam and oyster tissue by PCR. Int J Food Microbiol 111:81–86.
15. Mori Y, Notomi T (2009) Loop-mediated isothermal amplification (LAMP): a rapid, accurate, and cost-effective diagnostic method for infectious diseases. J Infect Chemother 15:62–69.
16. Notomi T, Okayama H, Masubuchi H (2000) Loop-mediated isothermal amplification of DNA. Nucleic Acids Res 28:E63.
17. Paul R, Siitonen A, Kärkkäinen P (1990) *Plesiomonas shigelloides* bacteremia in a healthy girl with mild gastroenteritis. J Clin Microbiol 28:1445–1446.
18. Lee AC, Yuen KY, Ha SY (1996) *Plesiomonas shigelloides* septicemia: case report and literature review. Pediatr Hematol Oncol 13:265–269.
19. Janda JM, Abbott SL (1993) Expression of hemolytic activity by *Plesiomonas shigelloides*. J Clin Microbiol 31:1206–1208.
20. Santos JA, González CJ, López TM (1999) Hemolytic and elastolytic activities influenced by iron in *Plesiomonas shigelloides*. J Food Prot 62:1475–1477.
21. Villarreal DM, Phillips CL, Kelley AM (2008) Enhancement of recombinant hemoglobin production in *Escherichia coli* BL21(DE3) containing the Plesiomonas shigelloides heme transport system. Appl Environ Microbiol 74:5854–5856.
22. Oldham AL, Wood TA, Henderson DP (2008) *Plesiomonas shigelloides* hugZ encodes an iron-regulated heme binding protein required for heme iron utilization. Can J Microbiol 54:97–102.
23. Ohtsuka K, Tanaka M, Ohtsuka T (2010) Comparison of detection methods for *Escherichia coli* O157 in beef livers and carcasses. Foodborne Pathog Dis 7:1563–1567.
24. Hara-Kudo Y, Niizuma J, Goto I (2008) Surveillance of Shiga toxin-producing *Escherichia coli* in beef with effective procedures, independent of serotype. Foodborne Pathog Dis 5:97–103.
25. Kaneko H, Kawana T, Fukushima E (2007) Tolerance of loop-mediated isothermal amplification to a culture medium and biological substances. J Biochem Biophys Methods 70:499–501.
26. Okada K, Chantaroj S, Taniguchi T (2010) A rapid, simple, and sensitive loop-mediated isothermal amplification method to detect toxigenic *Vibrio cholerae* in rectal swab samples. Diagn Microbiol Infect Dis 66:135–139.

17

Shigellosis Outbreak Associated with Contaminated Well Water in a Rural Elementary School: Sichuan Province, China, June 7–16, 2009

Fan He[1]❡, Ke Han[2]❡, Lunguang Liu[3]❡, Wei Sun[3], Lijie Zhang[4], Baoping Zhu[4], Huilai Ma[4]*

1 Zhejiang Provincial Center for Disease Control and Prevention, Hangzhou, People's Republic of China, **2** Guangdong Provincial Center for Disease Control and Prevention, Guangzhou, People's Republic of China, **3** Sichuan Provincial Center for Disease Control and Prevention, Chengdu, People's Republic of China, **4** Chinese Field Epidemiology Training Program, Chinese Center for Disease Control and Prevention, Beijing, People's Republic of China

Abstract

Objectives: We investigated a shigellosis outbreak in an elementary school to identify the source of infection, mode of transmission and risk factors for illness.

Methods: In a case-control investigation, we compared the source of drinking water, consumption of untreated well water and suspected food items, and hygienic habits between case-students and randomly selected asymptomatic control-students, frequency-matched by class on a 1:1 ratio.

Results: 18% of the 533 students and no teachers developed *Shigella*. 52%(44/85) of case-students and 17% (12/71) of control-students drank untreated well water (OR = 2.3, 95% CI = 1.1–5.8); 47% (n = 40/85) of case-students and 14% (10/71) of control-students drank untreated water from Well A (OR = 3.7, 95% CI = 1.3–11). The odds ratio increased with the amount of untreated Well A water consumed (p = 0.035, χ^2 test for trend). Rectal swabs from 5 of 6 case-students and water from Well A yielded *Shigella flexneri* 2b.

Conclusions: This shigellosis outbreak was caused by drinking untreated water from a well polluted by *Shigella flexneri* 2b.

Editor: Martyn Kirk, The Australian National University, Australia

Funding: This investigation was supported by the Program for Zhejiang Leading Team of Science and Technology Innovation, and the General Funds for Emergency Public Health Response from the Ministry of Health of China. The funders had no role in study design, data collection and analysis, decision to publish, or preparation of the manuscript.

Competing Interests: The authors have declared that no competing interests exist.

* E-mail: cfetpmhl@126.com

❡ These authors contributed equally to this article.

Introduction

Outbreaks of waterborne infection occur frequently in rural Chinese schools [1], [2]. According to data from the China Information System for Disease Control and Prevention [3], over 60 outbreaks of water-borne diseases, including hepatitis A, typhoid and cholera, were reported each year in rural Chinese schools during 2003–2009. More than 80% of these outbreaks were caused by contaminated well water.

On June 11, 2009, four patients with abdominal pain and diarrhea were admitted to a township hospital in Sichuan Province, China. The patients were all students at the same elementary school. Rectal swab samples from two of the patients were culture-positive for *Shigella*. Within three days, the number of reported cases increased to 32. We conducted an investigation to identify the source of infection, mode of transmission, and risk factors for this shigellosis outbreak. We also sought to elucidate the more general issues related to waterborne disease outbreaks in rural China.

Materials and Methods

We conducted this outbreak investigation immediately after the outbreak was reported on June 11. This investigation was in response to an acute public health emergency event, hence was exempted from ethics approval and informed consent.

A suspected shigellosis case was defined as onset of diarrhea (≥3 times per day), vomiting, or abdominal pain during June 5–25, 2009 in a teacher or student of the elementary school or resident who lived in close proximity to the school. A probable case was defined as onset of diarrhea (≥3 times per day) plus at least one of the following symptoms: fever (≥37.5°C), vomiting, or abdominal pain. A confirmed case was a suspected or probable case plus culture confirmation of *Shigella* infection from the stool specimens or rectal swabs.

For case finding, we systematically reviewed medical records at two private clinics and the township hospital. We reviewed medical records of patients with vomiting, diarrhea, abdominal pain and fever, and applied the case definitions to identify cases. We also asked the teachers to report illness in their students during

June 5–25. We also asked the teachers and staff to report their own and any family members' illness.

In a case-control investigation, we enrolled probable or confirmed case-students in Grade 4 or above, and conducted face-to-face interviews. Students below Grade 4 could not understand the questions adequately and were excluded. Controls were randomly selected among asymptomatic students on a 1:1 ratio, frequency matched by class. If any class had more case-students than asymptomatic students, then all asymptomatic students were selected as controls. We collected data about the onset time, symptoms and duration of illness, and history of exposure to suspected water and food items.

Rectal swabs or stool samples were collected from 97 case-students and 9 asymptomatic employees of the school cafeteria, and tested for *Vibrio cholerae, Staphylococcus aureus and Shigella*. We also collected 12 water samples (5 directly from Well A, 4 directly from Well B, 1 from a stagnant pool, 2 from the barreled water in the classrooms, and 5 from taps that drew water from Well A, 4 from taps that drew water from Well B) and tested for the same organisms. *Shigella* was also tested for in swab samples taken from the lunch boxes of 6 students, as well as from one student's wash basin and from the surfaces in the school cafeteria. We did serologically test among *Shigella* isolates of 6 cases and 1 untreated water directly from Well A. Laboratory testing was conducted in accordance with standard practices.

Univariate analysis (Student's t-test, Pearson chi-square test) was used to compare the age and sex distributions between the case- and control-students. Mantel-Haenszel chi-square test was used to assess risk of factors. The chi-square trend test was used to analyze dose-response relationships. Statistical analyses were performed using SPSS (version 15.0). Statistical significance was defined as $P<0.05$; all P-values were two-sided.

Results

Overall, we found 118 cases (21 suspected, 33 probable, and 64 confirmed), all among the 553 students (attack rate: 21%) and none among the 51 teachers and staff of the school. Also, no cases were found among the family members of the teachers and staff or the farmers living around the school. Among 118 case-students, 105 had diarrhea and only 73(62%) had at least 3 times per day. Other common symptoms included abdominal pain (82%), fever (75%), and vomiting (23%). Many patients reported their diarrhea as initially being bloody, then turning watery.

The first case-student had onset on June 7; the number of cases rose quickly, peaking on June 12. The epidemic curve suggested a common-source exposure. After the detection of the outbreak, the local public health authority disinfected the school's environment on June 12. Also, starting on June 11, water in the two water towers was chlorinated daily, and students were instructed not to drink water from the taps directly. Subsequently, the number of new cases declined (Figure 1).

The attack rate did not differ significantly between male and female students ($P=0.79$), but did differ between boarding (27%) and commuting students (19%, $P<0.05$). Of the 13 classes in the school, only 7 classes were supplied with barreled water because students in these classrooms agreed to pool money to pay for the barreled water; students in the other 6 classrooms did not want to pay for the barreled water; therefore those classrooms were not supplied with barreled water. 85% of the cases occurred in classrooms not supplied with barreled water during June 10–13. The attack rate was significantly higher in classrooms not supplied with barreled water (30%) than in those supplied with barreled water (13%) (RR = 2.4, 95% CI: 1.7–3.4). Case-students in

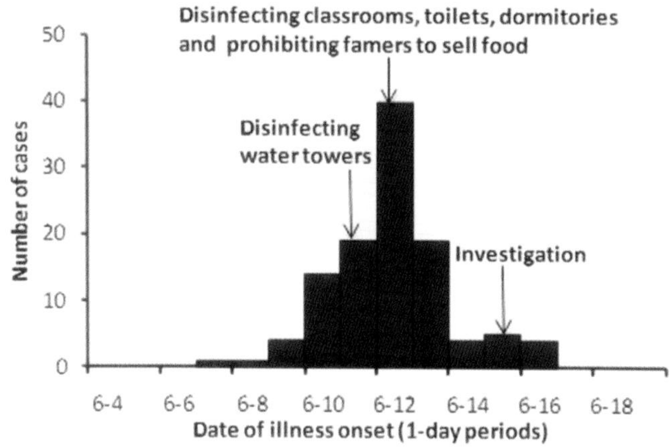

Figure 1. Epidemic curve. Epidemic curve for reported cases of Shigellosis by 1-day interval during a school outbreak, Sichuan Province, China, 2009.

classrooms with and without barreled water both peaked on June 12, suggesting that they had shared another common source of exposure.

We enrolled 85 cases-students and 71 control-students from 10 classrooms in the case-control study. During June 2–16, 52% of case-students drank untreated water compared with 17% of control-students (OR = 2.3, 95% CI: 1.1–5.8). Drinking untreated water from Well A was a significant risk factor for developing shigellosis (OR = 3.7, 95% CI: 1.3–11); moreover, the amount of untreated water from Well A consumed was associated with the risk of shigellosis in a dose-response fashion (Table 1).

Environmental investigation showed that, of the two wells the school owned, Well A was a shallow well (5 meters), constructed with stones, and was one meter away from a pond. Well B was a deep (30 meters), steel pipe well, drilled through the rock layer, and was 5 meters away from the pond. The sewage from the school and the surrounding farmers' residents was discharged directly into the pond, without treatment. Water from Well A and Well B was pumped into Tower A and Tower B, respectively, and was directly piped to the school's taps without treatment. The students reportedly drank untreated water frequently.

64 case-students were isolated Shigella positive. Laboratory serologically testing showed that, 5 case-students 1 untreated water directly from Well A yielded *Shigella flexneri* 2b. Other water and environmental samples, collected after chlorination and disinfection had taken place, tested negative for *Shigella*, *Vibrio cholera*, and *Staphylococcus aureus*.

Discussion

Shigellosis is a highly infectious diarrheal disease [4] that can lead to explosive, common-source [5], [6], [7], [8] or prolonged propagated epidemics [9]. Studies have linked unboiled water [10], [11], contaminated food [12], and household contacts [13] with shigellosis. In this investigation, we documented a school outbreak of shigellosis caused by drinking untreated water from a contaminated well.

In China, many private wells supplying water to schools are built in close proximity to pollution sources, including toilets, septic tanks, sewer ditches, lakes and ponds being discharged of sewage. Water from these wells is often not treated before being piped into schools. Consequently, waterborne outbreaks with

Table 1. Risks of shigellosis by exposure in 85 cases and 71 controls in the school, Sichuan Province, China, 2009.

Risk factors	Exposed(n)		Exposed(%)		OR	95%CI
	Cases	Controls	Cases	Controls		
Drinking water						
Untreated well water	44	12	52	17	2.3	1.1–5.8
Boiled water	40	39	47	55	1.4	0.60–3.3
Barreled purified water	42	49	49	69	1.4	0.47–4.2
Untreated water exposure						
Not drinking untreated water	39	55	46	78	Ref.	
Untreated Well A water	40	10	47	14	3.7	1.3–11
Untreated Well B water	10	8	12	11	0.40	0.08–2.1
Frequency of drinking untreated Well A water*						
Seldom	9	5	25	56	Ref.	
Usually	10	3	28	33	1.9	0.34–10
Always	17	1	47	11	9.4	0.95–94
Food exposures during June 8 to June 11						
Green beans	49	29	58	41	1.2	0.53–2.6
Potatoes	54	44	64	62	0.71	0.30–1.7
Stir-fried cucumber	33	27	39	38	1.7	0.73–3.8
Grass jelly	29	34	34	48	0.59	0.26–1.3
Cold noodles	43	38	51	54	1.1	0.48–2.4

NOTE.*Chi square for trend: $\chi^2 = 4.4$, $P = 0.035$.

various pathogens, such as hepatitis A, Shigella, Salmonella, and norovirus frequently occured [14], [15], [16].

During this outbreak, a substantial portion of the students in the 7 classrooms supplied with barreled water were still infected, and the epidemic curve suggested that these students shared another common exposure source with students in the 6 classrooms not supplied with barreled water. These infections might be due to the fact that, even though those 7 classrooms were supplied with barreled water, sometimes the water would run out, and the students had to drink the water from the taps. Also, the students washed their hands and faces and cleaned lunch boxes, and utensils using the tap water. Because shigella has very low infectious dose, those modes of exposure to the tap water might have caused the infections in the 7 classrooms supplied with barreled water.

Waterborne outbreaks also occurred frequently during the first half of the 20th century in Europe and North America [17]. After the implementation of community water treatment during the second half of the 20th century, waterborne infections declined sharply [18]. A major advantage of community water treatment is its cost-effectiveness, i.e., a successful implementation of this strategy can prevent infections by many different pathogens, as well as chemical agents.

In China, regulations on the location, design and construction of private wells exist. These regulations require that the location and design of wells serving as a source of drinking water need to be approved by public health authorities. However, these regulations are rarely implemented due to insufficient enforcement and lack of coordination between public health and educational departments. In this outbreak, the implicated well, Well A, was not only shallow (5 m), but also very close to a contaminated pond in which school and residential sewage is discharged. This is a gross violation of those regulations.

In light of the findings from this investigation, we recommend that all schools in China should be provided with municipal tap water whenever available. Inspections of all existing wells should be conducted, especially of those serving school children, who due to their young age are especially prone to waterborne communicable diseases; improperly constructed wells should be abandoned and filled up. Also, all water provided to school children should be treated and chlorinated. Additionally, sewage, especially that surrounding schools, should be treated properly before discharge to prevent drinking water sources from being polluted [19].

Acknowledgments

We are indebted to Robert E. Fontaine for his guidance during the outbreak investigation and for his comments and suggestions on data analysis and manuscript preparation.

Author Contributions

Conceived and designed the experiments: FH LL HM. Performed the experiments: FH KH LL WS. Analyzed the data: FH KH HM. Contributed reagents/materials/analysis tools: LZ. Wrote the paper: FH HM BZ.

References

1. Faruque AS, Teka T, Fuchs GJ (1998) Shigellosis in children: a clinico-epidemiological comparison between Shigella dysenteriae type I and Shigella flexneri. Ann Trop Paediatr 18: 197–201.
2. Mandomando I, Sigauque B, Valles X, Espasa M, Sanz S, et al. (2007) Epidemiology and clinical presentation of shigellosis in children less than five years of age in rural Mozambique. Pediatr Infect Dis J 26: 1059–1061.

3. LongDe Wang, Yu Wang, GongHuan Yang, JiaQi Ma, LiPing Wang, et al. (2012) China Information System for Disease Control and Prevention (CISDCP). Available: http://www.pacifichealthsummit.org/downloads/HITCaseStudies/Functional/CISDCP.pdf. Accessed: 2012 July 14.
4. Levine MM, DuPont HL, Formal SB, Hornick RB, Takeuchi A, et al. (1973) Pathogenesis of Shigella dysenteriae 1 (Shiga) dysentery. J Infect Dis 127: 261–270.
5. Egoz N, Shmilovitz M, Kretzer B, Lucian M, Porat V, et al. (1991) An outbreak of Shigella sonnei infection due to contamination of a municipal water supply in northern Israel. J Infect 22: 87–93.
6. Longfield R, Strohmer E, Newquist R (1983) Hospital-associated outbreak of Shigella dysenteriae type 2-Maryland. MMWR 32: 250–252.
7. Richen D, Lundrie P (1983) Epidemic of Shigellosis-Alberta. Can Dis Wkly Rep 9: 65–68.
8. Sorvillo FJ, Waterman SH, Vogt JK, England B (1988) Shigellosis associated with recreational water contact in Los Angeles County. Am J Trop Med Hyg 38: 613–617.
9. Mahoney FJ, Farley TA, Moriniere BJ, Winsor DK, Silberman RL, et al. (1991) Evaluation of an intervention program in the control of an urban outbreak of shigellosis. Am J Prev Med 7: 292–297.
10. Taylor DN, Bodhidatta L, Brown JE, Echeverria P, Kunanusont C, et al. (1989) Introduction and spread of multi-resistant Shigella dysenteriae I in Thailand. Am J Trop Med Hyg 40: 77–85.
11. Swaddiwudhipong W, Karintraratana S, Kavinum S (1995) A common-source outbreak of shigellosis involving a piped public water supply in northern Thai communities. J Trop Med Hyg 98: 145–150.
12. Hoge CW, Bodhidatta L, Tungtaem C, Echeverria P (1995) Emergence of nalidixic acid resistant Shigella dysenteriae type 1 in Thailand: an outbreak associated with consumption of a coconut milk dessert. Int J Epidemiol 24: 1228–1232.
13. Gaudio PA, Sethabutr O, Echeverria P, Hoge CW (1997) Utility of a polymerase chain reaction diagnostic system in a study of the epidemiology of shigellosis among dysentery patients, family contacts, and well controls living in a shigellosis-endemic area. J Infect Dis 176: 1013–1018.
14. Gao JX, Zhang J (2008) Analysis of the epidemiological characteristics and risk factors of typhoid and paratyphoid outbreak in China, 2004 to 2007. Disease surveillance 23: 698–701.
15. Yuan H, Cheng HJ, Li RH, Yang M, Liu WS, et al. (2004) Epidemiological investigation on outbreak of waterborne typhoid in a middle school. Strait J of Prev Med 10: 20–22.
16. Zhang LJ, Wang XJ, Bai JM, Fang G, Liu LG, et al. (2009) An outbreak of hepatitis A in recently vaccinated students from ice snacks made from contaminated well water. Epidemiol Infect 137: 428–433.
17. Ewald PW (1991) Waterborne transmission and the evolution of virulence among gastrointestinal bacteria. Epidemiol Infect 106: 83–119.
18. Centers for Disease Control and Prevention (1999) Ten Great Public Health Achievements - United States, 1900–1999. MMWR 48: 241–243.
19. World Health Organization (2012) Global costs and benefits of drinking-water supply and sanitation interventions to reach the MDG target and universal coverage. Available: http://www.who.int/water_sanitation_health/publications/2012/global_costs/en/index.html. Accessed: 2012 July 14.

Chromosomal and Plasmid-Encoded Factors of *Shigella flexneri* Induce Secretogenic Activity *Ex Vivo*

Christina Faherty[1], Jill M. Harper[2], Terez Shea-Donohue[2], Eileen M. Barry[1], James B. Kaper[3], Alessio Fasano[2]*, James P. Nataro[1]

1 Department of Medicine, Center for Vaccine Development, University of Maryland School of Medicine, Baltimore, Maryland, United States of America, **2** Mucosal Biology Research Center, University of Maryland School of Medicine, Baltimore, Maryland, United States of America, **3** Department of Microbiology and Immunology, University of Maryland School of Medicine, Baltimore, Maryland, United States of America

Abstract

Shigella flexneri is a Gram-negative, facultative intracellular pathogen that causes millions of cases of watery or bloody diarrhea annually, resulting in significant global mortality. Watery diarrhea is thought to arise in the jejunum, and subsequent bloody diarrhea occurs as a result of invasion of the colonic epithelium. Previous literature has demonstrated that *Shigella* encodes enterotoxins, both chromosomally and on the 220 kilobase virulence plasmid. The *Shigella* Enterotoxins 1 and 2 (ShET1 and ShET2) have been shown to increase water accumulation in the rabbit ileal loop model. In addition, these toxins increase the short circuit current in rabbit tissue mounted in Ussing chambers, which is a model for the ion exchange that occurs during watery diarrhea. In this study, we sought to validate the use of mouse jejunum in Ussing chamber as an alternative, more versatile model to study bacterial pathogenesis. In the process, we also identified enterotoxins in addition to ShET1 and ShET2 encoded by *S. flexneri*. Through analysis of proteins secreted from wildtype bacteria and various deletion mutants, we have identified four factors responsible for enterotoxin activity: ShET1 and Pic, which are encoded on the chromosome; ShET2 (encoded by *sen* or *ospD3*), which requires the type-III secretion system for secretion; and SepA, an additional factor encoded on the virulence plasmid. The use of mouse jejunum serves as a reliable and reproducible model to identify the enterotoxins elaborated by enteric bacteria. Moreover, the identification of all *Shigella* proteins responsible for enterotoxin activity is vital to our understanding of *Shigella* pathogenicity and to our success in developing safe and effective vaccine candidates.

Editor: Nicholas J. Mantis, Wadsworth Center, New York State Dept. Health, United States of America

Funding: This work was supported by NIH 5U19AI090873 and NIH R01-AI059223. The Center for Vaccine Development awarded the T32 Vaccinology Fellowship AI07524 to C.S.F. The funders had no role in study design, data collection and analysis, decision to publish, or preparation of the manuscript.

Competing Interests: The authors have declared that no competing interests exist.

* E-mail: afasano@mbrc.umaryland.edu

¤ Current address: Department of Pediatrics, University of Virginia School of Medicine, Charlottesville, Virginia, United States of America

These authors contributed equally to this work.

Introduction

Enteric infections resulting in diarrhea are prevalent throughout the developed and developing world. Children with frequent diarrheal episodes are at risk for life-long physical and mental defects [1]. While viruses and parasites cause a significant amount of diarrheal disease, bacterial pathogens, including the pathogenic strains of *Escherichia coli*, *Shigella*, and *Salmonella*, are a leading cause of diarrheal disease in the developing world [2]. Preventive and prophylactic measures have been difficult to develop and implement, making diarrheagenic bacteria a nuisance to public health and detrimental to the health of the affected populations. The lack of available animal models has been a hindrance to the process of vaccine and drug development.

Shigella species comprise a leading cause of diarrhea-associated morbidity and mortality in children under the age of five years in developing countries [3]. This age group is particularly susceptible to the effects of acute and chronic infections, although *Shigella* is clinically important in all age groups in the developing world. In addition to dehydration and the inability to absorb nutrients, children who are continuously exposed to pathogenic bacteria suffer from both physical and developmental milestone delays [1]. Stools from these children frequently contain multiple infectious organisms; however, *Shigella flexneri* 2a is the most prominent bacterial pathogen isolated from children suffering from diarrhea between the ages of 2 and 5 years [3]. Although the invasion process has been thoroughly dissected, the mechanisms by which *Shigella* induces secretory diarrhea are less defined. Like many other pathogenic bacteria, *S. flexneri* 2a possesses a type-III secretion system (T3SS) that produces several proteins required for invasion of intestinal cells. At least one T3SS effector has been identified as a putative toxin [4,5]. Most, if not all, pathogenic bacteria elaborate one or more toxins during the course of infection. These toxins have diverse activities that include, but are not limited to, colonization, proteolytic activity, cellular toxicity, and increasing intestinal secretion [6,7].

To date few studies have addressed the effects of extracellularly secreted bacterial products during *S. flexneri* 2a infection. Studies performed in the 1990s described two toxins produced by *S. flexneri* 2a, *Shigella* enterotoxin 1 (ShET1) and *Shigella* enterotoxin 2

(ShET2), that contribute to secretory activity in rabbit intestine *in vivo* and *in vitro* [4,8,9]. An epidemiological study of 383 *Shigella* isolates found that ShET1 was present in 30% of all *Shigella* isolates while ShET2 was present in 80% of isolates. Watery diarrhea is present in almost all shigellosis cases, and typically proceeds to dysentery. In fact in mild infections, watery diarrhea is the only clinical manifestation. [10,11]. ShET1 is encoded on the chromosome in the *she* pathogenicity island (PAI), and is only found in *S. flexneri* [8]. ShET2 is a T3SS effector encoded on the 220 kb invasion plasmid [5]. Previous studies reported the ability of bacterial supernatants prepared in iron-depleted medium to increase secretion in both Ussing chambers and the rabbit ileal loop model [4,8,9]. It was theorized that the secretion of ShET1 and ShET2 in the upper intestine (*e.g.* jejunum) would increase fluid secretion which, in turn, would facilitate the transit of bacteria to the colon, the site of invasion. This observation accounts for the watery diarrhea, as opposed to the scant bloody diarrhea, that occurs as a result of PMN infiltration at the site of invasion [12].

The overarching goal of this study was to validate mouse tissue as a useful model of intestinal secretion caused by exposure to secreted toxins. We also aimed at identifying all secreted factors that contribute to jejunal secretion to better define the mechanism of *Shigella*-induced diarrhea. *In vivo* intestinal secretion as a result of *S. flexneri* infection is difficult to study as the pathogen will only infect non-human primates at the natural site of infection [13]. Ussing chambers are a well-established system to define secretion from intestinal tissue *ex vivo*, and provide an alternative to *in vivo* studies [14]. Previous studies defined the response of rabbit jejunum to secreted *Shigella* toxins and recombinant proteins in the Ussing chambers [4,8,9]. We extended this secretory model to include mouse jejunum, which has proven to respond similarly to rabbit tissue. Herein we demonstrate the utility of mouse intestine as an affordable and informative model for defining secretory activity of bacterial toxins. Our study implicates both chromosomal and plasmid-encoded toxins as contributors to intestinal secretion caused by *S. flexneri* 2a. Identification of all of the enterotoxins encoded by *S. flexneri* is vital to our understanding of *Shigella* pathogenesis and may lead to targets suitable for drug and vaccine development.

Materials and Methods

Strains and Growth Conditions

Table 1 lists the bacterial strains and plasmids used in this study. Table 2 lists the enterotoxins expressed for each bacterial strain used in this study. Bacteria were routinely cultured at 37°C either in Luria-Bertani broth with aeration, or on tryptic soy broth plates with 1.5% agar and 0.025% Congo Red (CR; Sigma). Antibiotics were used at the following concentrations: kanamycin, 50 μg/ml; streptomycin, 50 μg/ml; and chloramphenicol, 5 μg/ml. Guanine supplementation (0.005%, Sigma) was used for strains harboring the Δ*guaBA* mutations (strain 1208S).

Mutant Construction

Strain 1377 (Δ*pic* and Δ*set1*AB) was constructed using a modification of the λ red linear recombination method [15] in which the entire *pic/set1*AB region was replaced with a kanamycin/sacB cassette. Selection for the mutation was performed using kanamycin. Sucrose sensitivity and PCR analysis verified that the mutation was achieved at the appropriate site. Strain 1380 is a spontaneous T3SS mutant, and was selected for by red/white colony screenings on CR plates. To construct 1522, the kanamycin/sacB cassette from 1377 was removed by a second linear recombination step in which the wildtype *pic/set1*AB locus was replaced back into the region of interest [16]. To construct 1542 the *pic/set1*AB locus with four point mutations to terminate transcription of *set1*A and *set1*B while maintaining transcription of *pic* was replaced back into the region of interest [16]. 1522 and 1542 were selected via sucrose resistance and screened for kanamycin sensitivity. DNA sequencing confirmed restoration of the wildtype or point mutation locus.

Strain BS796 (Δ*ospD3*) was constructed using the λ red linear recombination method as previously described [15]. PCR was used to amplify a chloramphenicol resistance cassette gene (cat) from pKD3 (Table 1) which had 5′ and 3′ overhangs identical to the 5′ and 3′ regions of *ospD3*. The sequence of the forward primer was 5′ – TGA AAG GAA TAT ATA CAT ATG CCA TCA GTA AAT TTA ATC CCA TCA AGG CAT ATG AAT ACC TCC TTA GTT CC –3′ and the sequence of the reverse primer was 5′ – ATC ACC ACG AGA TAA TAT TCA GCT TTT TAT ATT CTT CAT AAT TT CTA GTG TGT AGG CTG GAG CTG CTT C –3′. Chloramphenicol resistant recombinants were purified and screened via PCR using primers that annealed to unique regions upstream and downstream of *ospD3* to detect the size difference due to the insertion of the chloramphenicol cassette. For this PCR reaction, the forward primer sequence was 5′ – GCC ATC AAT CAT CCA AAG GG –3′ and the reverse primer sequence was 5′ – CGG AGG TAA CAG ACC AGA CG –3′. This mutant, in the BS766 background, was used as the donor strain for transduction of 2457T (the recipient) using P1L4 [17], and selection for chloramphenicol resistance generated BS796. The mutation was verified by PCR.

Animals Used in this Study

Female New Zealand White (NZW) rabbits were purchased from Charles River. Rabbits weighing between 2.3 and 3 kg were used in Ussing chamber experiments. Female C57BL/6 mice were purchased from the National Cancer Institute (Frederick, MD) and were used for Ussing experiments between 6 and 14 weeks of age.

Preparation of Bacterial Supernatants

Samples were prepared as follows for use in Ussing studies. Overnight cultures of bacteria were subcultured into 600 ml Luria-Bertani Broth (LB) with the appropriate antibiotic selection or nutrient supplementation required for each strain of *S. flexneri* (see strains and growth conditions). Cultures were grown at 37°C with shaking until the optical density (OD_{600}) reached 1.0. The bacteria were then pelleted by centrifugation at 5,000 rpm for 10 minutes at 4°C. Culture supernatants were subsequently filter-sterilized with a 0.45 μm vacuum filtration unit (Millipore) and stored at −20°C. The stored supernatants were thawed at 4°C and concentrated using the Centricon Plus-70 centrifugal filter devices with a molecular weight cutoff of 30 kD (Millipore), according to manufacturer's instructions. Concentrated proteins (averaging 30 μg/μl) were resuspended in 1X PBS to a final volume of 2 ml, and samples were stored at −80°C in 500 μl aliquots.

Preparation of Iron-depleted LB

In order to deplete the iron from LB, fifty grams of Chelex-100 resin (Bio-Rad) was added to 1 L of LB according to manufacturer's instructions and stirred for 2 hours, after which the solution was filtered through a 0.45 μM vacuum filter unit with receiver bottle (Millipore). $MgSO_4$ was added to a final concentration of 2 mM and $CaCl_2$ was added to a final concentration of 0.1 mM. All solutions were prepared with iron-free water in iron-free containers. The pH of the solution was adjusted to 7.4 with

Table 1. Strains and plasmids used in this study.

Name	Description	Reference
Strains		
2457T	Wildtype *S. flexneri* 2a	[36]
BS103	Plasmid-cured 2457T	[37]
BS652	2457T/*spa47::aadA*	[38]
1377	2457T/*pic/set1*AB*::aph-3*	[16]
1380	1377/type-III secretion system mutant	This study
1522	1377/*pic*$^+$/*set1*AB$^+$	[16]
1542	1377/*pic*$^+$	[16]
BS796	2457T/*ospD3::cat*	ATM; this study
1208S	2457T/Δ*guaBA*+Δ*set1*AB+Δ*ospD3*	[39]
	2457T/Δ*sepA*	BAM
E. coli HS	Commensal *E. coli*; Nal^r	[23]
Mutant Construction		
Strains		
BS766	2457T transformed with pKM208	[38]
Plasmids		
pKD3	oriR6K, *bla, cat*	[15]
pKM208	Temperature-sensitive *red-, gam-, lacI*-expressing plasmid driven by P_{Tac} promoter, *bla*	[15]

concentrated HCl. The iron-free LB was then filtered a second time through a 0.45 μM filter to ensure sterility. Medium was used immediately or stored at 4°C until use.

Ussing Chamber Studies

Assessment of secretory activity in response to secreted bacterial proteins was performed using jejunum mucosae stripped of muscle and mounted in Ussing chambers [18]. For rabbit jejunum 0.5206 cm^2 tissue was exposed for analysis in the Ussing chambers, while 0.1256 cm^2 tissue was exposed for mouse jejunum. While in the Ussing chambers, the tissue was short circuited every 50 s at 1 V (World Precision Instruments DVC, 1000 voltage clamp) and the short circuit current (Isc) was monitored continuously. The potential difference was measured using agar-salt bridges and electrodes. After equilibration of 0.126 cm^2 of tissue in 10 ml of Krebs' buffer (118 mM NaCl, 4.7 mM KCl, 1.2 mM KH2PO4, 1.2 mM MgSO4, 4.2 mM NaHCO3, 2 mM CaCl2, 10 mM glucose, 200 mM sulphinpyrazone and 10 mM Hepes, pH 7.4), a test for glucose absorption was conducted to assess the responsiveness of the tissue. To test the function of the sodium linked glucose transporter and, therefore, the integrity of the tissue, 20 mM glucose was added to the mucosal chamber while an iso-osmotic solution of mannitol was added to the serosal chamber; and Isc determined. The tissues were washed and allowed to equilibrate once more, after which 400 μl of concentrated secreted *Shigella* proteins were added to the mucosal chamber and 400 μl of PBS was added to the serosal chamber. Isc was measured for at least 30 minutes post-toxin addition; the change in Isc (ΔIsc) reflects the maximum change during this time course. Responses from two tissue segments exposed to secreted proteins from one mouse were averaged to yield a mean response per animal. Each sample was tested on a minimum of four animals. For every experiment, secreted proteins from wildtype 2457T served as a positive control. Values are expressed as mean ± standard error of the mean (SEM).

Table 2. Toxins expressed in the *Shigella flexneri* strains analyzed.

Strain	ShET1	Pic	ShET2	SepA
2457T	+	+	+	+
BS103	+	+	−	−
BS652	+	+	−	+
1377	−	−	+	+
1380	−	−	−	+
1522	+	+	+	+
1542	−	+	+	+
BS796	+	+	−	+
1208S	−	−	−	+
Δ*sepA*	+	+	+	−
E. coli HS	−	−	−	−

Congo Red Secretion Assay

The Congo red (CR) secretion assay was used to identify proteins secreted by the bacteria through the T3SS, and was performed as previously described [19]. Briefly, bacteria were grown to mid-log phase, resuspended in 1X PBS, and CR was added to a final concentration of 30 μg/ml. The bacteria were incubated at 37°C for 1 hour. After incubation, the bacteria were pelleted by centrifugation, and the supernatant was collected and filtered through a 0.22-μm-pore filter and stored at −20°C. The proteins in the supernatant represent the secreted proteins and were concentrated by trichloroacetic acid (TCA) precipitation. TCA pellets were resuspended in 50 μl sodium dodecyl sulfate (SDS) loading buffer for protein analysis and stored at −20°C. The bacterial pellets, representing the non-secreted proteins, were resuspended in 500 µl of SDS loading buffer and stored at −20°C.

Protein and Western Blot Analysis

For total protein analysis each sample was resolved by SDS-polyacrylamide gel electrophoresis (PAGE), and Coomassie blue stain was used to visualize total protein. For Western blot analysis proteins were transferred to a PVDF membrane and blocked with 10% dry milk in 1X PBS. IpaB was detected with mouse monoclonal anti-IpaB antibody (1:20,000 dilution) [20]. After washing, Alexa Fluor 700 goat anti-mouse immunoglobulin G (H+L) antibody (Molecular Probes) was added at a 1:3,000 concentration in PBS-Tween with 10% dry milk for 1 h. All washes of the PVDF membrane were performed with 1X PBST for 5 minutes at room temperature. Protein gels and Western blots were scanned using the Odyssey infrared detection system (Li-Cor).

Statistical Analysis

Two-tailed Student's t-tests or analysis of variance (ANOVA) were used to assess significance with $p<0.05$ considered to be significant.

Ethics Statement

This study was carried out in strict accordance with the recommendations in the Guide for the Care and Use of Laboratory Animals of the National Institutes of Health. The protocol was approved by the Institutional Animal Care and Use Committee (IACUC) at the University of Maryland at Baltimore (protocol #0111044). All efforts were made to minimize suffering during euthanasia of the mice.

Results

Iron-depletion of Medium does not Affect Enterotoxic Activity

Previous studies with enteroinvasive *E. coli* required iron depletion in order to detect an enterotoxin effect in the rabbit ileal loop model and increases in Isc in the Ussing chambers [21]. These iron-depleted conditions were continued with studies for *S. flexneri*; however, it was never determined if iron-depletion was required to induce enterotoxin expression in *S. flexneri*. In this study, we tested whether enterotoxic activity of *S. flexneri* 2457T was only apparent after preparation with iron-depleted media. Cultures were prepared with and without Chelex-100 resin, and the culture supernatants were processed as described in the Materials and Methods. Supernatants from 2457T cultures prepared with and without the iron chelator both resulted in a significant increase in Isc, and no significant difference was detected between the two conditions on rabbit tissue (Figure 1). The *Vibrio cholerae* toxin served as the positive control [22] whereas PBS and supernatants derived from the commensal *E. coli* HS strain, which does not produce any enterotoxic activity [23], were employed as the negative controls. These observations were confirmed in experiments with mouse tissue (data not shown). As a result of these experiments, we maintained normal growth conditions, without iron depletion, for analysis of the *S. flexneri* deletion mutants.

The Plasmid-cured Strain and a Type-III Secretion System Mutant Identify Loci of Putative Enterotoxin Genes

In order to corroborate and expand previous studies on the location (chromosome, virulence plasmid, or both) of genes encoding enterotoxic factors, we compared the plasmid-cured strain of *S. flexneri* (strain BS103) and a T3SS mutant (strain BS652) to wildtype 2457T. BS652 harbors a deletion in *spa47*, which encodes the ATPase that drives the T3SS. This mutation results in assembly of the T3SS apparatus but prevents secretion of T3SS effector proteins [24,25]. Therefore, proteins encoded on the virulence plasmid that do not require the T3SS for secretion are still present in the culture supernatants. *E. coli* HS served as a negative control for toxigenic activity. The protein profile of the concentrated supernatants for each strain is provided in Figure 2. High molecular weight proteins are encoded on both the chromosome and virulence plasmid, and represent the large autotransporter proteins encoded by the bacteria [26,27,28,29]. The smaller proteins present in the 2457T supernatants represent the effector proteins secreted by the T3SS [30].

Analysis of the concentrated supernatants on rabbit tissue in the Ussing chambers demonstrated that 2457T consistently induced an increase in Isc of approximately 100 $\mu A/cm^2$ while the enterotoxic signal triggered by strain BS103 was significantly lower compared to 2457T, with a consistent Isc of approximately 40 $\mu A/cm^2$ (Figure 3A). The data suggested that the chromosome harbors genes encoding enterotoxins. The ΔIsc of approximately 60 $\mu A/cm^2$ caused by strain BS652 was significantly lower than that induced by 2457T supernatants, but was also significantly higher than BS103 (Figure 3A). Since BS652 has a defective T3SS, the data indicated that there are two types of toxin contributions from the virulence plasmid. The first type is an effector secreted through the T3SS and the second type does not require the T3SS to be secreted. Based on the annotated sequence of the virulence plasmid and the appearance of supernatants on protein gel electrophoresis, we hypothesized that a high molecular weight autotransporter encoded on the plasmid would contribute to enterotoxin activity (see below). To develop a more practical and efficient *ex vivo* assay, we also performed analysis of the same strains on tissue isolated from mice. The supernatants were prepared and applied to the mouse jejunal tissue in the same manner as described for the rabbit jejunum. We found that 2457T, BS103, and BS652 induced similar changes in Isc in the mouse tissue as in the rabbit tissue (Figure 3B). Given the benefits of utilizing mouse tissue, we proceeded with mouse jejunum for the remainder of the experiments with 2457T supernatants serving as the positive control.

Identification of the Genes Encoding the Chromosomal Enterotoxin

In order to identify the toxins encoded on the chromosome, we first analyzed a deletion mutant of the previously implicated *set1*A and *set1*B genes, which encode ShET1 (strain 1377). Studies have demonstrated that in *S. flexneri* 2a the *pic* gene is encoded on the opposite strand of DNA from that encoding the *set1*AB region [16]. To ensure that all potential enterotoxic activity was removed from this region, mutant 1377 had the entire *pic/set1*AB region deleted. Strain 1377 produced a change in Isc of approximately 40 $\mu A/cm^2$ (Figure 4). Complementation of strain 1377 with the wildtype *pic/set1*AB locus replaced in strain 1522 restores enterotoxic activity to the same level as 2457T (Figure 4). The data therefore indicate that the chromosomal enterotoxic contribution arises from the ShET1/Pic region. Interestingly, when 1377 was complemented with *pic* alone in strain 1542, enterotoxic activity was restored to 2457T levels. In order to achieve complementation with *pic* alone, the locus was replaced with a cassette containing four point mutations that introduced stop codons in the *set1*A and *set1*B genes while maintaining the appropriate codons for *pic*. These data suggested that Pic is the

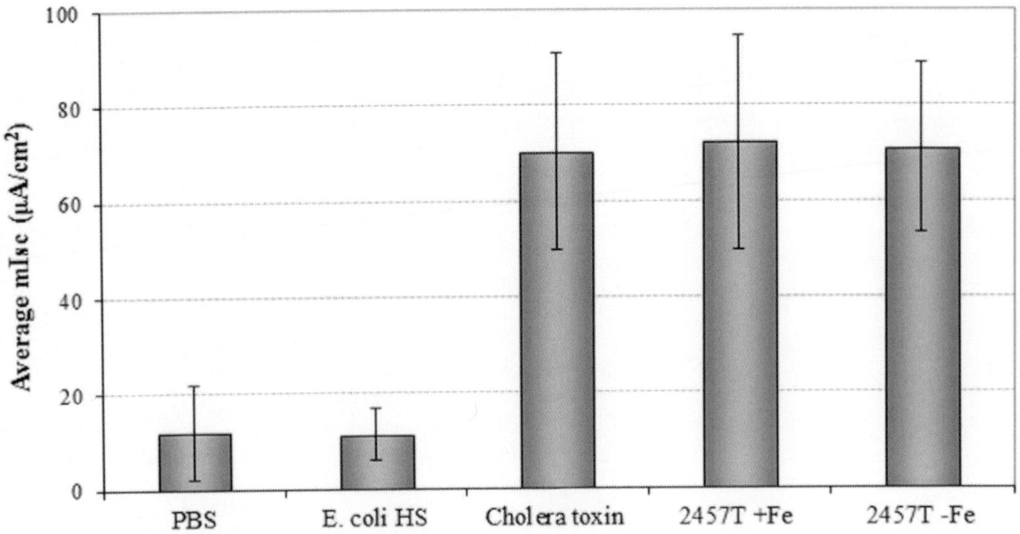

Figure 1. Iron depletion is not required for *S. flexneri* enterotoxin activity. The average change in short circuit current (μA/cm2) is plotted +/− the standard error for wildtype *S. flexneri* 2a strain 2457T with iron (+Fe) and without iron (-Fe). There is no significant difference between the two conditions. PBS and supernatant from *E. coli* HS served as negative controls while 40 μg of *Vibrio cholerae* toxin served as a positive control for inducing a change in Isc.

enterotoxin producing the greater contribution. Expression of *set1*AB alone, however, was sufficient to induce a significant

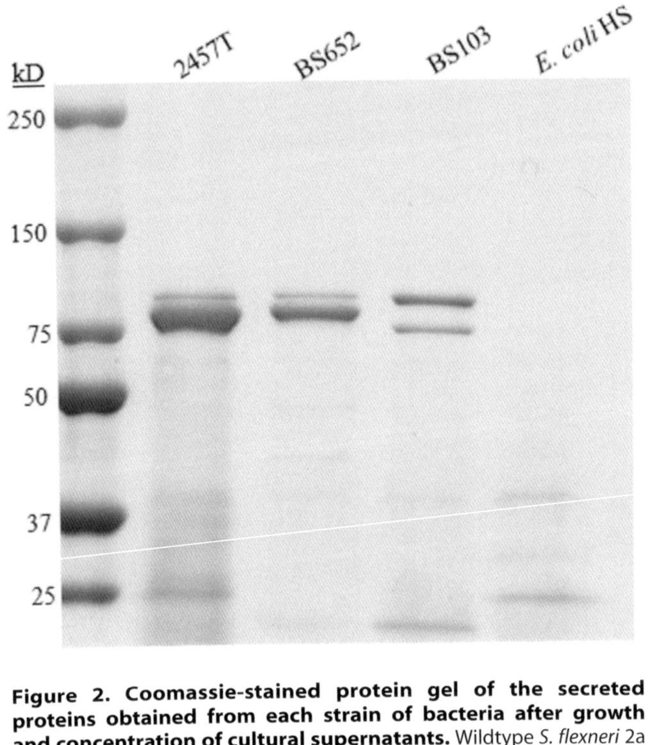

Figure 2. Coomassie-stained protein gel of the secreted proteins obtained from each strain of bacteria after growth and concentration of cultural supernatants. Wildtype *S. flexneri* 2a strain 2457T secretes the autotransporter proteins localized around 100 kD in addition to other type-III secretion system effector proteins at lower molecular weights. Strain BS652 has a defective T3SS but is still able to secrete the autotransporter SepA that is encoded on the virulence plasmid. Strain BS103 is the virulence plasmid-cured and therefore secrets only the chromosomal autotransporters. The negative control *E. coli* HS commensal strain secretes a minimal amount of protein.

change in Isc [8,9]. Therefore, we conclude that both Pic and ShET1 confer enterotoxic activity. Our data suggest that ShET1 and Pic are the chromosomally-encoded enterotoxins expressed under the culture conditions used in our experiments.

Identification of the Genes Encoding the Virulence Plasmid Enterotoxins

Given that strain BS652 is a T3SS mutant and that ShET2 has been identified as a T3SS effector protein, we next analyzed strain BS796, which harbors a mutation in *sen* (also called *ospD3*), the gene encoding ShET2. As shown in figure 5, a mutation in ShET2 resulted in approximately the same ΔIsc as a mutant with a defective T3SS (strain BS652), suggesting that the enterotoxin secreted by the T3SS was in fact ShET2.

Identification of Additional Enterotoxins Encoded by *Shigella flexneri*

The ΔIsc induced by strains 1380 and 1208S suggested that more enterotoxins were present in addition to Pic, ShET1, and ShET2. 1208S harbors a double mutation in ShET1 and ShET2. Strain 1380 is a spontaneous T3SS mutant of 1377 that was isolated by looking for white colonies on CR plates. PCR analysis for the *ospC1* to *ospD3* coding region (3.7 kb) revealed that 1380 still harbored the virulence plasmid (Figure 6A), and therefore was not a plasmid-cured strain of 1377. To verify that 1380 had a defective T3SS, a CR secretion assay was performed to ensure T3-secreted proteins were not present in supernatants. As shown in figure 6B, T3SS-specific secretion was significantly reduced in 1380, similar to the response in the *Δspa47* mutant (strain BS652). To confirm that secretion was T3SS-dependent, we performed Western blot analysis to detect the T3SS effector IpaB (Figure 6C); as expected, 1380 did not secrete IpaB. Therefore, we concluded that 1380 culture supernatants were deficient for Pic and ShET1 (due to the mutation), and ShET2 due to the lack of T3 effector secretion.

Strains 1208S and 1380 were analyzed using Ussing chambers to determine if some enterotoxic activity was retained despite removal or inadequate secretion of ShET1, Pic and, ShET2.

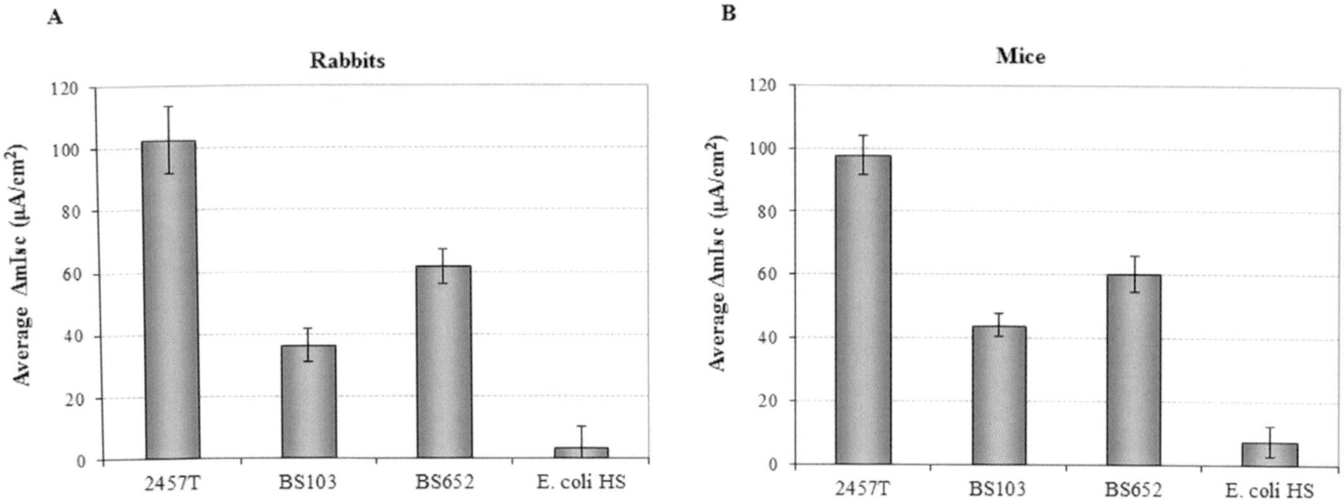

Figure 3. The *S. flexneri* chromosome and virulence plasmid encode enterotoxins that increase Isc in both rabbit and mouse tissue. The average change in short circuit current (mΔIsc, $\mu A/cm^2$) is plotted +/− the standard error for wildtype *S. flexneri* strain 2457T, the virulence plasmid-cured strain BS103, and the Δ*spa47* mutant strain BS652. Analysis of BS103 and BS652 revealed that both the chromosome and virulence plasmid encode enterotoxins. *E. coli* HS served as a negative control. Experiments were performed with intestinal tissue from rabbits (A) and mice (B). All differences are significant, with *p*-values <0.01.

Analysis of the secreted proteins from these strains demonstrated that enterotoxic activity was still present above *E. coli* HS levels (Figure 7A). These observations confirmed that *S. flexneri* encoded additional enterotoxins; and therefore, we proceeded to analyze a Δ*sepA* mutant generously provided by Dr. Beth McCormick. SepA is a Serine Protease Autotransporter of *Enterobacteriacae* (SPATE) that is encoded on the virulence plasmid [31]. This protein does not require the T3SS to be secreted, and therefore, served as a likely candidate to be the additional enterotoxin encoded on the virulence plasmid. The Δ*sepA* mutant elicited a ΔIsc significantly lower than wildtype (Figure 7A), indicating that SepA contributed to the enterotoxic activity.

Discussion

The mechanism by which *Shigella* causes watery diarrhea is currently unknown. Since secretogenic activity is a central hallmark of early disease progression, the goal of this study was to expand previous work on *Shigella*-induced secretion through the validation of a mouse jejunum model using Ussing chambers. By analyzing several *S. flexneri* mutants, we were able to characterize

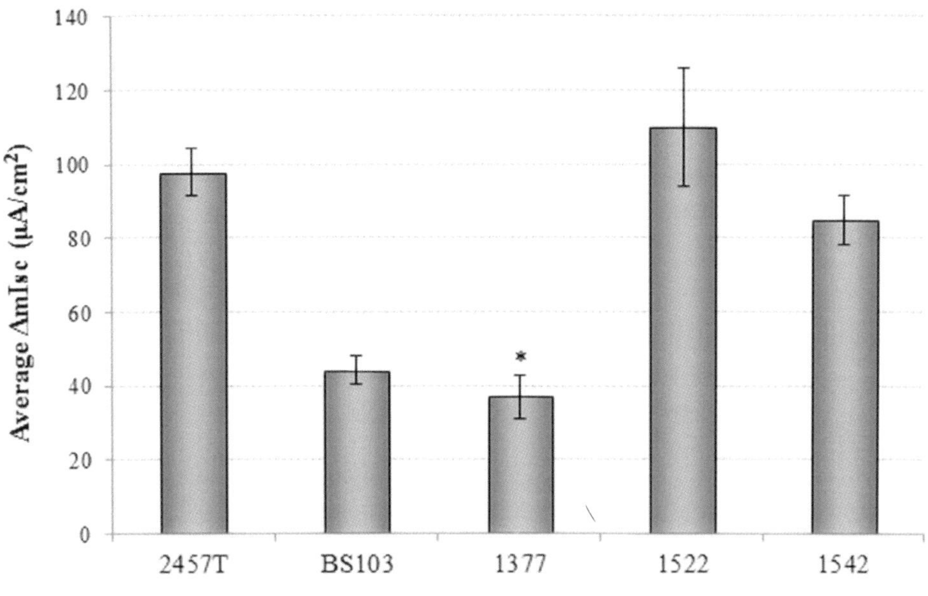

Figure 4. The *pic* and *set1AB* locus encodes the chromosomal toxins. Strain 1377 (Δ*pic*+Δ*set1AB*) had almost a 60% reduction in the change in short circuit current compared to wildtype 2457T. Complementation of the mutation in strain 1522 restores toxin activity to the same level as 2457T. In addition, addition of *pic* alone in strain 1542 restores ΔIsc to the same level as wildtype bacteria. The *p*-value difference between 2457T and 1377 is<0.001, as is the difference between 1377 and 1522 or 1542. There was no significant difference between 2457T, 1522, or 1542.

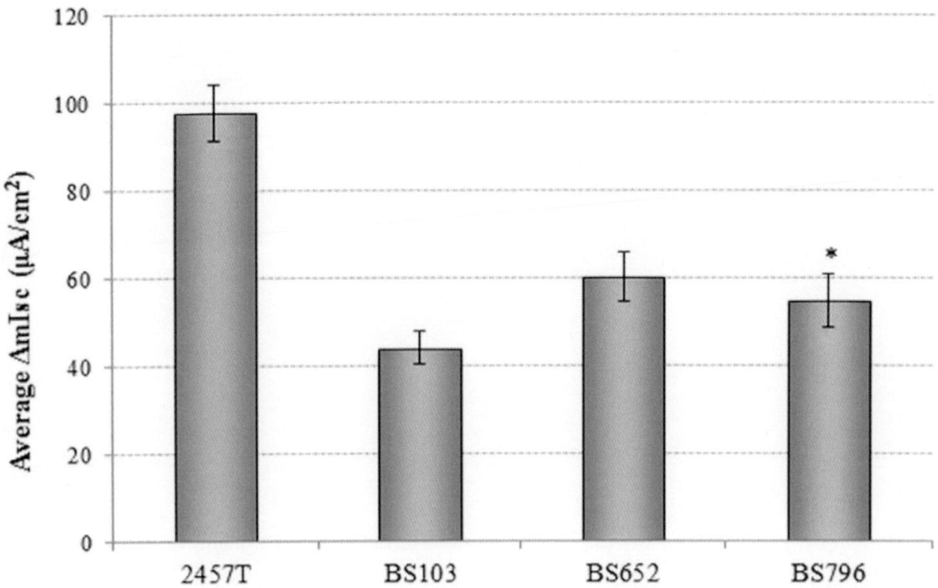

Figure 5. The type-III secretion system effector ShET2 (encoded by *sen* or *ospD3*) contributes to enterotoxin activity. A mutant that does not express ShET2 (BS796) causes the same change in short circuit current as the type-III secretion system mutant strain BS652. The *p*-value difference between 2457T and BS796 is$<$0.01. The data indicate that ShET2 is the type-III secretion system effector protein that contributes to enterotoxin activity.

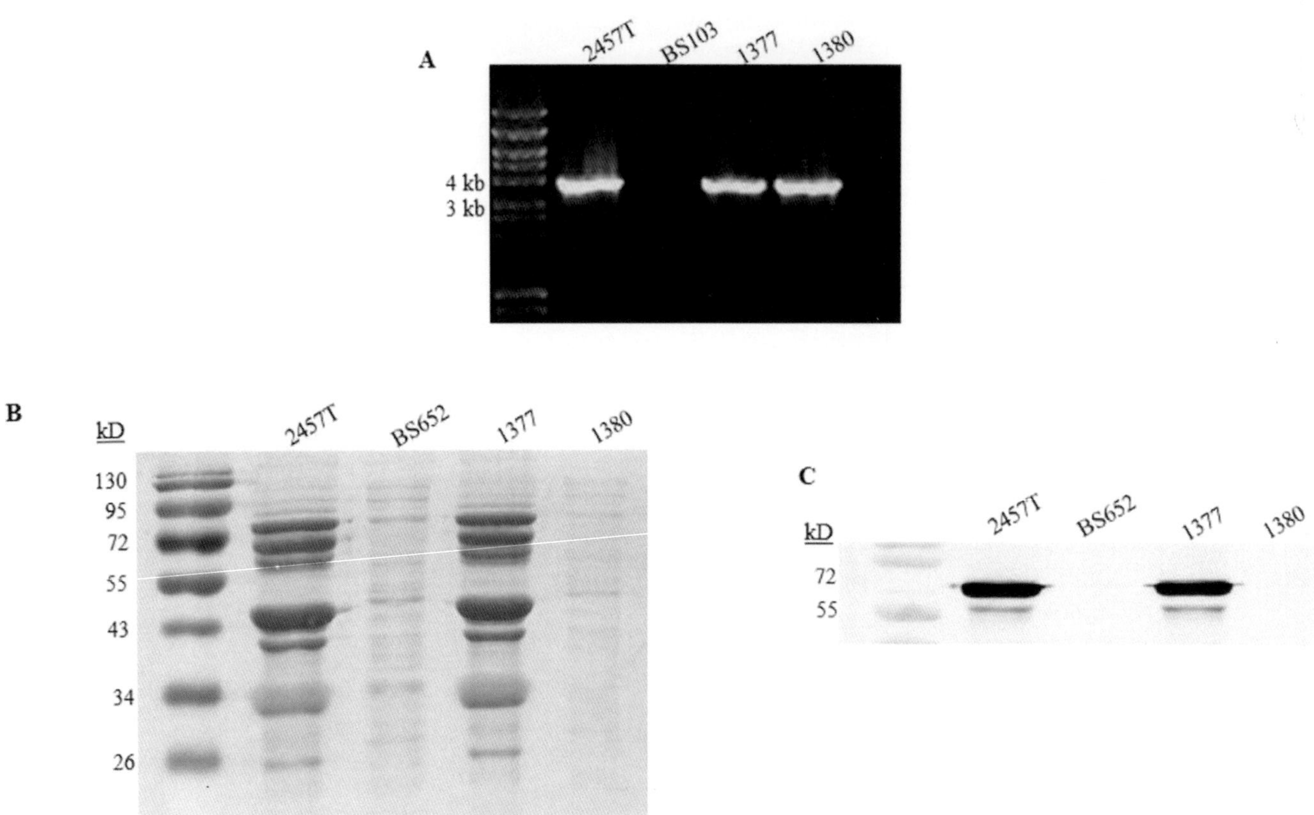

Figure 6. Strain 1380 has the virulence plasmid but a spontaneous mutation results in a defective T3SS. A: PCR analysis for the *ospC1* to *ospD3* coding region (3.7 kb) demonstrates presence of the virulence plasmid. The negative control is the plasmid-cured strain BS103. **B:** The Congo red secretion assay was performed, and the supernatants representing the secreted proteins were analyzed on an SDS-PAGE gel. The secretion profile of 2457T, BS652, 1377, and 1380 demonstrates that 1380 had a dysfunctional T3SS like the Δ*spa47* mutant (BS652). **C:** Western blot analysis of supernatants for IpaB. Secretion was only detected in the strains with a functional T3SS, strains 2457T and 1377.

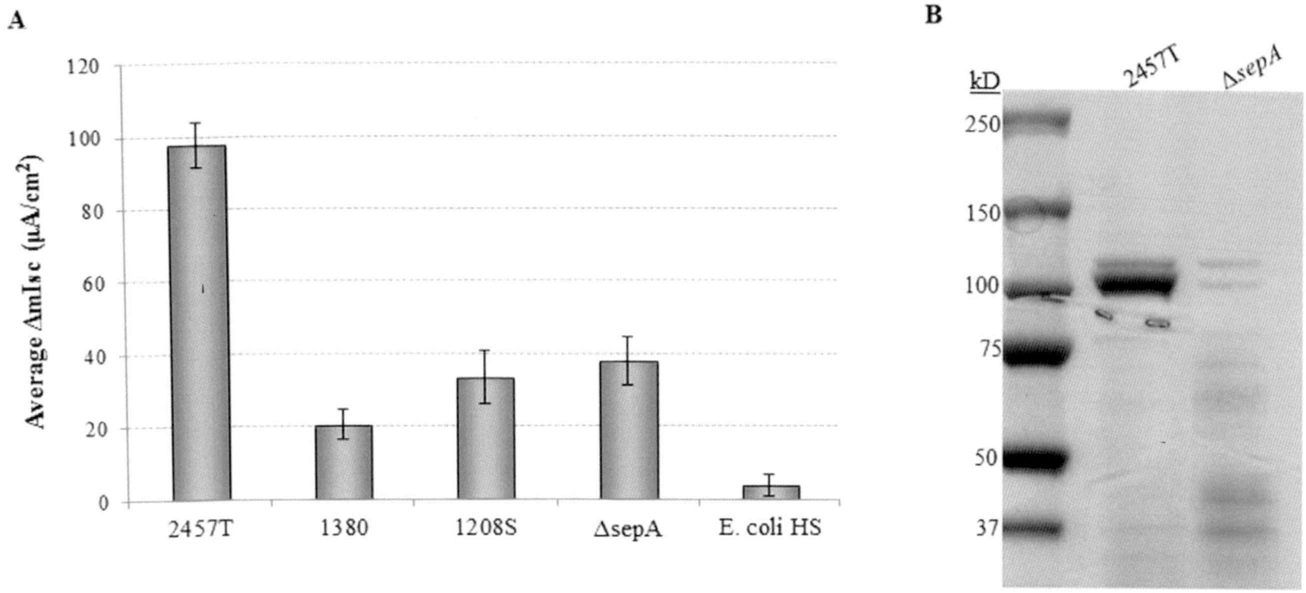

Figure 7. Additional *Shigella* proteins contribute to enterotoxin activity. A: Analysis of 1380 and 1208S verified that *S. flexneri* encodes enterotoxins in addition to Pic, ShET1, and ShET2. Analysis of a Δ*sepA* mutant demonstrated there was a significant decrease in the short circuit current, indicating that SepA contributed to enterotoxic activity. All 3 mutant strains have a significant increase in ΔIsc compared to *E. coli* HS with all *p*-values$<$0.01. **B:** Coomassie-stained protein gel of the secreted proteins obtained from the Δ*sepA* mutant after growth and concentration of cultural supernatants. SepA represents a large portion of the high molecular weight autotransporter proteins.

the genomic determinants encoding toxins capable of increasing intestinal secretion signals. Previous studies in the field were aimed at characterizing ShET1 and ShET2 as *Shigella* enterotoxins but did not extend the study to address the presence of additional toxins. In the previous studies, the toxins were cloned and artificially expressed in *E. coli*, and the purified proteins were applied to rabbit jejunum mounted in Ussing chambers [4,8,9]. While this approach was important to demonstrate that toxin addition alone was sufficient to induce changes in Isc, the higher level of protein expressed and possible alterations from production in *E. coli* could affect the amount of short circuit change detected. By using the natural host, our studies with *S. flexneri* mutants allowed us to dissect the specific contribution of each enterotoxin previously described (ShET1 and ShET2) and of those newly discovered by our studies (Pic and SepA) in causing *Shigella* electrolyte secretion in the small intestine. The use of the natural host can also address potential interactions that occur between toxins and other secreted proteins.

A major advance, and a central aspect of our studies compared to previous reports, was the utilization of mouse tissue in the Ussing chamber experiments. We chose C57BL/6 mice as we will perform additional studies to address the roles of these toxins in knockout mice on the same genetic background lacking specific pattern recognition pathways or secretory pathways to gain more insights on the mechanism of action *Shigella*-induced secretory diarrhea. In addition, female mice have less of a tendency to fight, which is important since fighting can affect the immune system and other bodily systems. For these reasons this strain of mice was ideal for our studies. We have validated this model against the previously reported rabbit model in order to use mouse intestinal tissue as a reliable and efficient assay for our current and future studies. Our results demonstrate that mouse jejunum in the Ussing chamber system is as responsive to *Shigella* toxins as rabbit jejunum. Although several models of shigellosis have been developed, including the nonhuman primate model, the guinea pig keratoconjunctivitis model, and the pulmonary shigellosis model, the models do not adequately measure the watery diarrheal phase of infection [32,33]. This study is the first to demonstrate secretogenic reactivity in an *ex vivo* mouse jejunum model to *Shigella* toxins.

The finding that the iron-depleted conditions were not necessary to study *Shigella* enterotoxic activities is an important aspect of this study. The iron-depleted medium that was initially utilized was based on the fact that these conditions were required to detect a change in Isc in studies with enteroinvasive *E. coli* [21]. Given the similarity between EIEC and *Shigella*, the iron-depleted conditions were continued into the *Shigella* studies [4,8,9]. In addition, supernatants isolated from a plasmid-cured strain of *S. flexneri* induced higher levels of water accumulation in the rabbit ileal loop model when the cultures were grown in the absence of iron [8]. However, another bacterial factor present in the culture supernatants, not ShET1, could have been affected by the iron limitation and enhanced water accumulation in the rabbit intestine. The data presented in figure 1 clearly demonstrate that iron-depletion is not required for Ussing chamber analysis of the *Shigella* enterotoxins. Whether iron limitation affects the efficacy of other *Shigella* proteins in the rabbit ileal loop analyses remains to be determined. Of course, use of other culture conditions could yield still more enterotoxins that may be produced *in vivo*.

Our mutant analysis strategy was instrumental in this study. We specifically chose to compare the plasmid-cured strain (BS103) and the Δ*spa47* mutant (BS652), a T3SS mutant that has been shown to be incapable of secreting T3SS effectors [24,25]. Based on the secretion profile in figure 2, the autotransporters encoded on the virulence plasmid were still secreted in this mutant. In recent years three proteins belonging to the Serine Protease Autotransporter of *Enterobacteriacae* (SPATE) family have been identified in *S. flexneri*: SepA, SigA, and Pic. SepA is non-T3SS effector encoded on the virulence plasmid. Although the substrate(s) of SepA has not been identified, a recent study associated SepA with diarrheal cases in

Mali [34]. SigA is encoded in the *she* pathogenicity island, and contributes to secretion in the rabbit ileal loop model [27]. Al-Hasani *et al.,* recently defined the structural protein fodrin as a target of SigA, implicating a role for this SPATE in cytoskeletal reorganization [35]. Finally, Pic is a mucinase that is encoded on the DNA strand directly opposite of the genes for ShET1. A recent study defined the substrate specificity of Pic, an immune system modulator [16]. Given the presence of the autotransporters in the culture supernatants and the association of these factors with diarrheal disease, we hypothesized that the SPATES could also contribute to enterotoxin activity. We therefore proceeded with our mutational analysis to determine if these SPATES had a role in inducing secretogenic activity.

Initially, analysis of BS103 and BS652 allowed us to determine if toxins were encoded on the chromosome and/or virulence plasmid. In addition, use of the Δ*spa47* mutant allowed us to demonstrate that the virulence plasmid harbored toxins that were T3-dependent and T3-independent since there was a significant increase in Isc compared to the plasmid-cured mutant (BS103) (figure 3). Based on our subtraction analysis, we conclude that three groups of toxins contribute to the increase in Isc: one group on the chromosome, one group on the virulence plasmid that requires the T3SS, and one group on the virulence plasmid that is secreted independently of the T3SS.

Further analysis indicated that the ShET1/Pic region is a major contributor of enterotoxin activity from the chromosome, which was confirmed by the analysis of the complementation of strain 1377 with ShET1-containing 1522 and ShET1-devoid 1542. Pic is transcribed on the opposite strand of DNA from the genes encoding ShET1, is only present in *S. flexneri,* and has been shown to target a wide range of leukocyte adhesion proteins [16]. How Pic contributes to secretogenic activity in our system and *in vivo* remains to be elucidated, and could function indirectly as an enterotoxin by affecting another protein. It is unclear in the previous literature whether or not the entire *pic* gene was present in the experiments in which the genes encoding ShET1 were cloned for expression and purification, but purified ShET1 has been shown to induce secretion in the rabbit ileal loop model [8,9]. Our studies indicate that the majority of the enterotoxic activity present in *Shigella* strain 2457T is due to Pic.

Comparison of BS103 and the Δ*spa47* mutant indicated the presence of an additional factor encoded on the virulence plasmid that affected Isc. The Δ*ospD3* mutant analysis confirmed that ShET2 is the T3SS effector responsible for enterotoxin activity, which agrees with previous literature [4]. In fact, Nataro *et al.* hypothesized that ShET2 was a T3SS effector protein since a signal peptide could not be detected [4]. Analysis of strains 1208S and 1380 also indicated there were additional enterotoxins encoded by *S. flexneri.* We chose to analyze a Δ*sepA* mutant since it is an autotransporter encoded on the virulence plasmid that has been shown to affect fluid accumulation in rabbit ileal loops [31] and to contribute to diarrhea in enteroaggregative *E. coli* [34]. The Δ*sepA* mutant caused a significant drop in Isc compared to wildtype bacteria (Figure 7A). The data demonstrate that SepA has enterotoxic activity; however, there may be two reasons as to why the mutation caused such a dramatic drop in Isc compared to wildtype bacteria. First, analysis of the concentrated proteins from the mutant demonstrates that a significant amount of SepA is secreted into the cultures (Figure 7B). Second, SepA may target the same eukaryotic protein or pathway as another enterotoxin to enhance the overall toxin effect. Given the fact that in our culture conditions the Δ*spa47* mutant had an approximate 20% increase in Isc compared to BS103, and that strain 1380 (with only SepA present) had approximately 20% increase compared to the negative control *E. coli* HS, we believe that the SepA contribution is approximately 20% in our system. As with Pic, SepA could function indirectly as an enterotoxin by affecting another protein. Further characterization of SepA will determine the role of this autotransporter protein in our system and *in vivo.*

In conclusion, our study confirms the enterotoxin activity of ShET1 and ShET2 from previous publications, validates the use of mouse jejunum in Ussing chamber analyses as a novel, more versatile and high-throughput bioassay for *Shigella* enterotoxic activity, and identifies additional *Shigella* proteins (Pic and SepA) that contribute to enterotoxin activity. The results obtained in this study may assist future studies for identification of eukaryotic protein targets. The fact that we have yet to identify a toxin-null mutant indicates there may be additional enterotoxin(s) encoded by *S. flexneri* that contribute to the overall watery component of *Shigella*-induced diarrhea. Despite this possibility, we are confident that we have demonstrated that ShET1/Pic, ShET2, and SepA are the factors that contribute most prominently to the changes in Isc in mouse jejunum in the Ussing chambers.

Acknowledgments

The authors would like to thank Dr. Anthony Maurelli, Uniformed Services University, and Dr. Beth McCormick, University of Massachusetts Medical School, for the bacterial strains used in this study. The authors would also like to thank Dr. Edwin Oaks, Walter Reed Army Institute of Research, for the IpaB antibody used in this study.

Author Contributions

Conceived and designed the experiments: CF JH JK AF JN. Performed the experiments: CF JH TSD. Analyzed the data: CF JH AF JN. Contributed reagents/materials/analysis tools: TSD EB AF JN. Wrote the paper: CF JH AF JPN.

References

1. Weisz A, Meuli G, Thakwalakwa C, Trehan I, Maleta K, et al. (2011) The duration of diarrhea and fever is associated with growth faltering in rural Malawian children aged 6–18 months. Nutr J 10: 25.
2. O'Ryan M, Prado V, Pickering LK (2005) A millennium update on pediatric diarrheal illness in the developing world. Semin Pediatr Infect Dis 16: 125–136.
3. Kotloff KL, Winickoff JP, Ivanoff B, Clemens JD, Swerdlow DL, et al. (1999) Global burden of *Shigella* infections: implications for vaccine development and implementation of control strategies. Bull World Health Organ 77: 651–666.
4. Nataro JP, Seriwatana J, Fasano A, Maneval DR, Guers LD, et al. (1995) Identification and cloning of a novel plasmid-encoded enterotoxin of enteroinvasive *Escherichia coli* and *Shigella* strains. Infect Immun 63: 4721–4728.
5. Farfan MJ, Toro CS, Barry EM, Nataro JP (2011) *Shigella* enterotoxin-2 is a type III effector that participates in *Shigella*-induced interleukin 8 secretion by epithelial cells. FEMS Immunol Med Microbiol 61: 332–339.
6. Henderson IR, Nataro JP (2001) Virulence functions of autotransporter proteins. Infect Immun 69: 1231–1243.
7. Schiavo G, van der Goot FG (2001) The bacterial toxin toolkit. Nat Rev Mol Cell Biol 2: 530–537.
8. Fasano A, Noriega FR, Maneval DR, Jr., Chanasongcram S, Russell R, et al. (1995) *Shigella* enterotoxin 1: an enterotoxin of *Shigella flexneri* 2a active in rabbit small intestine *in vivo* and *in vitro*. J Clin Invest 95: 2853–2861.
9. Fasano A, Noriega FR, Liao FM, Wang W, Levine MM (1997) Effect of *Shigella* enterotoxin 1 (ShET1) on rabbit intestine in vitro and in vivo. Gut 40: 505–511.
10. Farfan MJ, Garay TA, Prado CA, Filliol I, Ulloa MT, et al. (2010) A new multiplex PCR for differential identification of *Shigella flexneri* and *Shigella sonnei* and detection of *Shigella* virulence determinants. Epidemiol Infect 138: 525–533.
11. Niyogi SK (2005) Shigellosis. J Microbiol 43: 133–143.
12. Schroeder GN, Hilbi H (2008) Molecular pathogenesis of *Shigella* spp.: controlling host cell signaling, invasion, and death by type III secretion. Clin Microbiol Rev 21: 134–156.

13. Takeuchi A, Formal SB, Sprinz H (1968) Exerimental acute colitis in the Rhesus monkey following peroral infection with *Shigella flexneri*. An electron microscope study. Am J Pathol 52: 503–529.
14. Clarke LL (2009) A guide to Ussing chamber studies of mouse intestine. Am J Physiol Gastrointest Liver Physiol 296: G1151–1166.
15. Datsenko KA, Wanner BL (2000) One-step inactivation of chromosomal genes in *Escherichia coli* K-12 using PCR products. Proc Natl Acad Sci U S A 97: 6640–6645.
16. Ruiz-Perez F, Wahid R, Faherty CS, Kolappaswamy K, Rodriguez L, et al. (2011) Serine protease autotransporters from *Shigella flexneri* and pathogenic *Escherichia coli* target a broad range of leukocyte glycoproteins. Proc Natl Acad Sci U S A. 108: 12881–12886.
17. Maurelli AT, Curtiss R, 3rd (1984) Bacteriophage Mu d1(Apr lac) generates vir-lac operon fusions in *Shigella flexneri* 2a. Infect Immun 45: 642–648.
18. Sutton TL, Zhao A, Madden KB, Elfrey JE, Tuft BA, et al. (2008) Anti-Inflammatory mechanisms of enteric *Heligmosomoides polygyrus* infection against trinitrobenzene sulfonic acid-induced colitis in a murine model. Infect Immun 76: 4772–4782.
19. Bahrani FK, Sansonetti PJ, Parsot C (1997) Secretion of Ipa proteins by *Shigella flexneri*: inducer molecules and kinetics of activation. Infect Immun 65: 4005–4010.
20. Mills JA, Buysse JM, Oaks EV (1988) *Shigella flexneri* invasion plasmid antigens B and C: epitope location and characterization with monoclonal antibodies. Infect Immun 56: 2933–2941.
21. Fasano A, Kay BA, Russell RG, Maneval DR, Jr., Levin MM (1990) Enterotoxin and cytotoxin production by enteroinvasive *Escherichia coli*. Infect Immun 58: 3717–3723.
22. Burleigh DE, Borman RA (1997) Evidence for a nonneural electrogenic effect of cholera toxin on human isolated ileal mucosa. Dig Dis Sci 42: 1964–1968.
23. Levine MM, Bergquist EJ, Nalin DR, Waterman DH, Hornick RB, et al. (1978) *Escherichia coli* strains that cause diarrhoea but do not produce heat-labile or heat-stable enterotoxins and are non-invasive. Lancet 1: 1119–1122.
24. Tamano K, Aizawa S, Katayama E, Nonaka T, Imajoh-Ohmi S, et al. (2000) Supramolecular structure of the *Shigella* type III secretion machinery: the needle part is changeable in length and essential for delivery of effectors. EMBO J 19: 3876–3887.
25. Venkatesan MM, Buysse JM, Oaks EV (1992) Surface presentation of *Shigella flexneri* invasion plasmid antigens requires the products of the spa locus. J Bacteriol 174: 1990–2001.
26. Benjelloun-Touimi Z, Si Tahar M, Montecucco C, Sansonetti PJ, Parsot C (1998) SepA, the 110 kDa protein secreted by *Shigella flexneri*: two-domain structure and proteolytic activity. Microbiology 144 (Pt 7): 1815–1822.
27. Al-Hasani K, Henderson IR, Sakellaris H, Rajakumar K, Grant T, et al. (2000) The sigA gene which is borne on the she pathogenicity island of *Shigella flexneri* 2a encodes an exported cytopathic protease involved in intestinal fluid accumulation. Infect Immun 68: 2457–2463.
28. Henderson IR, Czeczulin J, Eslava C, Noriega F, Nataro JP (1999) Characterization of pic, a secreted protease of *Shigella flexneri* and enteroaggregative *Escherichia coli*. Infect Immun 67: 5587–5596.
29. Wagner JK, Heindl JE, Gray AN, Jain S, Goldberg MB (2009) Contribution of the periplasmic chaperone Skp to efficient presentation of the autotransporter IcsA on the surface of *Shigella flexneri*. J Bacteriol 191: 815–821.
30. Le Gall T, Mavris M, Martino MC, Bernardini ML, Denamur E, et al. (2005) Analysis of virulence plasmid gene expression defines three classes of effectors in the type III secretion system of *Shigella flexneri*. Microbiology 151: 951–962.
31. Benjelloun-Touimi Z, Sansonetti PJ, Parsot C (1995) SepA, the major extracellular protein of *Shigella flexneri*: autonomous secretion and involvement in tissue invasion. Mol Microbiol 17: 123–135.
32. Barman S, Saha DR, Ramamurthy T, Koley H (2011) Development of a new guinea-pig model of shigellosis. FEMS Immunol Med Microbiol 62: 304–314.
33. Pore D, Mahata N, Pal A, Chakrabarti MK (2011) Outer membrane protein A (OmpA) of *Shigella flexneri* 2a, induces protective immune response in a mouse model. PLoS One 6: e22663.
34. Boisen N, Scheutz F, Rasko DA, Redman JC, Persson S, et al. (2012) Genomic characterization of enteroaggregative *Escherichia coli* from children in Mali. J Infect Dis 205: 431–444.
35. Al-Hasani K, Navarro-Garcia F, Huerta J, Sakellaris H, Adler B (2009) The immunogenic SigA enterotoxin of *Shigella flexneri* 2a binds to HEp-2 cells and induces fodrin redistribution in intoxicated epithelial cells. PLoS One 4: e8223.
36. Formal SB, Dammin GJ, Labrec EH, Schneider H (1958) Experimental *Shigella infections*: characteristics of a fatal infection produced in guinea pigs. J Bacteriol 75: 604–610.
37. Maurelli AT, Blackmon B, Curtiss R, 3rd (1984) Loss of pigmentation in *Shigella flexneri* 2a is correlated with loss of virulence and virulence-associated plasmid. Infect Immun 43: 397–401.
38. Faherty CS, Maurelli AT (2009) Spa15 of *Shigella flexneri* is secreted through the type III secretion system and prevents staurosporine-induced apoptosis. Infect Immun 77: 5281–5290.
39. Kotloff KL, Simon JK, Pasetti MF, Sztein MB, Wooden SL, et al. (2007) Safety and immunogenicity of CVD 1208S, a live, oral DeltaguaBA Deltasen Deltaset *Shigella flexneri* 2a vaccine grown on animal-free media. Hum Vaccin 3: 268–275.

19

Waterborne Outbreak of Gastroenteritis: Effects on Sick Leaves and Cost of Lost Workdays

Jaana I. Halonen[1]*, Mika Kivimäki[1,2], Tuula Oksanen[1], Pekka Virtanen[3], Mikko J. Virtanen[4], Jaana Pentti[1], Jussi Vahtera[1,5]

1 Finnish Institute of Occupational Health, Helsinki, Finland, **2** Department of Epidemiology and Public Health, University College of London, London, United Kingdom, **3** Tampere School of Health Sciences, University of Tampere, Tampere, Finland, **4** Epidemiologic Surveillance and Response Unit, National Institute for Health and Welfare, Helsinki, Finland, **5** Department of Public Health, University of Turku, and Turku University Hospital, Turku, Finland

Abstract

Background: In 2007, part of a drinking water distribution system was accidentally contaminated with waste water effluent causing a gastroenteritis outbreak in a Finnish town. We examined the acute and cumulative effects of this incidence on sick leaves among public sector employees residing in the clean and contaminated areas, and the additional costs of lost workdays due to the incidence.

Methods: Daily information on sick leaves of 1789 Finnish Public Sector Study participants was obtained from employers' registers. Global Positioning System-coordinates were used for linking participants to the clean and contaminated areas. Prevalence ratios (PR) for weekly sickness absences were calculated using binomial regression analysis. Calculations for the costs were based on prior studies.

Results: Among those living in the contaminated areas, the prevalence of participants on sick leave was 3.54 (95% confidence interval (CI) 2.97–4.22) times higher on the week following the incidence compared to the reference period. Those living and working in the clean area were basically not affected, the corresponding PR for sick leaves was 1.12, 95% CI 0.73–1.73. No cumulative effects on sick leaves were observed among the exposed. The estimated additional costs of lost workdays due to the incidence were 1.8–2.1 million euros.

Conclusions: The prevalence of sickness absences among public sector employees residing in affected areas increased shortly after drinking water distribution system was contaminated, but no long-term effects were observed. The estimated costs of lost workdays were remarkable, thus, the cost-benefits of better monitoring systems for the water distribution systems should be evaluated.

Editor: Qamaruddin Nizami, Aga Khan University, Pakistan

Funding: This study was funded by the Academy of Finland (projects 124271, 124322, 129262, and 132944). Mika Kivimäki is supported by the BUPA Foundation, UK; and the New OSH ERA research programme. The funders had no role in study design, data collection and analysis, decision to publish, or preparation of the manuscript.

Competing Interests: The authors have declared that no competing interests exist.

* E-mail: jaana.halonen@ttl.fi

Introduction

Regardless of the developed systems for drinking water purification and distribution, and the active legislation towards safe water [1], microbial contamination of drinking water and waterborne infections keep occurring also in developed societies [2,3,4,5,6,7,8]. Large populations may become affected if public water systems are contaminated. These incidences may be due to system deficiencies, improper water treatment or contamination of one part of, or the whole, water supply [3,4,7]. In most developed countries with public water distribution systems, however, rapid actions for managing the incidences can be taken to limit the harms; clean water can often be provided by temporary arrangements and the distribution systems can be disinfected. Severities of the waterborne outbreaks are often evaluated by calculating excess cases or risk rates for morbidity among the exposed [2,4,5]. However, the effects of the waterborne infections on acute and cumulative sickness absences (*Campylobacter*, *Salmonella* and *Giardia* infections may also have long-term health effects [9,10,11,12]) and the related costs of lost workdays have rarely been determined [13].

In late November 2007 part of the municipal drinking water system in a Finnish town Nokia, a municipality participating in the Finnish Public Sector Study, was contaminated with wastewater effluent (including *Campylobacter* sp., Norovirus, *Giardia*, and *Salmonella* sp.) causing an outbreak of gastroenteritis [6]. In this study, we determined how this epidemic affected the sick leaves immediately and in the following year among employees of the Public Sector Study cohort who resided in Nokia. We hypothesized that employees living in the contaminated areas would be more affected than those living in the non-contaminated "clean" areas. We also estimated the additional costs of lost workdays for all branches of industry during the acute phase of the epidemic.

Methods

Ethics statement

All the register data obtained from the national registers were based on the legal permissions granted by institutes maintaining these registers, and data were analyzed anonymously. According to Finnish Personal Data Act (523/1999, Chapter 4, Section 14) [14], written consent was not needed for research that uses register data. The Coordinating Ethics Committee of Helsinki and Uusimaa Hospital District has approved the study.

The Finnish Public Sector Study cohort consists of employees working for 10 municipalities (including Nokia and neighbouring town Tampere) and 21 hospitals (including Tampere University Hospital). All men and women employed by these organizations for more than six months in any year between 1991 and 2005 were eligible for the cohort (n = 151 618). Of this cohort, 1789 members were employed and resided in Nokia during the outbreak (weeks 48/2007–8/2008 referred to as week of outbreak = 0, and weeks after +1, +2, etc. up to week +12) and formed the analytic sample of this study. Because in Finland female-dominated occupations are common in the public sector (nurses, kindergarten teachers, cleaners etc.) a majority of the study population were women. All information about cohort members' job contracts, age, sex and sick leaves was obtained from the employers' registers. For each day we obtained data on all sick leaves (due to own illness), and sick-child leaves (due to illness of a child <10 years), however, diagnoses for the illnesses were not available as they are not recorded by the employers. Sick days (up to 60 days) and sick-child days (allowed absence up to four days at one time) are paid by the employer and, thus, carefully recorded. Residential addresses of the cohort members and Global Positioning System (GPS)-coordinates of these addresses were obtained from Population Register Center. Coordinates of the buildings alongside the contaminated water line were in the National Institute for Health and Welfare. Using these coordinates the cohort members' residences we linked to the buildings to which contaminated drinking water was distributed. The locations of cohort participants' residences in relation to areas where contaminated and clean drinking water were supplied are shown in Figure 1.

The incidence has been described in detail previously [6]. In short, during maintenance work at the Nokia wastewater plant on November 28th 2007 (week 0) a valve connecting wastewater effluent line and drinking water line was accidentally opened, and in some areas inhabitants started to receive contaminated municipal drinking water (referred to as contaminated areas: inner pattern in Figure 1). This area was approximately 18 km^2 in size (whole town 347 km^2), and defined based on the addresses and GPS-coordinates of the buildings along the branch of the contaminated distribution system. Two days later, an increase in the number of patients with symptoms of gastroenteritis was observed at the local health care center. An estimated 450 m^3 of wastewater effluent had been mixed to the drinking water and distributed to the customers, until the water contamination was realized. Recommendation for boiling tap water was issued the same day, clean water distribution organized by municipal officials, the military, and volunteers was started, as well as increased chlorination of the distribution system. After the incident schools and day care centres were closed due to Christmas holiday on weeks +4 and +5. The last restrictions in water use were canceled on February 18th 2008 (week +12).

Statistical analyses

We calculated the weekly prevalence of study population taking at least one sick day or sick-child day during each week for seven weeks before, during, and 12 weeks after the incidence, separately for those living in the contaminated and clean areas. For contaminated and clean areas cumulative sick days per person year were also calculated for the 52 weeks following the incidence. This was because there is evidence of long-term health effects of *Campylobacter* infections (rheumatological complaints, symptoms of arthritis, inflammatory bowel disease) [9,10,15], *Giardia* infections (functional gastrointestinal diseases) [12], and *Salmonella* infections (inflammatory bowel disease) [15].

We calculated the prevalence ratios (PR) and 95% confidence intervals (CI) for weekly sickness absences using log-binomial regression analyses with GENMOD procedure of SAS [16], adjusting for age and sex. The reference period used in the analyses was the mean weekly prevalence of participants taking at least one sick day during the seven weeks prior to the incidence (weeks −7 to −1). The same method was used for the subgroup analyses of the cohort members consisting of those employed by schools and day care centers (n = 361). For them, the data included the location of their residence and workplace, and information of whether these were in the contaminated or clean area. Thus, we could estimate more explicitly the role of clean and contaminated areas in the sickness absences.

The additional cost of lost workdays on weeks 0 to +3 was estimated for the total number of employees residing in Nokia based on the number of additional (compared to reference period) personal and sick-child days per person among the cohort participants. The costs were estimated at 280 and 330 euros per day; the mean estimated costs of sickness absence for the service sector (200–250 €/day), industry (300–350 €/day) [17] and government employees (340–380 €/day) [18] in Finland. Of the total workforce in Nokia in 2007 (n = 10,719), 30% was employed by the government and 32% by industry. These estimations considered the contamination status of the residential area, and were calculated by sex (n of employed women in town = 5020, n of employed men in town = 5699) because the sex distribution of the analytic sample was skewed and women generally have higher rates of sick leaves than men [19].

Results

The total population in Nokia was 30 016 of which 9538 (32%) lived in the area of contaminated water distribution system. Correspondingly, of the 1789 cohort members 586 (33%) lived in the contaminated area. Of the study population 1419 (79.5%) were women, and the mean age was 45.9 years (standard deviation 9.4). The number of cohort members who worked at schools and day care centers in Nokia was 361, of which 174 lived and worked in the clean area, and 187 lived or worked, or both, in the contaminated area.

Sick leaves increased sharply after the contamination among those who lived in the contaminated area, but not among those living in the clean area for whom the prevalence returned back to the pre-incident level in three weeks (Figure 2). The prevalence of cohort members taking at least one sick day during the week immediately after the contamination (week +1) was 35%, whereas in the week before the contamination the corresponding figure was 10% (week −1). The prevalence of participants at sick-child leave also peaked in the contaminated area on week +1, being 4.3%, whereas the week before (week −1) the level was 1.3% (data not shown). The cumulative number of sick days grew at a faster rate during the first post-incident weeks among those who lived in the contaminated compared to clean area (Figure 3). However, later the curves for cumulative sick days developed similarly for the

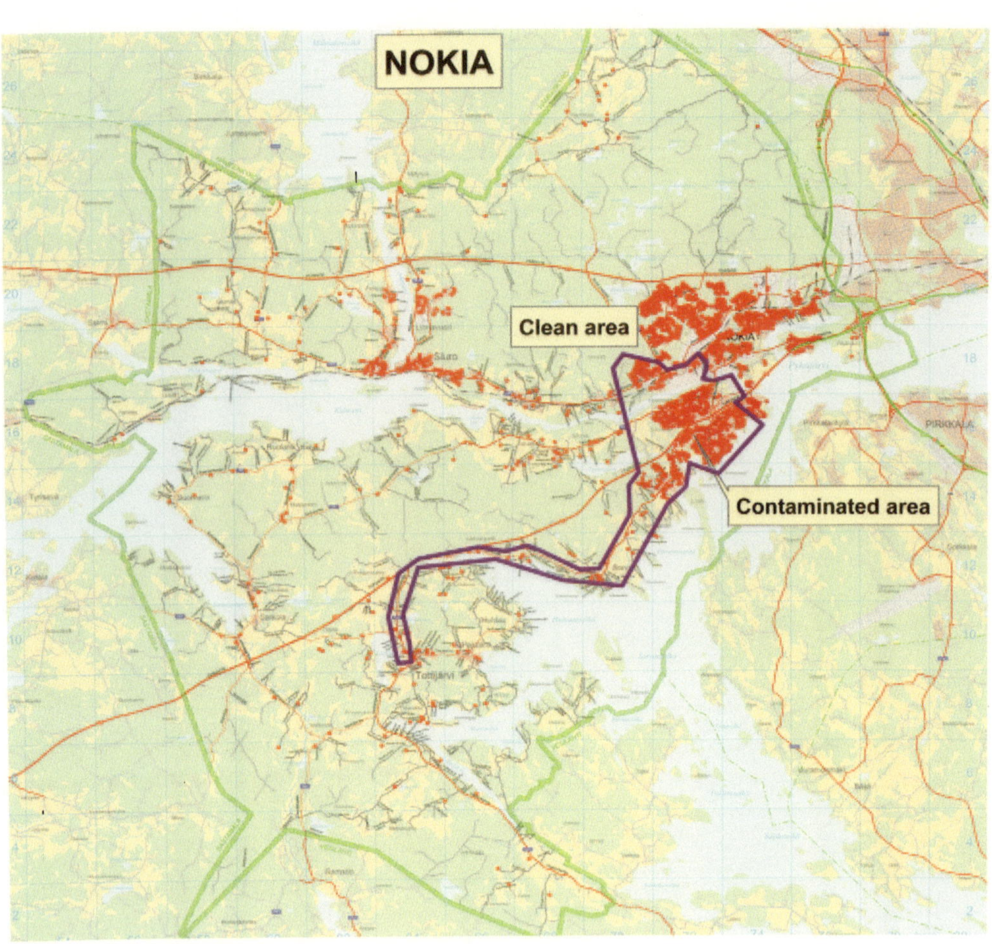

Figure 1. Distribution of cohort participants within areas receiving contaminated and clean drinking water. Dots in the inner pattern represent cohort participants' residences receiving contaminated water.

exposed and non-exposed and by the end of the year the difference had disappeared.

Compared to the reference period, the proportion of participants at sick leave in the contaminated area was the highest on the week following the incidence after which the prevalence ratio decreased gradually (Table 1). A slight increase in the sick leaves was observed also among those living in the clean area with the highest prevalence ratio for week +1. In the subgroup of personnel of schools and day care centers, we found that for those living and working in clean areas, the prevalence ratios for sick leaves remained at the same level after, compared to prior, the contamination (Table 2).

For the cost estimations we calculated weekly additional sick days (compared to the reference period) in this study population. For the clean and contaminated areas, the sum of additional sick

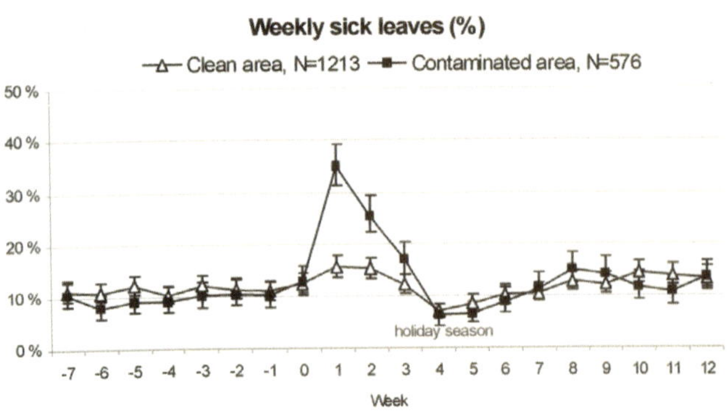

Figure 2. Weekly percentages of participants at sick leave before and after the contamination of water distribution system. Percentages are given by the contamination status of the participants' residence.

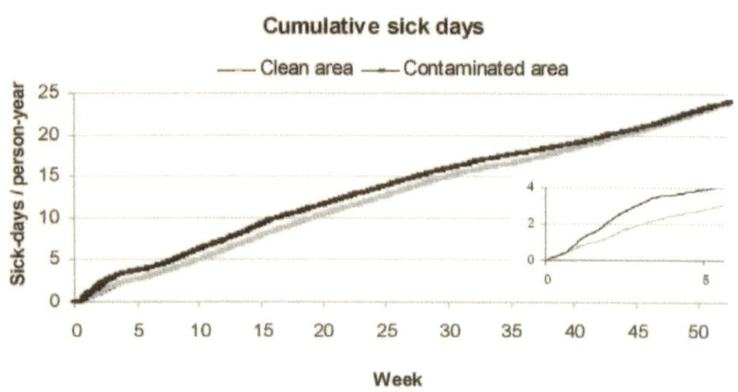

Figure 3. Cumulative sick days for the 52 weeks following the contamination by the contamination status of residence.

Table 1. Prevalence ratios (PR, 95% confidence intervals) for weekly sick leaves among public sector employees after the contamination of drinking water distribution system by contamination status of residence.

	Clean area (n = 1203[a])			Contaminated area (n = 586[b])		
Week	PR[c]	95% CI		PR[c]	95% CI	
−7 to −1 (ref)	1			1		
0	1.16	1.02	1.31	1.23	0.99	1.52
+1	1.41	1.23	1.61	3.54	2.97	4.22
+2	1.41	1.23	1.62	2.63	2.18	3.16
+3	1.17	1.01	1.36	1.88	1.52	2.31
+4–12	1.12	1.00	1.26	1.18	0.99	1.40

[a]Number of participants living in clean area;
[b]Number of participants living in contaminated area,
[c]Models adjusted for age and sex.

Table 2. Prevalence ratios (PR, 95% confidence intervals) of weekly sick leaves among the personnel of schools and day care centres after the contamination of drinking water distribution system by contamination status of residence and workplace.

	Clean area[a] (n = 174)			Contaminated area[b] (n = 187)		
Week	PR[c]	95% CI		PR[c]	95% CI	
−7 to −1 (ref)	1			1		
0	0.90	0.56	1.42	1.21	0.80	1.85
+1	1.12	0.73	1.73	3.43	2.58	4.55
+2	1.10	0.71	1.73	2.89	2.14	3.89
+3	1.03	0.67	1.58	1.36	0.93	2.00
+4–12	1.16	0.88	1.55	1.23	0.96	1.61

[a]Residence and workplace in the clean area;
[b]Residence or workplace, or both, in the contaminated area;
[c]Models adjusted for age and sex.

days per person on weeks 0 to +3 was 0.71 for women and 0.42 for men. Thus, the estimated auxiliary cost of lost workdays due to sick leaves among all employees residing in Nokia were 1.00–1.18 and 0.67–0.80 million euros for women and men, respectively. Similarly, the sum of additional sick-child days per person were 0.07 and 0.02, and the estimated cost of lost workdays 0.11–0.13 and 0.03–0.04 million euros for women and men, respectively. These resulted in a total of 1.8–2.1 million euros from lost workdays due to own illness and illness of one's child(ren).

Discussion

We studied the effect of microbial contamination of drinking water distribution system on sick leaves among public sector employees. Sick- and sick-child leaves were found to increase sharply after the contamination, and this increase was restricted to people either residing or working in the contaminated areas. However, 1-year accumulation of sick days was similar for exposed and unexposed suggesting the effects of the incidence were short-term. The estimated additional costs of lost workdays due to the incidence were 1.8–2.1 million euros.

Contaminations of water distribution systems in the scale of this study are rare, although some have been reported [2,4,20]. As far as we are aware, the effects of these incidences on sick leaves have scarcely been studied. We found that those residing in the contaminated area were heavily affected, while those residing and working in the clean areas were unaffected. The peak in the proportion of participants at sick leave was observed during the week after the contamination, which is in agreement with the peak in the detected cases of gastroenteritis related to this incidence [6]. This delay is also in line with other studies on waterborne outbreaks [21,22].

For the following year, we found no difference in the sick leave accruals between those living in the contaminated and clean areas during the incidence. This suggests the acute epidemic had no residual effects at a population level. Supporting evidence has been reported in regard of occurrence of reactive arthritis in this study area half a year after the incidence [23]. However, prior studies have shown that the effects of gastroenteritis from drinking water contaminated with *Campylobacter* may materialize later -with a delay of up to fifteen years- as increase in arthritis symptoms or inflammatory bowel disease [10,15,24], or in case of *Giardia* infection as functional gastrointestinal diseases [12]. Thus, we cannot exclude the possibility that the exposed may still be at increased risk of developing chronic conditions.

We estimated that the excess costs due to sick leaves related to this incidence was 1.8–2.1 million euros, a remarkable part of the total expenditure of the whole incidence that reaches possibly five to six million euros. The other expenses include e.g. the distribution of clean water for the inhabitants, cleaning of the water distribution system, and overtime work of the town and water works employees. As in occupational health in general [25], cost-benefit analyses are needed to estimate whether actions such as online monitoring systems of the water distribution networks would be beneficial in preventing and limiting the magnitude of waterborne outbreaks and all harms related to them. We found that only one study, almost two decades ago, has estimated costs of a waterborne gastroenteritis outbreak. The authors concluded the outbreak affecting 2000–3000 people caused costs of 1.6 million Danish krones (~215 000 euros in current exchange rate) [13]. However, the algorithm of this estimate was not reported, and because of the long delay between studies the comparison of the costs is difficult. We also found that sick leaves and sick-child leaves were more common among women than men, a finding in line with prior research [19]. Indeed, only a fourth of the costs of sick-child leaves were observed among men, which suggests that female-dominated sectors suffer considerably more from the illnesses of children than male-dominated sectors.

Major strengths of this study are the reliable and comprehensive records on the cohort members' sickness absences and information whether contaminated water was distributed to their residences. Additional information on the locations of workplaces for a sub-population of the cohort enabled us a more detailed examination of the differences in sick leaves between the exposed and non-exposed. One limitation of this study is that we could not determine the portion of the sick leaves that was actually related to the increase in infections of the digestive system because data on diagnoses were not available; however, it is unlikely that the observed short-term increase in the sick leaves is due to illnesses not related to the incidence. Because e.g. salaries and insurance costs vary by industry, we also emphasize that the calculations for the costs of sick leaves depend on the country and employer in question. Finally, due to differences in infrastructure and public services, the generalizability of these findings in less developed regions may be limited.

In summary, we have shown that the prevalence of sickness absences among public sector employees residing in affected areas increased considerably after drinking water distribution system was contaminated. The estimated costs of lost workdays were remarkable, thus, the cost-benefits of better monitoring systems for the water distribution systems should be evaluated.

Acknowledgments

The authors thank town of Nokia for providing the map of contaminated and clean areas to be used in this article.

Author Contributions

Conceived and designed the experiments: JIH MK TO JP JV. Analyzed the data: JIH JP MJV. Contributed reagents/materials/analysis tools: MK JP MJV JV PV. Wrote the paper: JIH TO JV. Critically reviewed the article: MV MJV JP PV.

References

1. Zacheus O, Miettinen IT (2011) Increased information on waterborne outbreaks through efficient notification system enforces actions towards safe drinking water. J Water Health 9: 763–772.
2. Yang Z, Wu X, Li T, Li M, Zhong Y, et al. (2011) Epidemiological survey and analysis on an outbreak of gastroenteritis due to water contamination. Biomed Environ Sci 24: 275–283.
3. Craun GF, Brunkard JM, Yoder JS, Roberts VA, Carpenter J, et al. (2010) Causes of outbreaks associated with drinking water in the United States from 1971 to 2006. Clin Microbiol Rev 23: 507–528.
4. Riera-Montes M, Brus Sjolander K, Allestam G, Hallin E, Hedlund KO, et al. (2011) Waterborne norovirus outbreak in a municipal drinking-water supply in Sweden. Epidemiol Infect 20: 1–8.
5. Daly ER, Roy SJ, Blaney DD, Manning JS, Hill VR, et al. (2009) Outbreak of giardiasis associated with a community drinking-water source. Epidemiol Infect 138: 491–500.
6. Laine J, Huovinen E, Virtanen MJ, Snellman M, Lumio J, et al. (2010) An extensive gastroenteritis outbreak after drinking-water contamination by sewage effluent, Finland. Epidemiol Infect 15: 1–9.
7. Brunkard JM, Ailes E, Roberts VA, Hill V, Hilborn ED, et al. (2011) Surveillance for waterborne disease outbreaks associated with drinking water—United States, 2007–2008. MMWR Surveill Summ 60: 38–68.
8. Breitenmoser A, Fretz R, Schmid J, Besl A, Etter R (2011) Outbreak of acute gastroenteritis due to a washwater-contaminated water supply, Switzerland, 2008. J Water Health 9: 569–576.
9. Locht H, Krogfelt KA (2002) Comparison of rheumatological and gastrointestinal symptoms after infection with Campylobacter jejuni/coli and enterotoxigenic Escherichia coli. Ann Rheum Dis 61: 448–452.
10. Garg AX, Pope JE, Thiessen-Philbrook H, Clark WF, Ouimet J (2008) Arthritis risk after acute bacterial gastroenteritis. Rheumatology (Oxford) 47: 200–204.
11. Mann EA, Saeed SA (2012) Gastrointestinal infection as a trigger for inflammatory bowel disease. Curr Opin Gastroenterol 28: 24–29.
12. Hanevik K, Dizdar V, Langeland N, Hausken T (2009) Development of functional gastrointestinal disorders after Giardia lamblia infection. BMC Gastroenterol 9: 27.
13. Laursen E, Mygind O, Rasmussen B, Ronne T (1994) Gastroenteritis: a waterborne outbreak affecting 1600 people in a small Danish town. J Epidemiol Community Health 48: 453–458.
14. Finnish Ministry of Justice (1999) Personal Data Act (523/1999). Available: http://www.finlex.fi/en/laki/kaannokset/1999/en19990523.pdf. Accessed 2012 15 Feb.
15. Gradel KO, Nielsen HL, Schonheyder HC, Ejlertsen T, Kristensen B, et al. (2009) Increased short- and long-term risk of inflammatory bowel disease after salmonella or campylobacter gastroenteritis. Gastroenterology 137: 495–501.
16. Spiegelman D, Hertzmark E (2005) Easy SAS calculations for risk or prevalence ratios and differences. Am J Epidemiol 162: 199–200.
17. Pohjola Pankki Oyj, (Company offering bank and insurance services) Sairauspoissaolokustannus [Sick leave costs]. Available: https://www.pohjola.fi/pohjola/yritys-ja-yhteisoasiakkaat/vakuutukset/vakuutustuotteet/henkilovakuutukset/sairauspoissaolokustannukset?id = 321811&srcpl = 4. Accessed 2012 16 Jan.
18. Lehtonen V Miten hallita sairauspoissaoloja? [in Finnish]. Available: http://www.vm.fi/vm/fi/04_julkaisut_ja_asiakirjat/01_julkaisut/06_valtion_tyomarkkinalaitos/miten_hallita_sairauspoissaoloja.pdf. Accessed 2011 15 Nov. Helsinki: Valtiovarainministeriö [Ministry of finance].
19. Bekker MH, Rutte CG, van Rijswijk K (2009) Sickness absence: A gender-focused review. Psychol Health Med 14: 405–418.
20. Koroglu M, Yakupogullari Y, Otlu B, Ozturk S, Ozden M, et al. (2011) A waterborne outbreak of epidemic diarrhea due to group A rotavirus in Malatya, Turkey. New Microbiol 34: 17–24.
21. Auld H, MacIver D, Klaassen J (2004) Heavy rainfall and waterborne disease outbreaks: the Walkerton example. J Toxicol Environ Health A 67: 1879–1887.
22. Public Health Agency of Canada (2000) Waterborne outbreak of gastroenteritis associated with a contaminated municipal water supply, Walkerton, Ontario, May–June 2000. Can Commun Dis Rep 26: 170–173.
23. Uotila T, Antonen J, Laine J, Kujansuu E, Haapala AM, et al. (2011) Reactive arthritis in a population exposed to an extensive waterborne gastroenteritis outbreak after sewage contamination in Pirkanmaa, Finland. Scand J Rheumatol 40: 358–362.
24. Bremell T, Bjelle A, Svedhem A (1991) Rheumatic symptoms following an outbreak of campylobacter enteritis: a five year follow up. Ann Rheum Dis 50: 934–938.
25. Burdorf A (2011) Do costs matter in occupational health? Occup Environ Med 68: 707–708.

Contribution of the Lipopolysaccharide to Resistance of *Shigella flexneri* 2a to Extreme Acidity

Mara Martinić, Anilei Hoare, Inés Contreras, Sergio A. Álvarez*

Departamento de Bioquímica y Biología Molecular, Facultad de Ciencias Químicas y Farmacéuticas, Universidad de Chile, Santiago, Chile

Abstract

Shigella flexneri is endemic in most underdeveloped countries, causing diarrheal disease and dysentery among young children. In order to reach its target site, the colon, *Shigella* must overcome the acid environment of the stomach. *Shigella* is able to persist in this stressful environment and, because of this ability it can initiate infection following the ingestion of very small inocula. Thus, acid resistance is considered an important virulence trait of this bacterium. It has been reported that moderate acid conditions regulate the expression of numerous components of the bacterial envelope. Because the lipopolysaccharide (LPS) is the major component of the bacterial surface, here we have addressed the role of LPS in acid resistance of *S. flexneri* 2a. Defined deletion mutants in genes encoding proteins involved in the synthesis, assembly and length regulation of the LPS O antigen were constructed and assayed for resistance to pH 2.5 after adaptation to pH 5.5. The results showed that a mutant lacking O antigen was significantly more sensitive to extreme acid conditions than the wild type. Not only the presence of polymerized O antigen, but also a particular polymer length (S-OAg) was required for acid resistance. Glucosylation of the O antigen also contributed to this property. In addition, a moderate acidic pH induced changes in the composition of the lipid A domain of LPS. The main modification was the addition of phosphoethanolamine to the 1′ phosphate of lipid A. This modification increased resistance of *S. flexneri* to extreme acid conditions, provide that O antigen was produced. Overall, the results of this work point out to an important role of LPS in resistance of *Shigella flexneri* to acid stress.

Editor: Ben Adler, Monash University, Australia

Funding: This work was supported by grant ADI-08/2006 from Comisión Nacional de Investigación Científica y Tecnológica (CONICYT; www.conicyt.cl)(Chile) and The World Bank and Fondo Nacional de Desarrollo Científico y Tecnológico (FONDECYT) grant 1100092. The funders had no role in study design, data collection and analysis, decision to publish, or preparation of the manuscript.

Competing Interests: The authors have declared that no competing interests exist.

* E-mail: salvarez@uchile.cl

Introduction

Species of the genus *Shigella* are the cause of shigellosis, a diarrheal disease that is endemic in developing countries [1]. The major site of *Shigella* pathology is the colon, where bacteria invade the intestinal mucosa, spread to the adjacent epithelial cells and cause much tissue damage, fluid secretion and inflammation, producing the clinical manifestations of shigellosis: diarrhea with blood and mucus [2]. Before colonization and invasion of the colonic mucosa, *Shigella* must overcome gastric acidity. In contrast to other bacterial enteric pathogens, such as *Vibrio cholerae* or *Salmonella* Typhi, species of *Shigella* are able to initiate infection of humans following ingestion of 10 to 100 bacteria, without neutralization of gastric acid [3–5]. For this reason, acid survival is considered an important pathogenic characteristic of these species [4].

Shigella has evolved sophisticated mechanisms for acid resistance that are induced under conditions of moderate acidity (pH 5.5) and are essential for its subsequent resistance to extreme acidity (pH 2.5). Two major acid-resistance pathways have been described in *Shigella*. The acid-resistance pathway 1, or oxidative system, is similar to that of *Escherichia coli* and requires complex media, oxidative growth and acid induction. This system is regulated by the RpoS sigma factor and the cyclic AMP receptor protein. The acid-resistance pathway 2, in turn, is a stationary-phase, glutamate-dependent pathway induced by growth in mildly acidic condition in the absence of oxygen [6–8]. A third system, which is induced in minimal media under fermentative conditions, has been described in *S. flexneri* 2457T [8].

Global gene expression profiling of the pH response in *S. flexneri* 2a [9], *E. coli* K-12 [10] and *Campylobacter jejunii* [11] has revealed a large number of genes that are differentially regulated by medium pH. The most pH-dependent genes were those involved in energy metabolism, as well as heat shock and oxidative stress genes. Also, pH differentially regulated a large number of periplasmic proteins and envelope components. This was not unexpected, since surface structures are exposed to the external pH and, thus, most probably play a role in the protective response of the cell to pH variations. Among *S. flexneri* pH-regulated genes, porin *ompF* and other outer membrane proteins genes were identified [9]. In *E. coli*, expression of transport proteins, redox modulators, chaperones and other membrane and periplasmic proteins was found to be pH-dependent [10], whereas in *C. jejunii*, capsular, flagellar and chemotaxis proteins expression was influenced by acid shock [11]. In *Helicobacter pylori*, acidity down-regulated 12 putative outer membrane proteins [12] and, in *Vibrio cholerae*, the OmpT porin was repressed by acid while the OmpU porin was required for acid resistance [13]. In addition, proteins involved in production of long fatty acids have been shown to be acid-induced in *Streptococcus mutans* [14,15] and *Lactobacillus lactis* [16]. In the latter, proteomic analysis revealed that several proteins involved in the biosynthesis of the cell wall and of capsular polysaccharides were regulated by the pH of the medium [16].

The lipopolysaccharide (LPS) is the major component of the outer membrane that mediates bacterial interaction with the environment; however, not much is known about the role that this complex glycolipid plays in resistance to extreme acidity. LPS is composed of three covalently-linked domains: lipid A, which is embedded in the outer membrane, the central oligosaccharide core and the O polysaccharide or O antigen (OAg), which is exposed to the bacterial surface. In *S. flexneri*, the OAg has two preferred chain lengths, a short OAg (S-OAg) of 11 to 17 repeat units and a very long OAg (VL-OAg) of about 90 repeat units. These chain lengths, or modal distributions, are controlled by the WzzB and Wzz_{pHS2} regulators, respectively [17,18]. Also, the addition of glucose residues to the OAg changes its conformation making it more compact and short [19].

It has been described that, under moderate acid conditions, the lipid A domain of LPS is modified by the addition of polar groups that vary between species. For instance, in *E. coli* and *Salmonella* Typhimurium, mildly acidic pH (6.0) activates the PmrAB two-component system. The PmrA transcription factor activates the expression of the *eptA* and *arnT* genes, which code for enzymes that attach phosphoethanolamine (PEtN) and L-amino arabinose (L-Ara4N), respectively, to the lipid A [20–25]. L-Ara4N is added to the 4′ phosphate of lipid A and sometimes to the 1′ phosphate, while PEtN can be attached to the 1 position. In *Salmonella*, but not in *E. coli*, PmrAB can be indirectly activated by low pH through the PhoPQ two-component system, which responds to low Mg^{2+} and Ca^{2+} and to low pH growth conditions [26,27]. PhoPQ activation results in addition of palmitate to form hepta-acylated lipid A, incorporation of 2-OH myristate at position 3′ and removal of 3-OH myristate from position 3 of lipid A [25,28]. In vivo, these changes in LPS structure are believed to contribute to bacterial resistance to antimicrobial peptides and to the moderate acidic environment found within macrophages [21,25,28,29].

With regard to the OAg, a few studies have suggested that the structure of this domain of LPS is modified in response to the pH of the medium. Delgado et al [30] reported that PmrAB activation in *S.* Typhimurium results in upregulation of the *cld* (wzz_{ST}) gene, increasing the L-OAg chain length distribution [30], whereas in *H. pylori*, exposure to low pH induced the expression of one unidentified gene related to OAg biosynthesis. A mutant lacking this gene was significantly more sensitive to acid stress (pH 3.5) than the wild-type strain. In addition, changes in the LPS electrophoretic profiles were observed [31]. The authors suggested that these modifications could contribute to the adaptation to resist extreme acidity, but this was not verified.

Together, these studies demonstrate that moderate low pH induce modifications of LPS in other enteropathogens, increasing their resistance to this environmental condition. However, they have not addressed whether these and/or other alterations of LPS structure play a role in resistance to extreme acid conditions. In this paper, we establish that both the OAg and the lipid A domains of *S. flexneri* LPS are modified by exposure to moderate acid conditions, we determine the nature of these modifications and show their importance in the acid-resistance phenotype of this pathogen.

Results

The O antigen contributes to acid resistance of *S. flexneri*

To ascertain whether the OAg is required for acid resistance, we constructed a deletion mutant of the *waaL* gene, which encodes the OAg ligase. The Δ*waaL* mutant (strain MSF1210) showed a rough LPS profile (devoid of OAg) in silver stained polyacrilamide gels (**Figure 1A**, lane 2). When this mutant was transformed with the intact *waaL* gene cloned in a multicopy plasmid (strain MSF1210/pMM112), an LPS profile showing the ladder corresponding to the

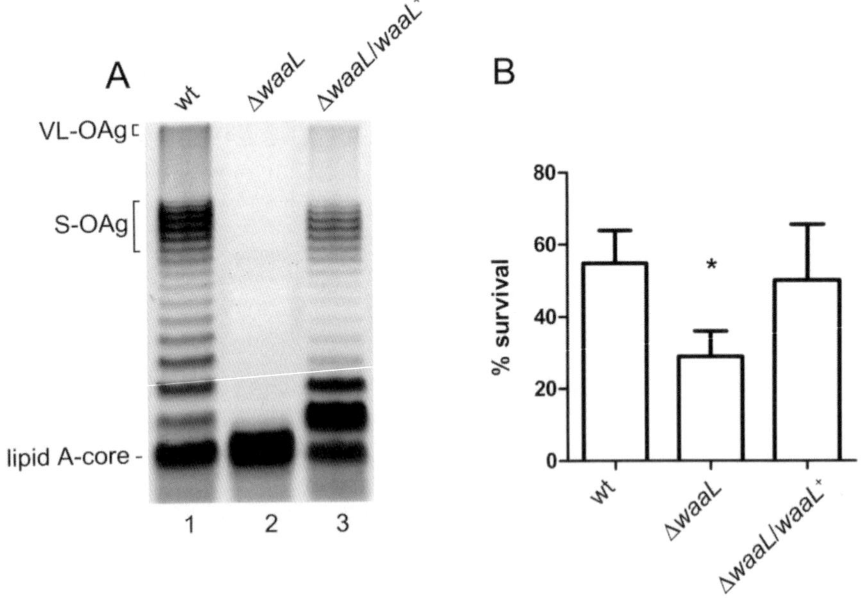

Figure 1. Contribution of the O antigen to *S. flexneri* 2a acid resistance. LPS profiles (A) and acid resistance (B) of S. *flexneri* 2457T (wt), MSF1210 (Δ*waaL*) and MSF1210/pMM112 (Δ*waaL*/*waaL*$^{+}$). LPS samples from equal numbers of bacterial cells (1×10^7 CFU) were loaded in each lane and were analyzed by Tricine-SDS-polyacrylamide gel electrophoresis on a 14% (w/v) acrylamide gel followed by silver staining. Brackets indicate the VL-OAg, the S-OAg and the lipid A-core region. For acid resistance assays, cells were grown overnight in citrate-buffered LB (pH 5.5) and diluted 1:1000 into the acid-challenge media. Survival is stated as a percentage of the inoculum. Averages±standard errors (error bars) are shown. Statistical significance was determined by a Student's *t* test. (*, $P < 0.05$).

OAg bands was observed (**Figure 1A**, lane 3). This profile was similar to that of the wild type (**Figure 1A**, lane 1). We compared the ability of the Δ*waaL* mutant and the wild-type 2457T to survive an exposure to pH 2.5 for 30 min, after overnight adaptation to pH 5.5, as described in Materials and Methods. As shown in **Figure 1B**, the mutant lacking OAg was significantly more sensitive to extreme acidity than the wild-type strain. The mutant harboring pMM112 recovered the ability to survive under this condition. A similar result was obtained for Δ*waaL* and Δ*waaL*/pMM112 derivatives of *S. flexneri* serotype 5a strain M90T (data not shown). Thus, the presence of polymerized OAg molecules increases resistance to extreme acidity of *S. flexneri* previously adapted to moderate acid pH.

The S-OAg is required for acid resistance

Because the results described above indicated that the OAg contributes to acid resistance, we investigated whether a particular length of the OAg molecules was required for this property. For this purpose, we constructed defined deletion mutants in genes *wzzB* (strain MSF102) and wzz_{pHS2} (strain MSF107), which encode proteins that regulate the S-OAg and VL-OAg chain length distributions, respectively. We also generated a double mutant lacking both regulators (strain MSF209). LPS was obtained and analyzed by SDS-PAGE and silver staining. As shown in **Figure 2A**, the Δ*wzzB* mutant was devoid of S-OAg but it produced VL-OAg (lane 2), whereas the Δwzz_{pHS2} mutant exhibited the opposite phenotype (lane 3). The double mutant showed a random distribution of OAg molecules (lane 4), in contrast to the wild type that produced both S-OAg and VL-OAg (lane 1). Transformation of the double mutant with each intact gene cloned in a multicopy plasmid restored the expression of the corresponding chain length (lanes 5 and 6). Acid resistance of each of these strains was assayed for 30 min at pH 2.5 after overnight adaptation to pH 5.5. As shown in **Figure 2B**, Δ*wzzB* and the double mutant (strains MSF102 and MSF209, respectively) were significantly more sensitive to extreme acid conditions, with survival levels less than 20% of the wild type. In contrast, the Δwzz_{pHS2} mutant (strain MSF107) showed acid resistance levels similar to the wild type. In accordance with these results, the double mutant transformed with a multicopy plasmid including the intact *wzzB* gene, but not the intact wzz_{pHS2} gene, recovered the wild-type levels of resistance to extreme acidity.

In order to ascertain whether the S-OAg chain length that is characteristic of *S. flexneri* 2a is required for acid resistance, strain MSF209 was transformed with multicopy plasmids expressing each OAg chain length regulator of *Salmonella* Typhimurium. Similar to *S. flexneri*, this bacterium shows a bi-modal distribution of the OAg expressing a long (L-)OAg of 16 to 35 repeat units regulated by Wzz_{ST} and a very long (VL-)OAg of more than 100 repeat units regulated by Wzz_{fepE} [32–36]. The *S. flexneri* double mutant expressing the heterologous chain regulators (strains MSF209/pMM110 and MSF209/pJC142) produced OAg modal lengths characteristic of *S.* Typhimurium (**Figure 2A**, lanes 7 and 8, respectively). The double mutant expressing any of the heterologous regulators showed acid resistance values significantly lower than those of the wild-type 2457T and of the mutant expressing *S. flexneri* WzzB (**Figure 2B**). Together, these results indicate that S-OAg distinctive of *S. flexneri* 2a is essential to confer acid resistance.

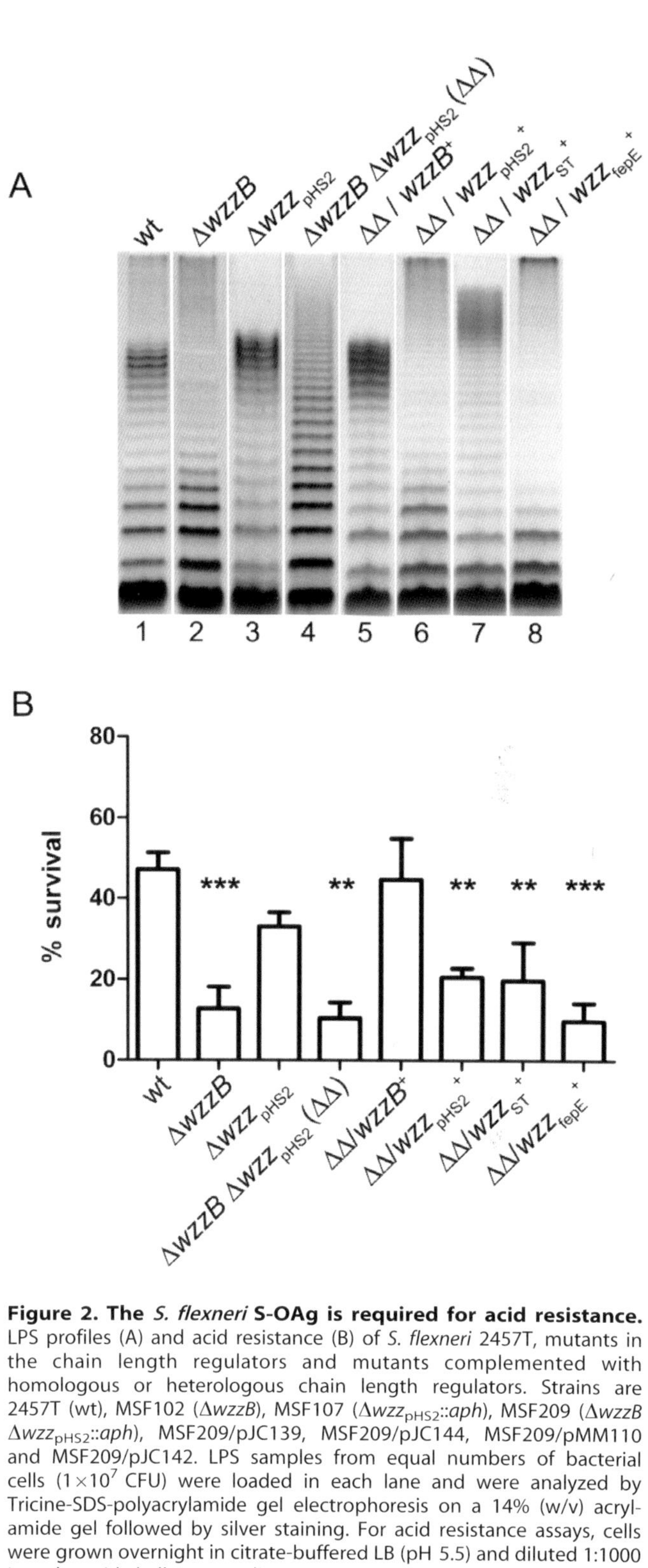

Figure 2. The *S. flexneri* S-OAg is required for acid resistance. LPS profiles (A) and acid resistance (B) of *S. flexneri* 2457T, mutants in the chain length regulators and mutants complemented with homologous or heterologous chain length regulators. Strains are 2457T (wt), MSF102 (Δ*wzzB*), MSF107 (Δwzz_{pHS2}::*aph*), MSF209 (Δ*wzzB* Δwzz_{pHS2}::*aph*), MSF209/pJC139, MSF209/pJC144, MSF209/pMM110 and MSF209/pJC142. LPS samples from equal numbers of bacterial cells (1×10^7 CFU) were loaded in each lane and were analyzed by Tricine-SDS-polyacrylamide gel electrophoresis on a 14% (w/v) acrylamide gel followed by silver staining. For acid resistance assays, cells were grown overnight in citrate-buffered LB (pH 5.5) and diluted 1:1000 into the acid-challenge media. Survival is stated as a percentage of the inoculum. Averages±standard errors (error bars) are shown. Statistical significance was determined by a Student's *t* test. (**, $P < 0.01$, ***, $P < 0.001$).

Glucosylation of the O antigen also contributes to acid resistance

The OAg of *S. flexneri* 2a is glucosylated in the last rhamnose residue [37]. It has been described that this modification affects the conformation of the polymer in such a way that LPS molecules containing glucosylated OAg are more compact and shorter than molecules of non-glucosylated OAg [38]. Because we found that the length of the OAg was critical to acid resistance (S-OAg), we decided to investigate whether the degree of glucosylation could also influence this property. To this end, we constructed a deletion mutant in the *gtrABII* operon encoding proteins responsible for glucosylation of the OAg. The electrophoretic profile of this mutant (strain MSF2743) showed OAg bands migrating slightly faster than those of the wild-type 2457T. This observation was more evident when the electrophoresis was performed on a longer polyacrylamide gel (**Figure 3A,** lanes 2 and 1, respectively). Acid resistance experiments showed that MSF2743 was about 50% more sensitive to pH 2.5 than the wild type. When this mutant was transformed with the intact *gtrABII* operon cloned in a multicopy plasmid, the acid resistant phenotype was restored to wild-type levels (**Figure 3B**).

A mild acidic condition modifies the LPS structure of *S. flexneri*

The mechanisms for resistance to extreme acidity are induced by previous adaptation to a moderate acidic pH [6–8]. In other enterobacteria, it has been demonstrated that this latter condition causes changes in the LPS structure [31]. We decided to investigate whether adaptation to pH 5.5 altered the LPS of *S. flexneri* 2a, and, if that was the case, whether these changes contributed to resistance to extreme acidity. We first compared the LPS profiles of bacteria grown at pH 7.0 and pH 5.5. As shown in **Figure 4**, the LPS of bacteria grown at pH 5.5 had a slightly lower mobility of the bands corresponding to S-OAg than bacteria grown at pH 7.0 (lanes 2 and 1, respectively). It was observed that at pH 5.5, this region contained lower amounts of OAg bands ranging from 11–15 units, but higher amounts of OAg bands of 16–18 units (see densitogram in **Figure 4**, upper right). In order to ascertain whether this modification was relevant to acid resistance, we performed acid-resistance assays using the Δ*wzzB* mutant (strain MSF102) transformed with plasmids containing site-directed mutations in the gene encoding the WzzB regulator (**Table 1**). When strain MSF102/pRMCD108 (mutation $WzzB_{(K267N)}$) was grown at pH 7.0, produced an LPS profile similar to that observed in the wild type grown at pH 5.5 (**Figure 5A**, compare lanes 2 and 3). In contrast, when strain MSF102/pRMCD127 (mutation $WzzB_{(M32T)}$) was grown at pH 5.5, it produced an LPS profile similar to the wild type grown at pH 7.0 (**Figure 5A**, compare lanes 1 and 4). Thus it was expected that, if the shift of the S-OAg that occurs at pH 5.5 was relevant to acid resistance, strain MSF102/pRMCD108 would be resistant to extreme acid pH without previous adaptation to pH 5.5. On the other hand, strain MSF102/pRMCD127 would be sensitive to acid even after adaptation.

The results showed that MSF102/pRMCD108 was as sensitive as the wild-type strain grown at pH 7.0 (non-adapted), whereas MSF102/pRMCD127 showed resistance levels similar to the wild-type grown at pH 5.5 (adapted) (**Figure 5B**). These results indicated that the change in the electrophoretic mobility of the S-OAg induced by moderate acidic conditions is not relevant to resistance to extremely acidic pH.

We also noticed that the OAg of bacteria grown at acid pH migrated as double bands (**Figure 4**, see densitogram lower right). The double bands were not attributable to glucosylated OAg molecules because they were also present in the Δ*gtrABII* mutant grown at pH 5.5 (data not shown). The double bands were more evident in the OAg molecules containing one, two, three and four repeat units and in the lipid A-core region. The double band in this region was also evident in LPS obtained form bacteria grown at pH 7.0, although it was much fainter than at pH 5.5 (compare lanes 1 and 2 in **Figure 4,** and lanes 1 and 3 in **Figure 5**). With these observations, we hypothesized that this modification actually occurred in the lipid A-core region and, as a consequence, the OAg profile appeared altered. In order to test this notion, we analyzed the LPS profiles of defined mutants in the polymerization or ligation of the OAg, and with different degrees of truncation of the outer core (Δ*waaD*, Δ*waaJ* and Δ*waaI*). The LPS patterns of the mutants and the structure of the LPS outer core [39,40] are shown in **Figures 6A and B**, respectively. The Δ*wzy* mutant exhibited the lipid A-core region substituted by one OAg unit (lanes 1 and 2), whereas the Δ*waaL* mutant synthesized only lipid A-core (lanes 3 and 4). The Δ*waaD* mutant showed a core region that migrated slightly faster than that of Δ*waaL* (lanes 5 and 6) consistent with the lack of the GlcNAc residue in the outer core (**Figure 6B**). Deletion of *waaJ* and *waaI* genes resulted in additional truncations of the core region (lanes 7 and 8; 9 and 10, respectively). The *waaJ* gene product adds Glc II while the *waaI* product adds the Gal residue to the outer core (**Figure 6B**). All strains exhibited the double band when grown at pH 5.5. These results indicated that the changes in the LPS structure by exposure to moderate acidic condition affected the lipid A and/or the inner core regions of LPS.

In *S.* Typhimurium, moderate acidic pH activates the PhoPQ two-component system. Phosphorylated PhoP activates expression of the *pagP* gene, encoding a protein responsible for the addition of palmitate to lipid A [25,41,42]. To define whether a similar regulation occurs in *S. flexneri*, we constructed a *phoP* deletion mutant and analyzed the LPS profiles of bacteria grown at pH 7.0 and 5.5. The results showed that double bands were still present in the Δ*phoP* mutant (data not shown). Thus, it was unlikely that the double bands were due to the addition of palmitate to lipid A.

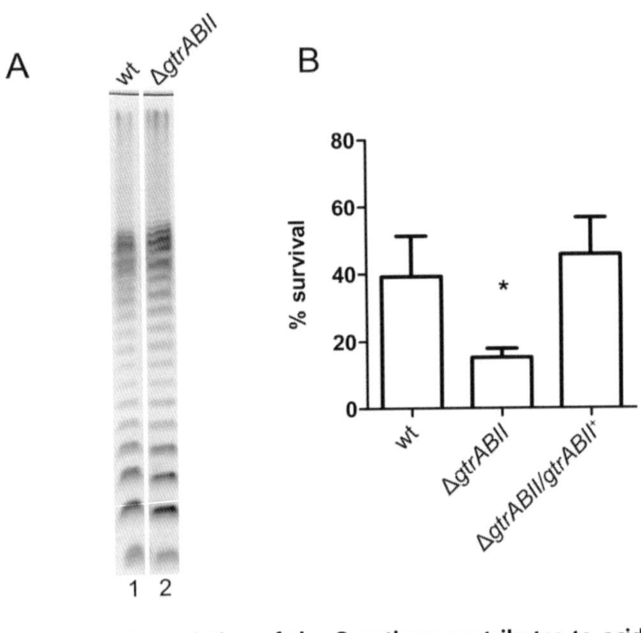

Figure 3. Glucosylation of the O antigen contributes to acid resistance. (A) LPS profiles of *S. flexneri* 2457T (wt) and MSF2743 (Δ*gtrABII*). LPS samples from equal numbers of bacterial cells (1×10^7 CFU) were loaded in each lane and were analyzed by Tricine-SDS-polyacrylamide gel electrophoresis on a 14% (w/v) acrylamide gel followed by silver staining. (B) Acid resistance of *S. flexneri* 2457T (wt), MSF2743 (Δ*gtrABII*) and MSF2743/pMM111 (Δ*gtrABII/gtrABII*$^+$). Cells were grown overnight in citrate-buffered LB (pH 5.5) and diluted 1:1000 into the acid-challenge media. Survival is stated as a percentage of the inoculum. Averages±standard errors (error bars) are shown. Statistical significance was determined by a Student's *t* test. (*, $P < 0.05$).

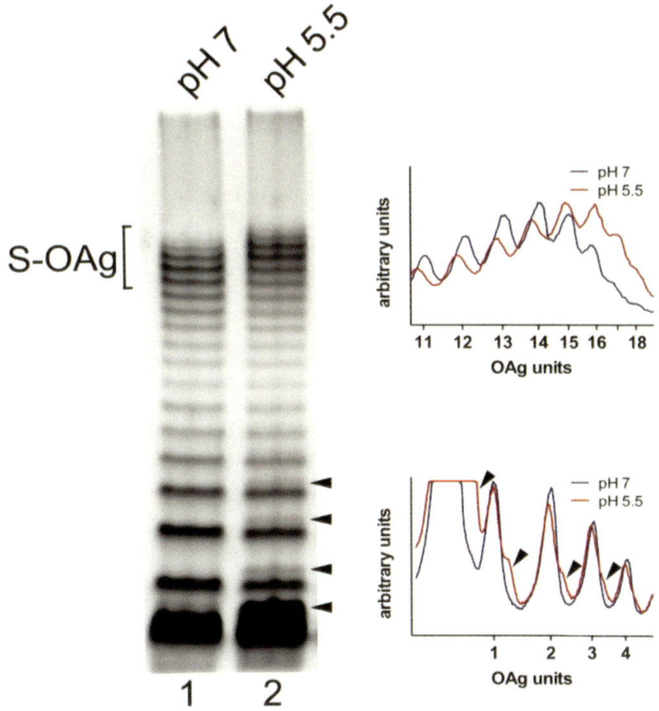

Figure 4. Effect of pH on LPS profiles from S. *flexneri* 2457T. Cells were grown at pH 7.0 or 5.5 and LPS samples were obtained. LPS samples from equal numbers of bacterial cells (1×10^7 CFU) were loaded in each lane and were analyzed by Tricine-SDS-polyacrylamide gel electrophoresis on a 14% (w/v) acrylamide gel followed by silver staining. Bracket shows the S-OAg region. Arrow heads point to the double bands observed in LPS from bacteria grown at pH 5.5. The right panels show the densitograms of the bands in the gel. Upper graph shows the bands corresponding to the S-OAg (11 to 18 units) and lower graph shows the bands corresponding to the Lipid A-core substituted with 1 to 4 units.

To elucidate the chemical nature of the modifications of lipid A, *S. flexneri* was grown in LB broth in the presence of ^{32}Pi, at pH 7.0 and pH 5.5. The ^{32}P-labelled lipid A was isolated and subjected to TLC as described in Materials and Methods. The results showed that *S. flexneri* grown at pH 7.0 produces lipid A molecules partially substituted with a second phosphate group (1-PP) and L-Ara4N (**Figure 7**, lane 1). In contrast, when bacteria were grown at pH 5.5 the lipid A was modified by the addition of PEtN, while 1-PP and L-Ara4N were not detected (**Figure 7**, lane 2). The chemical nature of these species was confirmed by analyzing the lipid A profiles of the Δ*arnT* mutant (strain MSF1650) and of the wild-type strain transformed with the *eptA* gene cloned in a multicopy plasmid (strain 2457T/pMM113) grown at pH 7.0. This strategy was used because we were unable to obtain an *eptA* mutant either by the Red swap methodology or by using the suicide vector pGP704 containing an internal region of the gene.

In strain 2457T/pMM113, spots corresponding to lipid A substituted with one and two molecules of PEtN (double) were observed. As in the wild type grown at pH 7.0, 1-PP and L-Ara4N were also detected (**Figure 7**, lane 3). This last spot was missing in the chromatogram of lipid A from strain MSF1650 (**Figure 7**, lane 4). Interestingly, in this mutant genetic background, PEtN was detected in lipid A from bacteria grown at pH 7.0. Finally, we analyzed lipid A obtained from a Δ*pmrA* mutant (strain MSF1666). As expected, this mutant lacked L-Ara4N; however, it was able to add PEtN to lipid A at pH 7.0 (**Figure 7**, lane 5).

Table 1. Evaluation of bacterial cell surface charge.

Strain (growth pH)	% Cytochrome C bound
2457T (7.0)	27.1±2.5
2457T (5.5)	8.8±2.4
2457T/pMM113 (7.0)	15.0±3.8

Values represent percent binding of cytochrome C after incubation with bacteria for 10 min at room temperature. Data are the means and standard deviations from two independent experiments run in duplicate.

A less negative bacterial surface charge is produced by lipid A modification under mild acidic condition

To evaluate whether the modifications of lipid A by the addition of polar groups alter the cell surface charge, we measured the cytochrome C binding affinity of the wild type cells grown at pH 7.0 and 5.5. The results (**Table 1**) showed that binding was lower when bacteria were grown at pH 5.5 that at pH 7.0, suggesting that addition of PEtN to lipid A at moderate acidic pH confers a less negative charge to the bacterial surface. To confirm this notion, cytochrome C binding affinity of the wild type cells overexpressing the *eptA* gene, grown at pH 7.0, was measured. As shown in **Table 1**, these cells bound about one half the amount of cytochrome C than the wild type grown under this condition.

Lipid A modifications induced under mild acidic conditions confer resistance to extreme acidity

To investigate whether the modification of the lipid A region induced by growth at pH 5.5 is involved in resistance to extreme acid conditions, we tested acid resistance of the wild-type strain transformed with pMM113. As shown in **Figure 8**, overexpression of the *eptA* gene significantly increased acid resistance after 30 and 60 min of exposure to pH 2.5, compared to the parental strain. This result indicates that the addition of PEtN to the lipid A region of LPS, induced by a moderate pH, contributes to *S. flexneri* resistance to extreme acid. In contrast, deletion of the *arnT* gene did not alter this property. As shown in **Figure 8**, the Δ*arnT* mutant (strain MSF1650) showed levels of acid resistance identical to the wild-type strain.

Finally, we transformed the Δ*waaL*, Δ*wzzB* and Δ*grtABII* mutants with plasmids pMM112 or pMM113 and assayed the acid resistance of the resulting strains. The results showed that the transformed strains were as sensitive to extreme acidity as the original mutants (data not shown), indicating that, even though lipid A modification contributes to acid resistance, the presence of glucosylated OAg is fundamental to this property.

Discussion

Remodelling of the bacterial envelope is an important strategy used by bacteria to adapt to stressful conditions. Global expression studies carried out in other enteropathogens have revealed that a great number of genes involved in the biosynthesis of surface structures are regulated by the pH of the environment [9–13]. In the present study, we investigated whether the lipopolysaccharide of *S. flexneri* 2a is modified by exposure to a moderate acidic pH, and if these modifications increase bacterial resistance to extreme acidity.

Our results clearly show that the presence of OAg is required for acid resistance, since a mutant that does not bind the polymer

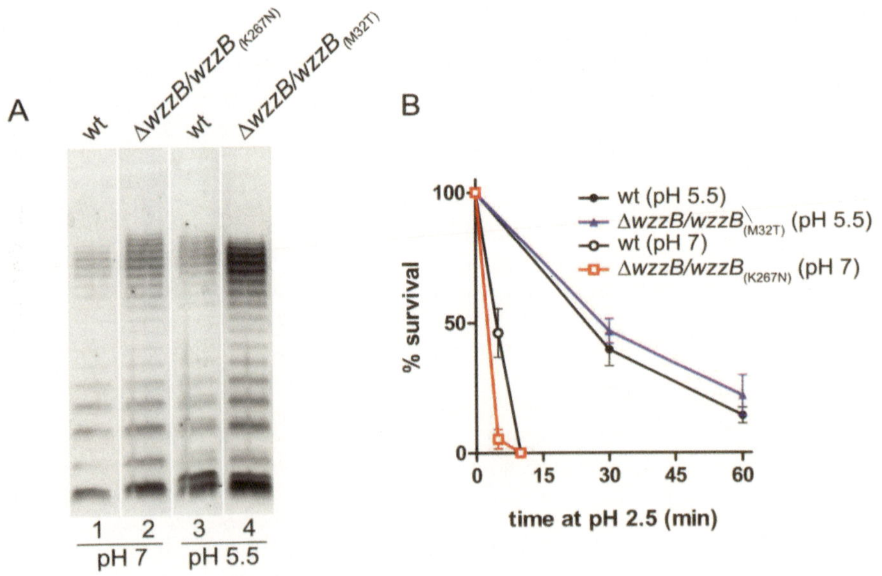

Figure 5. Changes in the electrophoretic mobility of the LPS induced by moderate acidic conditions are not relevant to resistance to extreme acid. LPS profiles (A) and acid resistance (B) of *S. flexneri* 2457T (wt) and MSF102 (Δ*wzzB*) transformed with plasmids pRMCD108 ($WzzB_{(K267N)}$) or pRMCD127 ($WzzB_{(M32T)}$). Bacteria were grown at pH 7.0 or 5.5 and LPS samples were obtained. LPS samples from equal numbers of bacterial cells (1×10^7 CFU) were loaded in each lane and were analyzed by Tricine-SDS-polyacrylamide gel electrophoresis on a 14% (w/v) acrylamide gel followed by silver staining. For acid resistance assays, cells were grown overnight in citrate-buffered LB (pH 5.5) and diluted 1:1000 into the acid-challenge media. Survival is stated as a percentage of counts at time zero. Averages±standard errors (error bars) are shown. Statistical significance was determined by the two-way ANOVA and Bonferroni post test. No significant differences were found in bacteria previously grown at pH 5.5 (closed symbols) or pH 7.0 (open symbols).

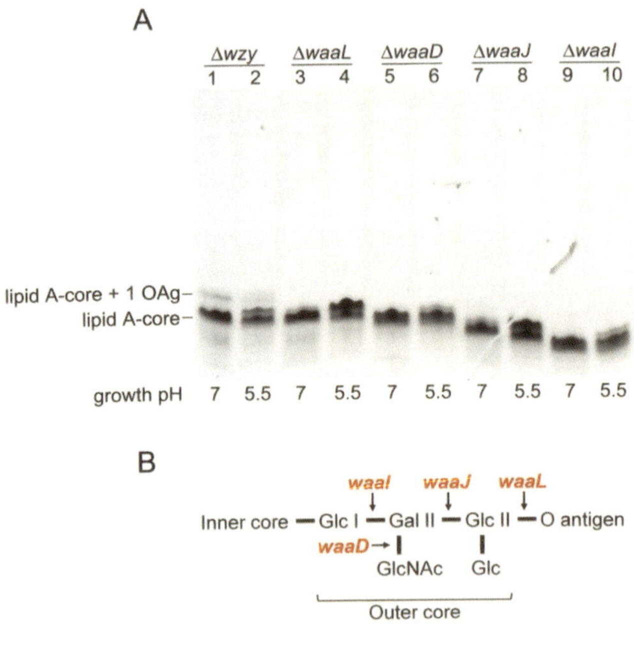

Figure 6. LPS profiles from S. *flexneri* mutants defective in O antigen and core synthesis and proposed structure of the outer core of *S. flexneri* 2a. (A) Bacteria were grown at pH 7.0 or 5.5. LPS samples from equal numbers of bacterial cells (1×10^7 CFU) were loaded in each lane and were analyzed by Tricine-SDS-polyacrylamide gel electrophoresis on a 14% (w/v) acrylamide gel followed by silver staining. The strains are MSF1749 (Δ*wzy*), MSF1210 (Δ*waaL*), MSF1144 (Δ*waaD*), MSF1009 (Δ*waaI*) and MSF1015 (Δ*waaJ*). (B) Genes encoding proteins involved in the addition of the different sugars during outer core biosynthesis are indicated in red.

to the lipid A-core was highly sensitive to pH 2.5, even after being adapted to pH 5.5. These results are consistent with the work of other authors, who demonstrated that the lack of OAg or diminished amount of this polysaccharide impaired the ability of *Rhizobium leguminosarum* biovar trifolii [43], *H. pylori* [31] and *Salmonella enterica* serovar Dublin [44] to grow or persist under acidic conditions. In an *E. coli* O157:H7, a strain closely related to *Shigella*, it has also been demonstrated the involvement of LPS in the resistance to organic acid [45]. Although the acid stress used in that study was different from our conditions (pH 4.5 versus pH 2.5), their results support our conclusion that the OAg is essential to acid resistance. More interestingly, we found that a particular length of the OAg, the S-OAg modal distribution, is required for resistance to extreme acidity. In contrast, neither the VL-OAg modal length nor OAg lengths characteristic of *S.* Typhimurium contributed significantly to this property.

McGowan et al [31] proposed that the OAg could act as a physical barrier to prevent entry of protons to the bacterial cell. Our results do not agree with this notion, because the mutant lacking VL-OAg (Δwzz_{pHS2}) was as resistant to extreme acid as the wild-type strain, meaning that LPS molecules of high molecular weight do not confer higher levels of resistance, as would be expected if the OAg polymer acted as a physical barrier for protons.

Another explanation for the role of the OAg in the acid stress response could be that the polysaccharide may be positively charged repelling protons from the surrounding medium. However, at the pH values used in this study, the –OH groups of the rhamnose residues in the *S. flexneri* OAg are protonated and neutral [46] and, hence, they do not confer a positive charge to the OAg molecules. On the other hand, the amide group in the N-acetylglucosamine residue is deprotonated and neutral at the pH values used here. In consequence, the OAg would not be charged

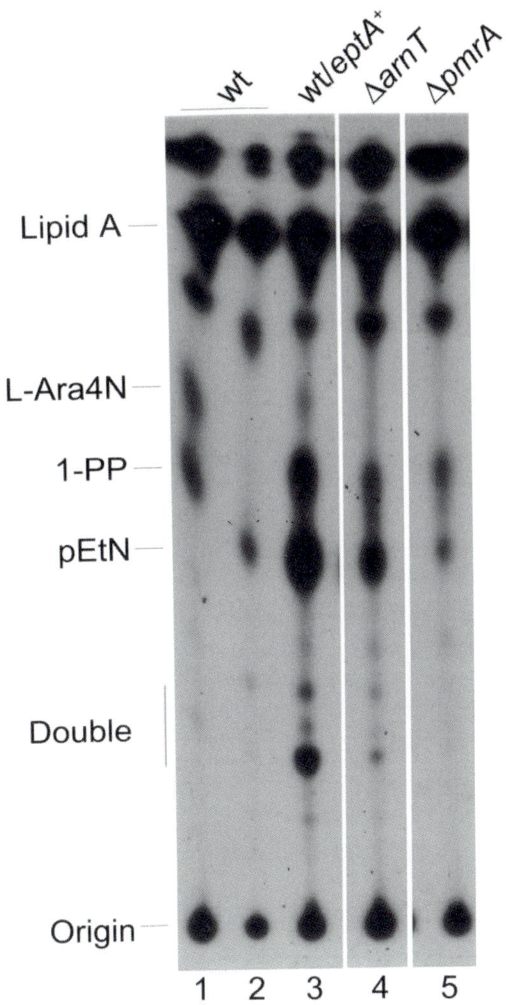

Figure 7. Effect of pH on lipid A modifications in *S. flexneri*. ^{32}P-labelled lipid A was isolated from bacteria grown in N-minimal medium at pH 7.0 (lanes 1, 3, 4 and 5) or 5.5 (lane 2). Lipid A species were resolved by TLC with the solvent system chloroform/pyridine/88% formic acid/water (50:50:16:5, v/v). The strains are 2457T (wt), 2457T/pMM113 (wt/*eptA*$^+$), MSF1650 (Δ*arnT*) and MSF1666 (Δ*pmrA*).

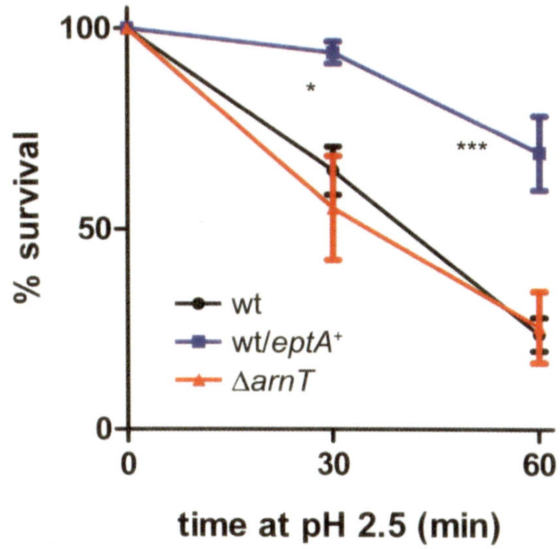

Figure 8. Effect of lipid A modifications on acid resistance of *S. flexneri*. The strain are 2457T (wt), 2457T/pMM113 (wt/*eptA*$^+$) and MSF1650 (Δ*arnT*). Cells were grown overnight in citrate-buffered LB (pH 5.5) and diluted 1:1000 into the acid-challenge media. Survival is stated as a percentage of counts at time zero. Averages±standard errors (error bars) are shown. Statistical significance was determined by. the two-way ANOVA and Bonferroni post test (*, $P<0.05$, ***, $P<0.001$).

under the conditions of this study and, thus, it would not act as an electrostatic barrier for the influx of protons.

Because it is known that moderate acidic conditions produce changes in the expression of outer membrane proteins [47,48] and that the absence of some porins affects resistance to acidic pH [49,50], we propose that the presence of OAg, in particular the S-OAg modal length, may be necessary for assembly or function of a protein in the bacterial envelope required for acid resistance. In support of this idea, it has been suggested that a preferential association between certain outer membrane proteins and LPS molecules of a particular length may occur [35]. For example, the IcsA protein, involved in actin polymerization that allows *S. flexneri* spreading between epithelial cells, requires the presence of S-OAg to be assembled at one pole of the bacterial surface [35, 51 52]. Alternatively, or in addition, synthesis of S-OAg may slow down polymerization of very long OAg molecules (VL-OAg), which could mask a membrane protein needed for acid resistance. In this context, our previous work [53] demonstrated that the two *Shigella* chain-length regulators compete to control the degree of O antigen polymerization; hence, increase in one modal length results in a parallel decrease in the other.

Our results also show that glucosylation of the OAg contribute to acid resistance. Our data indicates that this modification is also present in bacteria grown under standard conditions (LB, pH 7.0), in agreement with a previous study conducted by West et al [19]. Interestingly, these authors demonstrated that glucosylation of the OAg is required for the proper function of the Type Three Secretion System (T3SS) of *S. flexneri*, because glucosylated OAg is more compact and short than non-glucosylated LPS, allowing a proper exposure of the needle complex [38]. Additionally, a more compact and dense OAg favours the interaction between OAg molecules, contributing to stabilize the outer membrane [54] and protecting it from the damage caused by acidic pH and entry of protons. Given all these observations, we speculate that glucosylated OAg containing mainly S-OAg molecules is required for optimal functioning of one or more proteins that contribute to the acid stress response.

The current work also demonstrates that moderate acidic pH induces modifications in the lipid A region of *S. flexneri*. Previous work by Gibbons et al [29] showed that lipid A of *S.* Typhimurium is covalently modified by the addition of acyl and/or polar substituents in response to low Mg^{2+} concentrations and mild acidic pH. Under these conditions, lipid A was derivatized with phosphoethanoamine (PEtN), aminoarabinose (L-Ara4N), 2-hydroxymyristate and/or palmitate moieties. It is believed that these modifications confer resistance to cationic antimicrobial peptides by masking negative phosphate groups with positively charged moieties [55–58]. In *E. coli* K12 W3110, lipid A is modified in response to growth under acidic but no low Mg^{2+} conditions. The main change is the addition of PEtN to the phosphate molecule at position 1 of N-acetyl glucosamine. The addition of two PEtN to each phosphate molecule at positions 1 and 4 was also detected in a small fraction of lipid A molecules. In contrast to *S.* Typhimurium, no L-Ara4N was detected. At pH 7.5, lipid A was mainly unmodified or, a low fraction of molecules, carried a 1-PP group [29,59].

Our results demonstrate that similar modifications occur in *S. flexneri*. As in *E. coli*, the main change induced at pH 5.5 was the addition of PEtN to lipid A, whereas L-Ara4N was not detected. In contrast, at pH 7.0 the lipid A molecules were derivatized with 1-PP and L-Ara4N. The regulatory pathways involved in these modifications also appear to be different to *E. coli* and *S.* Typhimurium, because a Δ*pmrA* mutant lacked L-Ara4N but it was able to add PEtN to lipid A, showing a chromatographic profile similar to Δ*arnT*. This result suggests that modification of lipid A with PEtN in response to acid pH is not mediated by the PmrAB system. Future work will be needed to uncover the regulatory system involved in this modification.

The presence of L-Ara4N does not seem to add to extreme acid resistance. In contrast, addition of PEtN to lipid A protects *S. flexneri* from extreme acid pH. It has been reported that PEtN lipid A modification reduces the net charge of the phosphate group from −1.5 to −1 at neutral pH [54]. Here we demonstrate that addition of PEtN confers a less negative charge to bacterial surface. We speculate that at pH 2.5 the presence of positively charged amine groups increases the net charge to reach positive values. Thus, we hypothesize that lipid A modification with polar substituents generate an electrostatic barrier that acts repelling protons and diminishing their influx to the bacterial cytoplasm.

To our knowledge, this is the first report that addresses the role of LPS in resistance of *S. flexneri* to extreme acid conditions. Our data demonstrate that both modification of the lipid A region and the presence of glucosylated OAg molecules containing the S-OAg modal length are required to confer *S. flexneri* its high level of acid resistance. Our results strengthen the hypothesis proposed by others [35,38] that, during evolution of *S. flexneri* as a successful pathogen, selection of preferred OAg chain lengths and glucosylation of the polysaccharide was optimized. LPS modifications that occur in response to environmental conditions contribute to adaptation of bacteria to the different stages of infection.

Materials and Methods

Bacterial strains, plasmids, media and growth conditions

Table 2 summarizes the properties of the bacterial strains and plasmids used in this study. Bacteria were grown at pH 7.0 in Luria-Bertani medium (LB, 10 g/l Bacto tryptone, 5 g/l Bacto yeast extract, 5 g/l NaCl) or in citrate-buffered LB medium

Table 2. Strains and plasmids used in this study.

Strain or plasmid	Relevant properties[a]	Source or reference
S. flexneri		
2457T	wild-type strain	ISP[b]
MSF107	2457T Δwzz_{pHS2}::*aph*, Km^R	[50]
MSF102	2457T Δ*wzzB*	[50]
MSF209	2457T Δ*wzzB* Δwzz_{pHS2}::*aph*, Km^R	[50]
MSF1749	2457T Δ*wzy*	This study
MSF1210	2457T Δ*waaL*	This study
MSF1144	2457T Δ*waaD*	This study
MSF1009	2457T Δ*waaI*	This study
MSF1015	2457T Δ*waaJ*	This study
MSF2743	2457T Δ*gtrABII*	This study
MSF1650	2457T Δ*arnT*	This study
MSF1666	2457T Δ*pmrA*	This study
Plasmids		
pKD46	*bla* PBAD *gam bet exo* pSC101 *ori*TS	[57]
pKD4	*bla* FRT *aph* FRT PS1 PS2 *ori*R6K	[57]
pCP20	*bla cat* cI857 λP_R *flp* pSC101 *ori*TS	[58]
pGEM-T-Easy	TA cloning vector, Ap^R	Promega
pJC139	*S. flexneri* 2457T *wzzB* cloned into pGEM-T-Easy Ap^R	[63]
pJC142	*S.* Typhimurium LT2 wzz_{fepE} cloned into pGEM-T-Easy Ap^R	[67]
pMM110	*S.* Typhimurium LT2wzz_{LT2} cloned into pGEM-T-Easy, Ap^R	This study
pJC144	*S. flexneri* 2457T wzz_{pHS2} cloned into pGEM-T-Easy, Ap^R	[66]
pMM112	*S. flexneri* 2457T *waaL* cloned into pGEM-T-Easy, Ap^R	This study
pMM113	*S. flexneri* 2457T *eptA* cloned into pGEM-T-Easy, Ap^R	This study
pCC1	Single copy cloning vector, oriII, oriV, Cm^R	EPICENTRE
pMM111	*S. flexneri* 2457T *gtrABII* cloned into pCC1, Cm^R	This study
pRMCD108	$WzzB_{(K267N)}$	[68]
pRMCD127	$WzzB_{(M32T)}$	[68]

[a]Km^R, kanamycin resistant; Ap^R ampicillin resistance; Cm^R, chloramphenicol resistance.
[b]ISP, Institute of Public Health, Santiago, Chile.

(pH 5.5). Ampicillin (100 μg/ml), kanamycin (50 μg/ml), and chloramphenicol (20 μg/ml) were added when appropriate.

Mutagenesis of waaD, waaJ, waaI, waaL, gtrABII, arnT and pmrA genes

Mutagenesis was performed by the Red/Swap method to create chromosomal mutations by homologous recombination using PCR products [60]. *Shigella flexneri* 2a strain 2457T containing pKD46, which expresses the λ Red recombinase system, was transformed with PCR products that were generated using as template plasmid pKD4, which contains the FRT-flanked kanamycin-resistance gene (*aph*). Primers were designed according to the DNA sequence available for the *S. flexneri* 2457T strain. Each primer pair also carried 30 bases that were homologous to the edge of the gene targeted for disruption. The sequences of the oligonucleotide primers are shown in **Table 3**. The kanamycin-resistant transformants were replica plated in the absence of antibiotic selection at 37°C and finally assayed for ampicillin sensitivity to confirm loss of pKD46. To obtain non-polar deletion mutants, the antibiotic resistance gene was removed by transforming the gene replacement mutants with pCP20, which encodes the FLP recombinase [61]. Correct insertional gene replacements and the deletion of the antibiotic gene cassettes were confirmed by PCR.

Construction of expression plasmids

DNA fragments containing the *S. flexneri* 2457T *waaL*, *arnT*, *eptA*, *gtrABII* genes and *S.* Typhimurium LT2 wzz_{ST} were obtained by PCR. The amplicons were cloned into pGEM-T Easy as recommended by the supplier, except for *gtrABII* operon that was cloned into the one copy vector pCC1 (**Table 1**).

LPS analysis

Culture samples were adjusted to an optical density at 600 nm of 2.0 in a final volume of 100 μl. Then, proteinase K-digested whole-cell lysates were prepared as described previously [62], and LPS was separated on 12% (w/v) acrylamide gels using a Tricine-sodium dodecyl sulfate (SDS) buffer system [63]. Gel loadings were normalized so that each sample represented the same number of cells. Gels were silver stained by a modification of the procedure of Tsai & Frasch [64]. Densitometry analysis was performed using the UN-SCANT-IT gel software (Silk Scientific).

Acid resistance assay

For acid-resistance assays bacteria were aerobically grown overnight in LB (pH 7.0) or citrate-buffered LB (pH 5.5) media. Cultures grown to stationary phase were diluted 1:1000 into 5 ml of E medium (0.2 g/l $MgSO4 \cdot 7H_2O$, 2 g/l citric acid monohydrate, 10 g/l $K_2HPO_4 \cdot 3\ H_2O$, 3.5 g/l $NaNH_4HPO_4 \cdot 4H_2O$), acidified with HCl to pH 2.5. This medium was supplemented with 0.2% glucose as carbon source, 20 μg/ml aspartic acid and 20 μg/ml nicotinic acid. The pH 2.5 cultures were incubated at 37°C with shaking; acid challenge was stopped at 0 and 30 min by dilution in LB and cell viability was immediately determined by plating appropriate dilutions in LB plates in triplicate. At least

Table 3. Primers used in this study.

primers	Sequence (5′-3′)	purpose
W_sf_waaL1	acctcaacattatttttctctctcgagaaacatatgaatatcctccttag	*waaL* deletion
W_sf_waaL2	cttgtttttcatcgctaataataagccggcgtgcaggctggagctgcttc	*waaL* deletion
Sf_waaL-1	atttaacggcggcactggat	*waaL* cloning into pGEM-T Easy
Sf_waaL-2	tcactacagttgggatggcg	*waaL* cloning into pGEM-T Easy
Fwr WgtrABII	tgtaaagtacacatctataggtgtgctgaagtgcaggctggagctgcttc	*gtrABII* deletion
Rev WgtrABII	Cctttttctctgatagttttattatcacccatatgaatatcctccttag	*gtrABII* deletion
SfgtrABII- HindIII (1)	cccaagcttggggcgagcaaaatcgatgcgat	*gtrABII* cloning into pCC1
SfgtrABII- HindIII (2)	cccaagcttgggtgaaaaagggaggcgctcttt	*gtrABII* cloning into pCC1
1149	ggctacactgtctccagcttcatcc	*wzz*ST cloning into pGEM-T Easy
1150	gagcaccatccggcaaagaagcttac	*wzz*ST cloning into pGEM-T Easy
eptA (1)	ccggggcgaaagaggttatg	*eptA* cloning into pGEM-T Easy
eptA (2)	cgccagaatcagtccctgca	*eptA* cloning into pGEM-T Easy
Wzysf_A	tcaataacttccctatttttaacatcctttattttgctcccatatgaatatcctccttag	*wzy* deletion
Wwzysf_B	Ctgattattggtggtggtggaagattactggagccatgtgtaggct	*wzy* deletion
W_sf_waaD1	gttgataaaataatatttacggttactcctcatatgaatatcctccttag	*waaD* deletion
W_sf_waaD2	ttcaaaccaattatgaataacctcttcgaagtgtaggctggagctgcttcg	*waaD* deletion
W_sf_waaJ1	gattttaaacatcttactcaatttaaagatcatatgaatatcctccttag	*waaJ* deletion
W_sf_waaJ2	acctttcataacattatatttaattgctgtgtgtaggctggagctgcttcg	*waaJ* deletion
W_sf_waaI1	tctcaactcaatgatagtgacatcatccttcatatgaatatcctccttag	*waaI* deletion
W_sf_waaI2	gaagcatttttctttataatactttaaatagtgtaggctggagctgcttcg	*waaI* deletion
arnT (H1+P1)	gtagtcgctgatgaaatcggtacgttaccttatcggcatcgtgcaggctggagctgcttc	*arnT* deletion
arnT (H2+P2)	gttagccagatcatttgggacgatactgaatcagcaccagcatatgaatatcctccttag	*arnT* deletion
WpmrA (1)	gagtgagtaaatgaaaattctgattgttgaagacgatacggtgcaggctggagctgcttc	*pmrA* deletion
WpmrA (2)	gattcaattagttttcctcattcgcgaccagcatatagcccatatgaatatcctccttag	*pmrA* deletion

Underline indicates the region that anneals to the 5′ or 3′ end of the antibiotic resistance cassette used for the mutagenesis.

three repetitions were performed for each experiment. Acid resistance was calculated as percent survival, taking the bacterial counts obtained at time 0 as 100%.

Analysis of ^{32}Pi labelled lipid A

An overnight culture grown at 37°C on LB was diluted 1000-fold into 5 ml of fresh LB medium at pH 7.0 or 5.5. Labelling was started by addition of 5 μCi/ml of $^{32}H_3PO_4$ (Chilean Commission of Nuclear Energy), and allowed to continue growing overnight at 37°C with shaking. The ^{32}P-labeled bacteria were collected by centrifugation and washed twice with 5 ml of phosphate-buffered saline (PBS), pH 7.4. The bacterial pellets were resuspended in 0.8 ml of PBS and the lipid A fractions were extracted as described by Zhou et al [65]. The lipid A samples were dissolved in chloroform/methanol (4:1, v/v), and several microliters (5,000 cpm per lane) were applied to the origin of a Silica Gel 60 TLC plate. The ^{32}P-labelled lipid A species were resolved with the solvent system chloroform/pyridine/88% formic acid/water (50:50:16:5, v/v). The plate was developed by autoradiography.

Cytochrome C binding assay

An overnight culture grown at 37°C on LB was diluted 1000-fold into 5 ml of fresh LB medium at pH 7.0 or 5.5. Bacteria were collected by centrifugation and washed twice with 10 mM phosphate buffer (PB), pH 6.8. Bacterial pellets were resuspended in 1 ml of PB and the $OD_{600\ nm}$ was measured. Then, samples were diluted to 5 OD units and 30 μl of cytochrome C (10 mg/ml in PB) were added to 1.2 ml of bacterial suspensions. Samples were incubated for 10 min at room temperature and then centrifuged for 2 min at 13,000 rpm. The supernatants (1 ml) were recovered and the $OD_{530\ nm}$ was measured.

Aknowledgments

We thank Renato Morona and Luisa Van Den Bosch for the gift of plasmids pRMCD127 and pRMCD108. We thank Carla Delporte for her help with the TLC experiments and Carlos Santiviago for helpful discussions.

Author Contributions

Conceived and designed the experiments: MM SAA IC. Performed the experiments: MM AH SAA. Analyzed the data: MM AH SAA IC. Wrote the paper: MM SAA IC.

References

1. Kotloff KL, Winickoff JP, Ivanoff B, Clemens JD, Swerdlow D, et al. (1999) Global burden of *Shigella* infections: implications for vaccine development and implementation of control strategies. Bull W H O 77: 651–666.
2. Schroeder GN, Hilbi H (2008) Molecular pathogenesis of *Shigella* spp.: controlling host cell signaling, invasion, and death by type III secretion. Clin Microbiol Rev 21: 134–156.
3. Blaser MJ, Newman LS (1982) A review of human salmonellosis: I. Infective dose. Rev Infect Dis 4: 1096–1106.
4. Gorden J, Small PLC (1993) Acid resistance in enteric bacteria. Infect Immun 61: 364–367.
5. Audia JP, Webb CC, Foster JW (2001) Breaking through the acid barrier: an orchestrated response to proton stress by enteric bacteria. Int J Med Microbiol 29: 97–106.
6. Lin J, Lee IS, Frey J, Slonczewski JL, Foster JW (1995) Comparative analysis of extreme acid survival in *Salmonella typhimurium*, *Shigella flexneri*, and *Escherichia coli*. J Bacteriol 177: 4097–4104.
7. Foster JW (2004) *Escherichia coli* acid resistance: tales of an amateur acidophile. Nat Rev Microbiol 2: 898–907.
8. Jennison AV, Verma NK (2007) The acid-resistance pathways of *Shigella flexneri* 2457T. Microbiology 153: 2593–2602.
9. Cheng F, Wang J, Peng J, Yang J, Fu H, et al. (2007) Gene expression profiling of the pH response in *Shigella flexneri* 2a. FEMS Microbiol Lett 270: 12–20.
10. Maurer LM, Yohannes E, Bondurant SS, Radmacher M, Slonczewski JL (2005) pH regulates genes for flagellar motility, catabolism, and oxidative stress in *Escherichia coli K-12*. J Bacteriol 187: 304–319.
11. Reid AN, Pandey R, Palyada K, Whitworth L, Doukhanine E, et al. (2008) Identification of *Campylobacter jejuni* genes contributing to acid adaptation by transcriptional profiling and genome-wide mutagenesis. Appl Environ Microbiol 74: 1598–1612.
12. Merrell DS, Goodrich ML, Otto G, Tompkins LS, Falkow S (2003) pH-regulated gene expression of the gastric pathogen *Helicobacter pylori*. Infect Immun 71: 3529–3539.
13. Merrell DS, Bailey C, Kaper JB, Camilli A (2001) The ToxR-mediated organic acid tolerance response of *Vibrio cholerae* requires OmpU. J Bacteriol 183: 2746–2754.
14. Quivey RG Jr., Faustoferri R, Monahan K, Marquis R (2000) Shifts in membrane fatty acid profiles associated with acid adaptation of *Streptococcus mutans*. FEMS Microbiol Lett 189: 89–92.
15. Fozo EM, Quivey RG Jr. (2004) Shifts in the membrane fatty acid profile of *Streptococcus mutans* enhance survival in acidic environments. Appl Environ Microbiol. 70: 929–936.
16. Budin-Verneuil A, Pichereau V, Auffray Y, Ehrlich D, Maguin E (2007) Proteome phenotyping of acid stress-resistant mutants of *Lactococcus lactis* MG1363. Proteomics 7: 2038–2046.
17. Morona R, Van den Bosch L, Manning PA (1995) Molecular, genetic, and topological characterization of O-antigen chain length regulation in *Shigella flexneri*. J Bacteriol 177: 1059–1068.
18. Stevenson G, Kessler A, Reeves PR (1995) A plasmid-borne O-antigen chain length determinant and its relationship to other chain length determinants. FEMS Microbiol Lett 125: 23–30.
19. West NP, Sansonetti P, Mounier J, Exley RM, Parsot C, et al. (2005) Optimization of virulence functions through glucosylation of *Shigella* LPS. Science 307: 1313–1317.
20. Helander IM, Kilpeläinen I, Vaara M (1994) Increased substitution of phosphate groups in lipopolysaccharides and lipid A of the polymyxin-resistant pmrA mutants of *Salmonella typhimurium*: a 31P-NMR study. Mol Microbiol 11: 481–487.
21. Nummila K, Kilpeläinen I, Zähringer U, Vaara M, Helander IM (1995) Lipopolysaccharides of polymyxin B-resistant mutants of *Escherichia coli* are extensively substituted by 2-aminoethyl pyrophosphate and contain aminoarabinose in lipid. A. Mol Microbiol 16: 271–278.
22. Gunn JS, Ryan SS, Van Velkinburgh JC, Ernst RK, Miller SI (2000) Genetic and functional analysis of a PmrA-PmrB-regulated locus necessary for lipopolysaccharide modification, antimicrobial peptide resistance, and oral virulence of *Salmonella enterica* serovar Typhimurium. Infect Immun 68: 6139–6146.
23. Zhou Z, Ribeiro AA, Lin S, Cotter RJ, Miller SI, et al. (2001) Lipid A modifications in polymyxin-resistant *Salmonella typhimurium*: PmrA-dependent 4-amino-4-deoxy-L-arabinose, and phosphoethanolamine incorporation. J Biol Chem 276: 43111–43121.
24. Lee H, Hsu FF, Turk J, Groisman EA (2004) The PmrA-regulated *pmrC* gene mediates phosphoethanolamine modification of lipid A and polymyxin resistance in *Salmonella enterica*. J Bacteriol 186: 4124–4133.
25. Gunn JS (2008) The *Salmonella* PmrAB regulon: lipopolysaccharide modifications, antimicrobial peptide resistance and more. Trends Microbiol 16: 284–290.
26. García Véscovi E, Soncini FC, Groisman EA (1996) Mg^{2+} as an extracellular signal: environmental regulation of *Salmonella* virulence. Cell 84: 165–174.
27. Bearson BL, Wilson L, Foster JW (1998) A low pH-inducible, PhoPQ-dependent acid tolerance response protects *Salmonella typhimurium* against inorganic acid stress. J Bacteriol 180: 2409–2417.
28. Ernst RK, Guina T, Miller SI (2001) *Salmonella typhimurium* outer membrane remodeling: role in resistance to host innate immunity. Microbes Infect 3: 1327–1334.
29. Gibbons HS, Kalb SR, Cotter RJ, Raetz CR (2005) Role of Mg^{2+} and pH in the modification of *Salmonella* lipid A after endocytosis by macrophage tumour cells. Mol Microbiol 55: 425–440.
30. Delgado MA, Mouslim C, Groisman EA (2006) The PmrA/PmrB and RcsC/YojN/RcsB systems control expression of the *Salmonella* O-antigen chain length determinant. Mol Microbiol 60: 39–50.
31. McGowan CC, Necheva A, Thompson SA, Cover TL, Blaser MJ (1998) Acid-induced expression of an LPS-associated gene in *Helicobacter pylori*. Mol Microbiol 30: 19–31.
32. Bastin DA, Stevenson G, Brown PK, Haase A, Reeves PR (1993) Repeat unit polysaccharides of bacteria: a model for polymerization resembling that of ribosomes and fatty acid synthetase, with a novel mechanism for determining chain length. Mol Microbiol 7: 725–734.
33. Batchelor RA, Alifano P, Biffali E, Hull SI, Hull RA (1992) Nucleotide sequences of the genes regulating O-polysaccharide antigen chain length (rol) from *Escherichia coli* and *Salmonella typhimurium*: protein homology and functional complementation. J Bacteriol 174: 5228–5236.

34. McClelland M, Sanderson KE, Spieth J, Clifton SW, Latreille P, et al. (2001) Complete genome sequence of *Salmonella enterica* serovar Typhimurium LT2. Nature 413: 852–856.
35. Morona R, Daniels C, Van Den Bosch L (2003) Genetic modulation of *Shigella flexneri* 2a lipopolysaccharide O antigen modal chain length reveals that it has been optimized for virulence. Microbiology 149: 925–939.
36. Murray GL, Attridge SR, Morona R (2003) Regulation of *Salmonella typhimurium* lipopolysaccharide O antigen chain length is required for virulence; identification of FepE as a second Wzz. Mol Microbiol 47: 1395–1406.
37. Allison GE, Verma NK (2000) Serotype-converting bacteriophages and O-antigen modification in *Shigella flexneri*. Trends Microbiol 8: 17–23.
38. West NP, Sansonetti P, Mounier J, Exley RM, Parsot C, et al. (2005) Optimization of virulence functions through glucosylation of *Shigella* LPS. Science 307: 1313–1317.
39. Jin Q, Yuan Z, Xu J, Wang Y, Shen Y et al (2002) Genome sequence of *Shigella flexneri* 2a: insights into pathogenicity through comparison with genomes of *Escherichia coli* K12 and O157. Nucleic Acid Res 30: 4432–4441.
40. Kaniuk NA, Vinogradov E, Li J, Monteiro MA, Whitfield C (2004) Chromosomal and plasmid-encoded enzymes are required for assembly of the R3-type core oligosaccharide in the lipopolysaccharide of *Escherichia coli* O157:H7. J Biol Chem 279: 31237–31250.
41. Bishop RE, Gibbons HS, Guina T, Trent MS, Miller SI, et al. (2000) Transfer of palmitate from phospholipids to lipid A in outer membranes of gram-negative bacteria. EMBO J 19: 5071–5080.
42. Raetz CR, Reynolds CM, Trent MS, Bishop RE (2007) Lipid A modification systems in gram-negative bacteria. Annu Rev Biochem 76: 295–329.
43. Chen H, Gartner E, Rolfe BG (1993) Involvement of Genes on a Megaplasmid in the Acid-Tolerant Phenotype of *Rhizobium leguminosarum* Biovar Trifolii. Appl Environ Microbiol 59: 1058–1064.
44. Thomsen LE, Chadfield MS, Bispham J, Wallis TS, Olsen JE (2003) Reduced amounts of LPS affect both stress tolerance and virulence of *Salmonella enterica* serovar Dublin. FEMS Microbiol Lett 228: 225–231.
45. Barua S, Yamashino T, Hasegawa T, Yokoyama K, Torii K et al (2002) Involvement of surface polysaccharides in the organic acid resistance of Shiga Toxin-producing *Escherichia coli* O157:H7. Mol Microbiol. 43: 629–640.
46. Sinnott ML (2007) Carbohydrate Chemistry and Biochemistry: Structure and Mechanism. The Royal Society of Chemistry, Cambridge UK. 705 p.
47. Huang YJ, Tsai TY, Pan TM (2007) Physiological response and protein expression under acid stress of *Escherichia coli* O157:H7 TWC01 isolated from Taiwan. J Agric Food Chem 55(17): 7182–91.
48. Merrell DS, Goodrich ML, Otto G, Tompkins LS, Falkow S (2003) pH-regulated gene expression of the gastric pathogen *Helicobacter pylori*. Infect Immun 71: 3529–3539.
49. Merrell DS, Bailey C, Kaper JB, Camilli A (2001) The ToxR-mediated organic acid tolerance response of *Vibrio cholerae* requires OmpU. J Bacteriol 183: 2746–2754.
50. Sato M, Machida K, Arikado E, Saito H, Kakegawa T, et al. (2000) Expression of outer membrane proteins in *Escherichia coli* growing at acid pH. Appl Environ Microbiol 66: 943–947.
51. Sandlin RC, Goldberg MB, Maurelli AT (1996) Effect of O side-chain length and composition on the virulence of *Shigella flexneri* 2a. Mol Microbiol 22: 63–73.
52. Van den Bosch L, Manning PA, Morona R (1997) Regulation of O-antigen chain length is required for *Shigella flexneri* virulence. Mol Microbiol 23: 765–775.
53. Carter JA, Jiménez JC, Zaldívar M, Alvarez SA, Marolda CL, et al. (2009) The cellular level of O-antigen polymerase Wzy determines chain length regulation by WzzB and Wzz_{pHS-2} in *Shigella flexneri* 2a. Microbiology 155: 3260–3269.
54. Nikaido H (2003) Molecular basis of bacterial outer membrane permeability revisited. Microbiol Mol Biol Rev 67: 593–656.
55. Gunn JS, Ryan SS, Van Velkinburgh JC, Ernst RK, Miller SI (2000) Genetic and functional analysis of a PmrA-PmrB-regulated locus necessary for lipopolysaccharide modification, antimicrobial peptide resistance, and oral virulence of *Salmonella enterica* serovar Typhimurium. Infect Immun 68: 6139–6146.
56. Tamayo R, Choudhury B, Septer A, Merighi M, Carlson R, et al. (2005) Identification of *cptA*, a PmrA-regulated locus required for phosphoethanolamine modification of the *Salmonella enterica* serovar typhimurium lipopolysaccharide core. J Bacteriol 187: 3391–3399.
57. Perez JC, Groisman EA (2007) Acid pH activation of the PmrA/PmrB two-component regulatory system of *Salmonella enterica*. Mol Microbiol 63: 283–293.
58. Herrera CM, Hankins JV, Trent MS (2010) Activation of PmrA inhibits LpxT-dependent phosphorylation of lipid A promoting resistance to antimicrobial peptides. Mol Microbiol 76: 1444–1460.
59. Touzé T, Tran AX, Hankins JV, Mengin-Lecreulx D, Trent MS (2008) Periplasmic phosphorylation of lipid A is linked to the synthesis of undecaprenyl phosphate. Mol Microbiol 67: 264–277.
60. Datsenko KA, Wanner BL (2000) One-step inactivation of chromosomal genes in *Escherichia coli* K-12 using PCR products. Proc Natl Acad Sci U S A 97: 6640–6645.
61. Cherepanov PP, Wackernagel W (1995) Gene disruption in *Escherichia coli*: Tc^R and Km^R cassettes with the option of Flp-catalyzed excision of the antibiotic-resistance determinant. Gene 158: 9–14.
62. Hitchcock PJ, Brown TM (1983) Morphological heterogeneity among *Salmonella* lipopolysaccharide chemotypes in silver-stained polyacrylamide gels. J Bacteriol 154: 269–277.
63. Lesse AJ, Campagnari AA, Bittner WE, Apicella MA (1990) Increased resolution of lipopolysaccharides and lipooligosaccharides utilizing tricine-sodium dodecyl sulfate-polyacrylamide gel electrophoresis. J Immunol Methods 126: 109–117.
64. Tsai CM, Frasch CE (1982) A sensitive silver stain for detecting lipopolysaccharides in polyacrylamide gels. Anal Biochem 119: 115–119.
65. Zhou Z, Lin S, Cotter RJ, Raetz CR (1999) Lipid A modifications characteristic of *Salmonella typhimurium* are induced by NH4VO3 in *Escherichia coli* K12. Detection of 4-amino-4-deoxy-L-arabinose, phosphoethanolamine and palmitate. J Biol Chem 274: 18503–18514.
66. Carter JA, Blondel CJ, Zaldívar M, Álvarez SA, Marolda CL, et al. (2007) O-antigen modal chain length in *Shigella flexneri* 2a is growth-regulated through RfaH-mediated transcriptional control of the *wzy* gene. Microbiology 153: 3499–3507.
67. Bravo D, Silva C, Carter JA, Hoare A, Álvarez SA, et al. (2008) Growth-phase regulation of lipopolysaccharide O-antigen chain length influences serum resistance in serovars of *Salmonella*. J Med Microbiol 57: 938–946.
68. Daniels C, Morona R (1999) Analysis of *Shigella flexneri wzz* (Rol) function by mutagenesis and cross-linking: *wzz* is able to oligomerize. Mol Microbiol 34: 181–194.

Concurrent Outbreak of Norovirus Genotype I and Enterotoxigenic *Escherichia coli* on a U.S. Navy Ship following a Visit to Lima, Peru

Victor E. Gonzaga[1], Mariana Ramos[1], Ryan C. Maves[1], Randal Freeman[2], Joel M. Montgomery[1]*

1 United States Naval Medical Research Unit Six (NAMRU-6), Lima, Peru, **2** United States Army, El Paso, Texas, United States of America

Abstract

An outbreak of norovirus (NoV) genotype I and Enterotoxigenic *Escherichia coli* (ETEC) occurred among US Navy Ship personnel following a visit to Lima, Peru, in June 2008. Visiting a specific area in Lima was significantly associated with illness. While ETEC and NoV are commonly recognized as causative agents of outbreaks, co-circulation of both pathogens has been rarely observed in shipboard outbreaks.

Editor: Patricia V. Aguilar, University of Texas Medical Branch, United States of America

Funding: This study was supported by grant AFHSC-GEIS, work unit number 847705 82000 25GB B0016. The views expressed in this article are those of the authors and do not necessarily reflect the official policy or position of the Department of the Navy, Department of Defense, nor the U.S. Government. The funders had no role in study design, data collection and analysis, decision to publish, or preparation of the manuscript.

Competing Interests: The authors have declared that no competing interests exist.

* E-mail: jmontgomery@ke.cdc.gov

Introduction

The discovery of novel gastrointestinal viruses has prompted the global health community to reevaluate their epidemiological perspective on the common causes of gastroenteritis. Norovirus (NoV) is responsible for approximately 50% of all food-borne gastroenteritis outbreaks in the United States [1]. Outbreaks related to NoV have usually been reported in closed settings [2,3]. Currently, there are five recognized NoV genogroups, of which three (I,II and IV) are known to cause illness in humans [4]. NoV infection often presents as acute-onset vomiting, watery non-bloody diarrhea with abdominal cramps and nausea. The incubation period ranges from 24–48 hours and is typically transmitted through direct person-to-person contact or through the oral fecal route [4]. For this reason NoV is frequently associated with large outbreaks within military populations and on military and civilian ships, reaching attack rates as high as 60% [2]. Several studies have attempted to estimate the prevalence of NoV and other viral infections among diarrheal cases in Latin America [5,6] but the knowledge is still limited and much more information is needed to fully understand the burden of illness. Co-circulation of NoV with enterotoxigenic *Escherichia coli* (ETEC) as cause of outbreaks has been poorly described on the literature [7]. On June 30th, 2008 an outbreak of a gastrointestinal illness occurred aboard a US Navy ship in the port of Lima. Several days prior to the outbreak, numerous personnel visited tourist destinations and restaurants throughout Lima. An investigation was conducted to identify the etiologic agent, to evaluate factors associated with the outbreak and to provide recommendations to the ship's commander on how to control the current and prevent future outbreaks.

Methods

The study protocol was approved by the U.S. Naval Medical Research Unit Six (NAMRU-6) Institutional Review Board in compliance with all applicable Federal regulations governing the protection of human subjects. NAMRU-6's IRB determined that this project did not meet the definition of human subject research and waived the need for consent; therefore we could proceed without further review by IRB. This study was based on a response to an outbreak of Norovirus in a ship and involved testing of human specimens previously obtained by the ship's medical staff.

An unmatched case-control study was conducted among crew members on June 30th, 2008. A case was defined as an individual within the crew with a history of vomiting and/or diarrhea from June 21st until July 10th, 2008. One control per case was randomly selected from the unaffected crew population. A self administered questionnaire was completed by both cases and controls. Socio-demographic, clinical and epidemiological variables were assessed, including history of contact with ill individuals, hand washing behaviors and exposure to a specific location known as "Pizza Alley", which was frequently reported by cases during preliminary descriptive studies. Stool and emesis samples were collected from eleven symptomatic patients and tested for evidence of bacterial, parasitic and NoV infection. Light microscopy was used for parasite identification, while conventional culture procedures were used for bacterial identification, followed by multiplex PCR to differentiate pathogenic strains of *E. coli* [8]. Real time RT-PCR was employed to detect NoV using primers and probes for the polymerase gene of both genotypes I and II (GI and GII), as previously described [9]. Initial RNA extracts were purified prior to direct sequencing on an ABI Prism 3130 sequencer (Applied

Biosystems) using cycle sequencing dye terminator chemistry (Perkin-Elmer, Foster City, CA). Sequences were compared against published sequences using NCBI's Basic Local Alignment Search Tool (BLAST; available at http://www.ncbi.nlm.nih.gov/blast/Blast.cgi). Odds ratios (OR) and 95% confidence intervals (CI) were calculated using bivariate and multivariate logistic regression analysis in STATA 11.0.

Results

One hundred and thirty individuals of the 230 total crewmembers were interviewed on July 1st, 2008 (response rate: 57%; 65 cases: 65 controls). NoV GI was identified in 1 emesis sample and 9/11 (82%) stool samples. Enterotoxigenic *E. coli* (ETEC) was also detected by PCR in 8/11 (73%) stool samples, although cultures for *E. coli* were negative. Of the 11 samples tested, 6 were positive to both ETEC and NoV. All symptomatic individuals had been treated with ciprofloxacin prior to sample collection. Viral sequence was 96% homologous to NoV GI. The clinical attack rate was 28.3%; mean age of individuals was 28.7 years; 85.3% were male. We observed no difference in mean age and gender between groups ($p = 0.6$ and $p = 0.07$, respectively). The peak of the outbreak occurred 7 days after the index case began with symptoms (Figure 1). Most frequent symptoms included diarrhea (93.9%), nausea (66.2%), abdominal cramps (65.3%) and vomiting (40%). Mean duration of symptoms was 2.7 ± 1.4 days. Several factors associated with illness were identified in the bivariate analysis (Table 1). We separately evaluated the consumption of particular food such as vegetables, fruits, raw fish or seafood; however, no association was observed. Only two variables remained significant in the multivariate analyses, after adjusting for contact with a case and self-reporting of hand washing after being in contact with a case. Factors associated with an increased risk of infection included, visiting a specific location ("Pizza Alley") in Lima (OR = 8.04, IC95% 1.22 to 52.73; $p = 0.03$). Consumption of only bottled water during the visit to Peru was shown to be highly protective against infection (OR = 0.01, IC95% 0.001 to 0.17; $p = 0.001$).

Discussion

This study describes a gastrointestinal outbreak which occurred on a US Navy ship in the port of Callao, Peru. Although NoV GI and ETEC were both identified as etiological agents in the early phase of the outbreak, it is likely that NoV was the source of the outbreak in the secondary wave based upon its mechanism of transmission. Retrospective investigations have identified NoV GI as the cause of outbreaks and single infections among populations of several South and Central American countries [3,5], including a recent extensive outbreak which occurred in Antofagasta, Chile [10]. This is the first description of an outbreak related to infection with NoV GI in Peru and, to our knowledge, the first outbreak of NoV reported on a US naval ship in South America. With the exception of one study conducted in Denmark, outbreaks linked to dual infections of NoV and ETEC have been limited and poorly described [7]. Although we were unable to collect control samples, which may have helped to better define the role of ETEC in this outbreak, our data suggests NoV was likely the primary cause of illness in the later cases due to its short incubation period and daily presentation of new cases several days after leaving port, suggesting person-to-person transmission. Unlike NoV, there is some evidence suggesting that ETEC is not readily transmitted via fomites [11], this may be due to a shorter half-life of the pathogen in the environment. However, ETEC and NoV have been shown to be co-associated in individuals with diarrhea and among cases in outbreaks [10,12]. The dual role of these pathogens in outbreaks and illness should be carefully evaluated in future investigations.

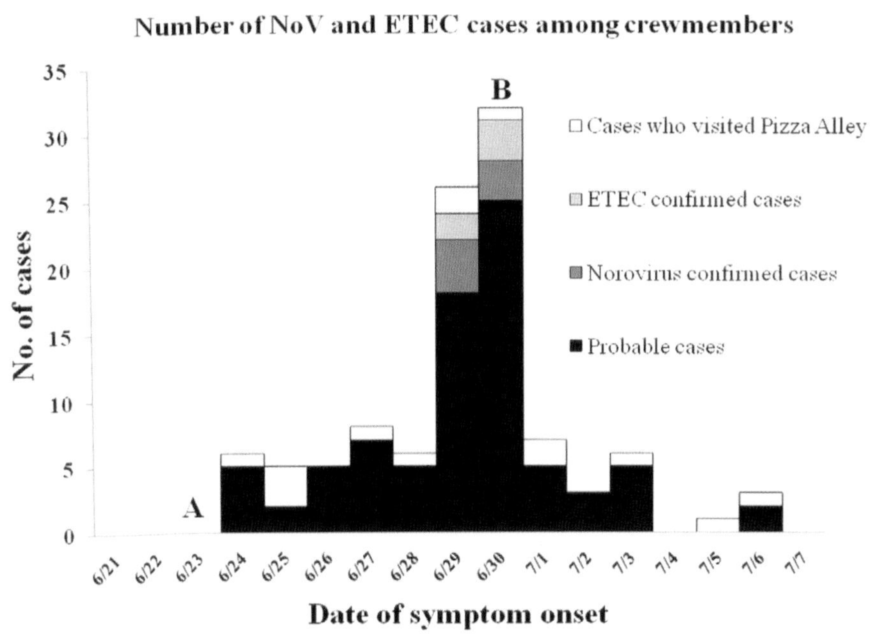

Figure 1. Number of cases of acute gastroenteritis among 230 members of the crew showing the evolution of the outbreak of NoV GI and ETEC in a US Navy ship. A. Crew members visited several locations during their visit to Lima, including "Pizza Alley" a location of many restaurants, bars and nightclubs. B. Control measures included: thorough cleaning of all ship surfaces with a 5% bleach solution, reinforcement of the importance of proper hand washing, provision of hand sanitizers (alcohol hand gel) in each room, recommendation to only consumed cooked foods (including vegetables) and requirement for any crewmember to report to the ships infirmary in the event they develop symptoms of gastroenteritis.

Table 1. Exposures and activities associated with acute gastroenteritis.

Exposure or activity	Case patients (n = 65)	Control patients (n = 65)	OR (95%CI)	P
Age (median; range)	28 (23–32)	30 (24–33)	-	0.49
Gender: male	59 (90.8%)	52 (80%)	0.39 (0.14 to 1.12)	0.08
Bivariate analysis				
Visiting a specific area in Lima¶	14/28 (50%)	5/48 (10.42%)	8.60 (2.62 to 28.15)	<0.001
Having contact with a case§	36 (56.25%)	14 (21.88%)	4.59 (2.12 to 9.93)	<0.001
Consumption of vegetables during their stay in Lima€	57 (87.69%)	50 (76.92%)	2.62 (1.01 to 6.80)	0.05
Participating in a humanitarian mission to Ventanilla*	5 (7.69%)	7 (10.77%)	0.69 (0.20 to 2.29)	0.54
Hand washing after using the ship's gym	52 (86.67%)	57 (90.48%)	0.68 (0.22 to 2.10)	0.5
Hand washing after having had contact with a case§	31 (48.44%)	43 (68.25%)	0.43 (0.21 to 0.89)	0.02
Hand washing after using the restroom	3 (4.69%)	7 (10.77%)	0.40 (0.10 to 1.65)	0.20
Consumption of bottled water during stay in Lima	5 (7.69%)	40 (62.50%)	0.05 (0.01 to 0.14)	<0.001
Multivariate analysis				
Visiting a specific area in Lima¶	-	-	8.04 (1.22 to 52.73)	0.03
Consumption of bottled water during stay in Lima	-	-	0.01 (0.001 to 0.17)	0.001

NOTE: OR, odds ratio; CI, 95% confidence intervals.

¶Numerous crewmembers (including the index cases(s)) visited several locations during their visit to Lima, including "Pizza Alley," a location of many restaurants, bars and nightclubs.

§i.e. Sharing a berthing facility, being in close proximity during daily activities, etc.

€Both cooked and uncooked vegetables.

*Ventanilla is a low income area of Lima near the Port of Callao, Peru. A group of crewmembers conducted housing construction and renovation during one day of their deployment to Lima, as part of a humanitarian assistance mission.

NoV infection is a frequent cause of diarrhea and vomiting among travelers to developing countries [13] and has been widely recognized as an important cause of outbreaks on US military and civilian ships [2,14]. Although outbreaks on US Navy ships are not typically associated with visits to high-risk ports for traveler's diarrhea [14], our findings demonstrate that NoV has the potential to be introduced into a ship following personnel visits to a foreign port during deployed missions. Precautions among the ship's personnel (i.e., health education on food safety and proper food and hand hygiene) should be reinforced prior to entering port cities. Precautions should also include avoiding the consumption of beverages prepared with unknown source water, including ice, during these visits. The protective role of consuming bottled water observed in our study may have been related to individuals who were less likely to engage in risky behaviors such as ingestion of uncooked foods or poor hand hygiene, both of which are known to be linked to and propagate food-borne outbreaks. Personnel should be encouraged to drink only bottled beverages, consume thoroughly washed or cooked foods and routinely wash their hands prior to eating.

In this outbreak, the primary infection (i.e., index case(s)) likely occurred during their visit to a specific area in Lima, with subsequent person-to-person and fomite transmission (i.e., hand rails, bunks, etc.). Although the initial disinfection of the ship probably removed the majority of the surface contamination, repeated contamination of these surfaces likely occurred, as 28% of the crewmembers were symptomatic and moving throughout the ship. Persistence of NoV is among the most significant contributing factors for shipboard outbreaks, as surfaces can remain contaminated for lengthy periods of time facilitating transmission of the infection to naïve individuals. Thus, various prevention measures should be considered to minimize dissemination of this virus during shipboard outbreaks. Such measures may include, a shipboard outbreak response program which could allow implementation of rapid and effective control measures during gastrointestinal outbreaks (i.e., proper disinfection guidelines), informational materials providing symptomatic individuals with guidance on personal hygiene and recommendations on temporary self-isolation/movement restriction, informational materials for asymptomatic individuals on how to prevent illness during an outbreak (i.e., hand hygiene, etc.) and installation of alcohol hand gel dispensers in key locations. Finally, surveillance and identification of gastrointestinal viruses, including NoV GI, during gastrointestinal outbreaks and among individuals suffering from gastrointestinal illness should be considered, to better define the epidemiology and burden of illness caused by these viruses and their interaction with other pathogens (e.g., ETEC) in developing countries, particularly in South America.

Acknowledgments

We thank the Norovirus working group at Universidad Peruana Cayetano Heredia, especially to Dr. Robert Gilman, Daniel Velasquez, Sonia Apaza and Susan Espetia for their laboratory support. We also want to thanks Maruja Bernal and Carmen Lucas for their support by testing samples for bacteria and parasites, respectively.

Author Contributions

Conceived and designed the experiments: VG MR JMM RM. Performed the experiments: VG MR JMM. Analyzed the data: MR JMM VG. Contributed reagents/materials/analysis tools: RM MR JMM VG. Wrote the paper: MR VG JMM RM RF.

References

1. Widdowson MA, Sulka A, Bulens SN, Beard RS, Chaves SS, et al. (2005) Norovirus and foodborne disease, United States, 1991–2000. Emerg Infect Dis 11: 95–102.
2. McCarthy M, Estes MK, Hyams KC (2000) Norwalk-like virus infection in military forces: epidemic potential, sporadic disease, and the future direction of prevention and control efforts. J Infect Dis 181 Suppl 2: S387–391.

3. Vidal R, Solari V, Mamani N, Jiang X, Vollaire J, et al. (2005) Caliciviruses and foodborne gastroenteritis, Chile. Emerg Infect Dis 11: 1134–1137.
4. CDC (2010) Norovirus: Technical Fact Sheet.
5. Castilho JG, Munford V, Resque HR, Fagundes-Neto U, Vinje J, et al. (2006) Genetic diversity of norovirus among children with gastroenteritis in Sao Paulo State, Brazil. J Clin Microbiol 44: 3947–3953.
6. Ferreira MS, Xavier MP, Fumian TM, Victoria M, Oliveira SA, et al. (2008) Acute gastroenteritis cases associated with noroviruses infection in the state of Rio de Janeiro. J Med Virol 80: 338–344.
7. Ethelberg S, Lisby M, Bottiger B, Schultz AC, Villif A, et al. (2010) Outbreaks of gastroenteritis linked to lettuce, Denmark, January 2010. Euro Surveill. pp 15.
8. Guion CE, Ochoa TJ, Walker CM, Barletta F, Cleary TG (2008) Detection of diarrheagenic Escherichia coli by use of melting-curve analysis and real-time multiplex PCR. J Clin Microbiol 46: 1752–1757.
9. Trujillo AA, McCaustland KA, Zheng DP, Hadley LA, Vaughn G, et al. (2006) Use of TaqMan real-time reverse transcription-PCR for rapid detection, quantification, and typing of norovirus. J Clin Microbiol 44: 1405–1412.
10. Galeno H Gastrointestinal disease outbreak in Antofagasta.
11. Levine MM, Rennels MB, Cisneros L, Hughes TP, Nalin DR, et al. (1980) Lack of person-to-person transmission of enterotoxigenic Escherichia coli despite close contact. Am J Epidemiol 111: 347–355.
12. Ko G, Garcia C, Jiang ZD, Okhuysen PC, Belkind-Gerson J, et al. (2005) Noroviruses as a cause of traveler's diarrhea among students from the United States visiting Mexico. J Clin Microbiol 43: 6126–6129.
13. Apelt N, Hartberger C, Campe H, Loscher T. The Prevalence of Norovirus in returning international travelers with diarrhea. BMC Infect Dis 2010 May 25 10: 131.
14. Thornton S, Davies D, Chapman F, Farkas T, Wilton N, et al. (2002) Detection of Norwalk-like virus infection aboard two U.S. Navy ships. Mil Med 167: 826–830.

22

In Vivo Comparison of Two Human Norovirus Surrogates for Testing Ethanol-Based Handrubs: The Mouse Chasing the Cat!

Syed A. Sattar*, Mohammad Ali, Jason A. Tetro

Center for Research on Environmental Microbiology (CREM), University of Ottawa, Ottawa, Ontario, Canada

Abstract

Human noroviruses (HuNoV), a major cause of acute gastroenteritis worldwide, cannot be readily cultured in the lab. Therefore, a feline calicivirus (FCV) is often used as its surrogate to, among other things, test alcohol-based handrubs (ABHR). The more recent laboratory culture of a mouse norovirus (MNV) provides an alternative. While MNV is closer to HuNoV in several respects, to date, no comparative testing of FCV and MNV survival and inactivation on human hands has been performed. This study was designed to address the knowledge gap. The rates of loss in viability during drying on hands were −1.91 and −1.65% per minute for FCV and MNV, respectively. When the contaminated skin was exposed for 20 s to either a commercial ABHR with 62% (v/v) ethanol or to 75% (v/v) ethanol in water, FCV infectivity was reduced by <1 $\log_{10}$ while that of MNV by nearly 2.8 $\log_{10}$. Extending the contact time to 30 s reduced the FCV titer by almost 2 $\log_{10}$ by both test substances and that of MNV by >3.5 $\log_{10}$ by the commercial ABHR while 75% ethanol did not show any noticeable improvement in activity as compared to the 20 s contact. An 80% (v/v) aqueous solution of ethanol gave only a 1.75 $\log_{10}$ reduction in MNV activity after 20 s. The results show significant differences in the ethanol susceptibility of FCV and MNV in contact times relevant to field use of ABHR and also that 62% ethanol was a more effective virucide than either 75% or 80% ethanol. These findings indicate the need for a review of the continuing use of FCV as a surrogate for HuNoV.

Editor: Herman Tse, The University of Hong Kong, Hong Kong

Funding: The authors have no support or funding to report.

Competing Interests: The authors have declared that no competing interests exist.

* E-mail: ssattar@uottawa.ca

Introduction

Human noroviruses (HuNoV) remain the most common cause of acute viral gastroenteritis (AVG) with 6 million clinical cases and 200,000 deaths/year worldwide [1]. Outbreaks of HuNoV are frequent in healthcare [2], community settings [3] and onboard cruise ships [4]; nosocomial outbreaks can close hospital wards [5]. The virus is shed in feces and in vomitus [6] and is relatively stable outside hosts [7,8].

Since laboratory culture of HuNoV is difficult, the feline calicivirus (FCV) is often used as its surrogate in testing, among other things, microbicides [9,10]. However, FCV may be unsuitable for this purpose due its higher acid sensitivity and also because it is normally a respiratory pathogen in felines [11].

The successful *in vitro* culture of a murine norovirus (MNV) now provides an alternative to FCV [12]; MNV is similar in acid resistance to HuNoV and also causes in mice a disease highly reminiscent of AVG in humans [12]. These factors, and a closer genetic kinship to HuNoV, could make MNV a better surrogate for testing microbicides, including alcohol-based handrubs (ABHR).

Comparative studies between MNV and FCV have been published; however, they have focused either on the environmental survival of the viruses [11,13] or compared the activity of chemicals against FCV and MNV in *in vitro* settings [14–16]. There has been no documented comparison of the activity of ethanol and ethanol-based ABHR against FCV and MNV using an *in vivo* test protocol. The information gained from such a comparison would allow for a better understanding of the choice of surrogate for HuNoV. This study was designed to fill the knowledge gap.

Materials and Methods

ABHR tested

The concentrations of ethanol used are given as volume/volume (v/v). The ABHR tested were one commercial gel with 62% ethanol as the only listed active, and aqueous ethanol solutions at 75% and 80%.

Subjects

This study was approved by the Ottawa Hospital Research Ethics Board (OHREB) under protocol #2000289-01H: The use of Fingerpads of Adult Volunteers to Investigate the Germicidal Activity of Handwash and Handrub Agents. Persons (20–60 years in age), were briefed on the project and those willing to participate gave signed consent. Each subject then received microbicide-free personal care items for use starting a one week before the first day of participation in the study. Six subjects were used in each comparative test.

Viruses

Strain F9 of FCV (ATCC #VR-782) was received from Dr. S. Bidawid (Health Canada, Ottawa, ON) and MNV Type 1 was a gift from Dr. H.W. Virgin (Washington Univ., St. Louis, MO).

Host cells

CrFK cells (ATCC CCL-94) and RAW 267.4 cells (ATCC #TIB-71) were also obtained from Dr. Bidawid and were used to grow and plaque assay FCV and MNV, respectively.

Preparation of virus pools

Monolayers of both types of cells were grown at 36±1°C in Eagle's minimal essential medium (MEM; Invitrogen, Burlington, ON, Canada) with 10% fetal bovine serum (FBS; Invitrogen Burlington, ON, Canada), 2% L-Glutamine (Invitrogen), and 2% of 7.5% sodium bicarbonate ($NaHCO_3.7H_2O$) in 75 cm^2 plastic flasks (Sarstedt, Saint-Leonard, QC, Canada).

Each monolayer separately received 200 µL of FCV or MNV and the flasks were held for one h at 36±1°C for virus adsorption. Ten mL of MEM supplemented with 2% FBS was added to each flask and reincubated at 36±1°C till nearly 80% of each monolayer showed virus-induced cytopathology. The flasks were then subjected to three freeze-thaw cycles for virus release, their contents centrifuged at 1,000×*g* for ten minutes and the supernatant was pooled and then aliquoted for storage at −80°C.

Soil load

All virus inocula contained a soil load to simulate the presence of feces or vomitus. A 340-µl volume of virus suspension was mixed with 35 µl 5% Tryptone (BD Difco; Mississauga, ON, Canada), 25 µl of 5% bovine serum albumin (BD Difco; Mississauga, ON, Canada), and 100 µl of 0.4% mucin (type 1) from bovine submaxillary glands (Sigma, St. Louis, MO), all in sterile normal saline in phosphate buffer (pH 7.2) with a total protein content roughly equal to that in 5% FBS [17]. The final concentration of the virus was approximately 10^7 plaque-forming units (PFU)/mL.

Plaque assays

The plaque assay methods for FCV and MNV were as described previously by Wobus et al. [18] and Bidawid et al [12], respectively. Briefly, host cell monolayers were prepared in 12-well cluster plates (Corning; Fisher, Ottawa, ON, Canada) in 2 mL of growth medium (supplemented MEM with 10% FBS) in each well and incubated at 36±1°C in a 5% CO_2 atmosphere for 16–18 h. The medium was aspirated and 0.1 mL of the virus sample diluted in Earle's Balanced Salt Solution (EBSS; Invitrogen) was placed separately in each of at least three wells. Each plate also included two wells as negative controls (0.1 mL EBSS only) and one well as positive control (0.1 mL of undiluted virus). The inoculated plates were incubated one h for virus adsorption. Each well then received 2 mL of an agar overlay and reincubated for plaque formation for 18 and 36 hours for FCV and MNV, respectively. The monolayers were then fixed and stained for PFU as described [18].

Inoculating fingerpads

The subject's hands were first inspected to ensure freedom from any apparent damage. The subject then removed all ornaments from the hands and forearms and washed the hands with a non-medicated soap, rinsed them with running tap water (~40°C) and dried them with a paper towel. Five mL of 70% ethanol was put into the subject's cupped hands for rubbing over both hands till dry. The pad of each digit was pressed against the mouth of an empty 2.0 mL cryovial (Sarstedt, St. Leonard, QC, Canada) for a circular indentation to place the inoculum at its centre. The subject then sat with the hands inside a laminar-flow hood to receive the virus. A virus inoculum of 10 µl was placed on each fingerpad using a positive-displacement pipette.

The air temperature and relatively humidity in the lab during the experiments ranged between 22–26°C and 45–55%, respectively.

Virus elution

The digit to be eluted was placed over the mouth of a cryovial containing 1 mL of the eluent consisting of EBSS supplemented with 0.1% Tween-80 (Sigma-Aldrich, Oakville, ON, Canada), which neutralized the test solution through dilution and disaggregated viral clumps to provide a more realistic assessment of inactivation. The vial was inverted with the digit still in place and the eluent brought into contact with the contaminated area for 10 seconds followed by 20 full inversions. The 10-second contact and the inversion steps were performed once more. The vial was then turned upright and the surface of the skin was firmly scraped against the inside rim of the vial in a downward motion. Each fingerpad was inspected to ensure that the skin was free of any visible liquid. The skin of each pad was decontaminated by pressing it against a paper towel soaked in domestic bleach (1,000 ppm available chlorine) for 3 minutes. The subject then washed both hands with plain soap and dried them thoroughly before leaving the lab.

Testing virus survival

Both thumbpads received 10 µL of the test virus in soil load and the inocula eluted immediately representing the 'zero-time' control or the number of PFU placed on each digit. Each fingerpad then received 10 µL of the virus and observed for drying. The inocula were eluted from two randomly-selected fingerpads (one left and one right) simultaneously after 20, 30 and 40 min.

Virucidal activity of test formulations and controls

This procedure was based on the standard #E-1838-10 of ASTM International [17]. Briefly, both thumbpads received 10 µL of the test virus and the inoculum was eluted immediately and simultaneously from both (see below) and the thumbpads decontaminated; this represented the 'zero-time' control or the number of PFU placed on each digit. Each fingerpad then received 10 µL of virus and the subject kept the hands still in a laminar flow hood with the blower on till the inocula were visibly dry. Two randomly-selected fingerpads were eluted at this stage for the 'baseline value' or the PFU that survived the drying.

To test for virucidal activity, at least two randomly-selected fingerpads (one from each hand) were exposed simultaneously to 1.0 mL of the test substance or control fluid in a 2-mL cryovial by placing each fingerpad separately over the mouth of a vial and inverting to bring the fluid into contact with the skin for the required contact time. The fingerpad was then eluted as described above but the liquid remaining on the skin was not scraped off. The virus inoculation, drying, exposure and elution steps were repeated for the remaining fingers. The fingerpads were decontaminated with diluted bleach and washed as mentioned above.

Data Analysis

For virus survival, regression analysis was performed to determine a rate of decay for each virus. Rates of decay were compared between viruses using a one-way Analysis of Co-Variance (ANCOVA). For virus inactivation experiments, six replicates were performed for each inactivation test and statistically analyzed using the Analysis of Variance (ANOVA) test with post-hoc Tukey Honestly Significant Difference (HSD) analysis.

Results

Virus survival on hands

Survival of the viruses on the fingerpads was normalized to a percentage survival to demonstrate the comparative decay in the viability of the viruses. Three samples for each time point and each virus were analyzed to ensure proper regression and ANCOVA analysis could be performed. As shown in Figure 1, virus survival was negatively associated with time. FCV viability was reduced at a rate of 1.91 percent per minute ($r^2 = 0.82$). MNV reduction was 1.65 percent per minute ($r^2 = 0.64$). Using the one-way ANCOVA test, the two rates of decay were not found to be significantly different ($F = 0.61$; $p = 0.44$).

Inactivation of FCV and MNV by ethanol-based ABHR and Ethanol

Six subjects for each concentration and contact time were used to allow for proper statistical analyses. Fig. 2A and 2B show the reduction in the viability of both viruses after 20 s and 30 s of contact, respectively. At 20 s, both levels of ethanol produced a<1 $\log_{10}$ reduction in FCV infectivity, while the reductions in MNV infectivity was almost 3 $\log_{10}$. Increasing the contact time to 30 s enhanced the reduction in FCV infectivity to about 2 $\log_{10}$ irrespective of the ethanol concentration. Whereas there appeared to be no significant difference between the activities of 62% and 75% ethanol against MNV at 20 s (Figure 2A), a difference was noted between the activities of the two ethanol concentrations with a contact time of 30 s (Figure 2B). However, the results of ANOVA and Tukey analyses were inconclusive due to variations in the data.

We thus compared the activities of three concentrations of ethanol against MNV at a contact time of 20 seconds. The results (Fig. 3) showed 62% ethanol was better than 75% ethanol ($p<0.01$ ANOVA; $p<0.01$ Tukey HSD) and that both concentrations showed better activity than the 80% solution ($p<0.01$ ANOVA; $p<0.01$ Tukey HSD).

Discussion

This is the first report on comparative testing of the survival on skin and ethanol resistance of the two leading surrogates for HuNoV under conditions that closely mimic actual field use.

Our findings suggest that, the ability of the two viruses to survive on the hands of adults over the normal drying time [19]) was not significantly different. However, the time-associated reduction did demonstrate the necessity to perform reduction calculations using the baseline value (i.e. dried virus) as the starting point rather than the zero time.

The commercial product chosen claimed only one active ingredient, ethanol, with no other antimicrobial activity from the excipients. Other commercial products with higher concentrations of alcohol were found to be a mixture of ethanol and isopropanol, which was outside the scope of this study. Moreover, several formulations contained other excipients such as organic acids, which could bias the study and thus were not included. The choice of an aqueous ethanol solution was to ensure that only ethanol was the active to be tested. It should be noted here that non-alcohol-based formulations usually also are aqueous with only one active ingredient. However, the actives are often a quaternary-ammonium compounds (quats), which are weak in their activity against non-enveloped viruses in particular.

There have been several studies focusing on the resistance of FCV or MNV to various alcohol solutions [10,20,21]. However, there has been little consistency between the methods, the test materials, the viral challenge and the contact time. This has unfortunately led to confusion with respect to the use of ABHR and a plethora of comments and claims of activity that may not be entirely accurate for field use. The *in vivo* method used in this study is a standard of ASTM International [17] and it is recommended by the World Health Organization [22] for testing ABHR against human pathogenic viruses. It has been used previously for studies focusing on the *in vivo* evaluation of virucidal activity of antiseptics [19,23–25]. The test gives data comparable to that with the whole-hand method [19,24], while permitting a more thorough inspection of the hands of the

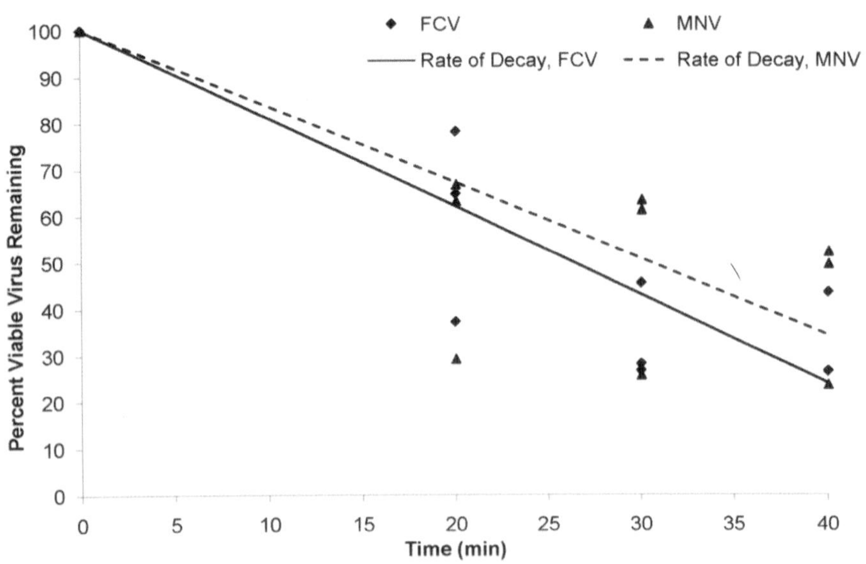

Figure 1. Survival of FCV (◆) and MNV (■) on human skin. Ten µL of virus in soil load was placed on the fingerpads of volunteers and allowed to dry. After 20, 30 or 40 minutes, the virus was eluted off the fingerpads and enumerated using plaque assays. Lines of decay were calculated using regression analysis and determined to be 1.91 percent per minute for FCV ($r^2 = 0.82$) and 1.65 percent per minute for MNV ($r^2 = 0.64$). Analysis of Co-Variance (ANCOVA) testing of the two regression lines demonstrated no significant difference between the two viruses ($F = 0.61$; $p = 0.44$).

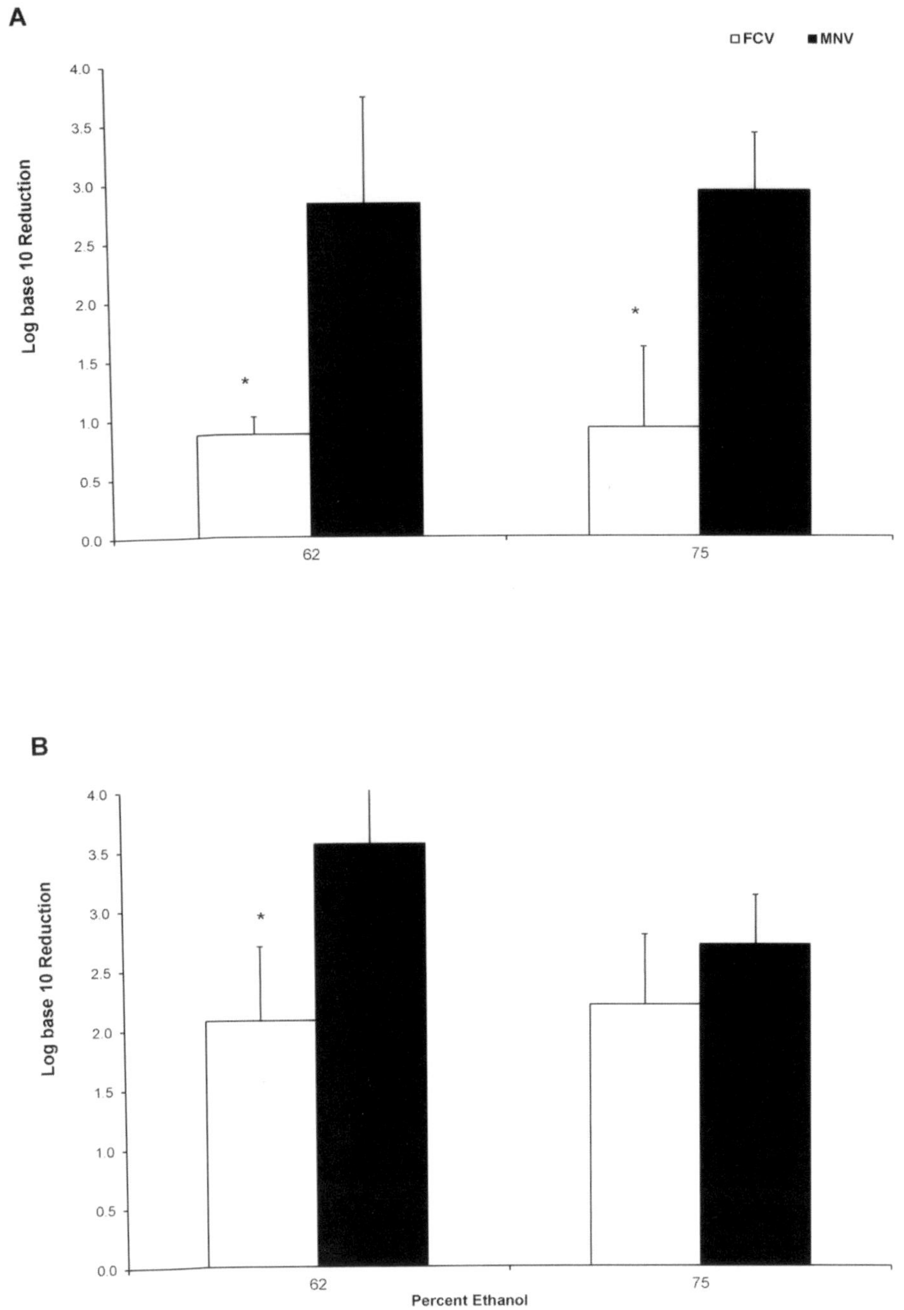

Figure 2. Reduction in the viability of FCV and MNV after contact with ethanol. Virus reduction was observed after 20 s (A) or 30 s (B) contact time with a commercial ABHR (62% ethanol) and an aqueous solution of 75% (v/v) ethanol on the fingerpads of adult subjects (n = 6). Significant difference between FCV and MNV ($p<0.01$) indicated by asterisks.

subjects for any damage, thus making their experimental contamination virtually risk-free. Further, much smaller volumes of virus pools are required for the fingerpad method while allowing for replicates and controls being tested on the same subject in any given sitting. Perhaps the most useful aspect of this test is the ability to control the contact time precisely. In this study, contact times were at their lowest 20 seconds, which is perhaps the shortest time tested yet may be the most accurately representative of field use [20].

Since ABHR are no-rinse formulations, they are expected to inactivate pathogens *in situ* to achieve hand antisepsis. In view of this, the test substance remaining on the fingerpads at the end of the contact time was not scraped off but allowed to remain there for subsequent elution to better represent field use.

Even though ABHR are meant for use on hands free of visible contamination, a certain level of soiling of hands is inevitable during casual contact with the environment. The soil load added to the virus inocula was to represent this low level of organic and inorganic contamination on the skin, the potential protection it could afford to handborne pathogens and the ability of the tested formulations to achieve virus inactivation in its presence.

The observed differences between the susceptibilities of the two viruses to ABHR in general may be due to the structural properties

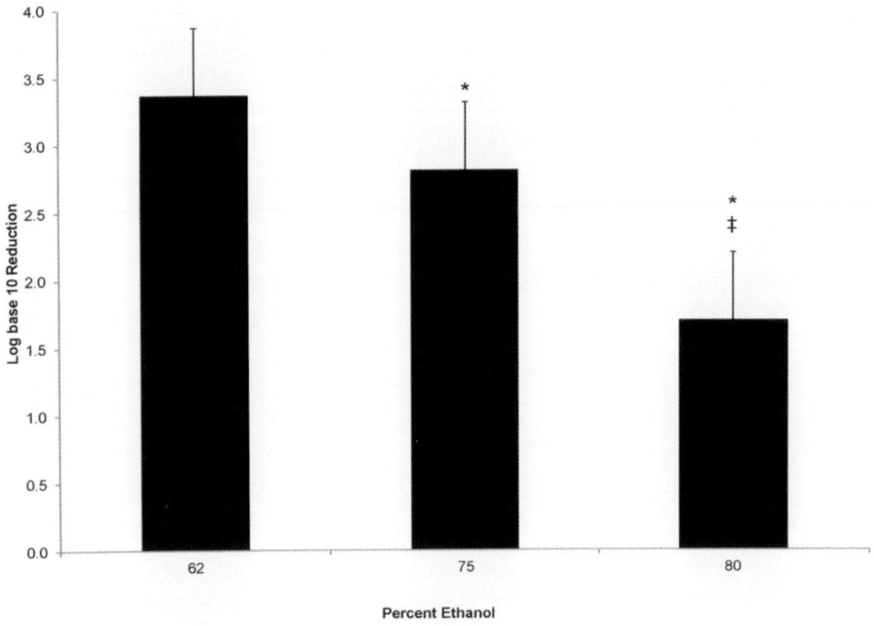

Figure 3. Reduction of MNV after 20 second contact with ethanol. MNV reduction was observed after 20 s contact time with one of either a commercial ABHR (62% ethanol), 75% ethanol or 80% aqueous ethanol solution on the fingerpads of adult subjects (n = 6). Significant differences were observed between both 62% and 75% ($p<0.01$) and 80% ($p<0.01$) indicated by asterisks (*). A significant difference was also seen between 75% and 80% ($p<0.01$) indicated by the double dagger (‡).

of the viral capsid. Ethanol is well known for its ability to destabilize water and hydrophilic amino acids [26]. The cell receptor binding motif of FCV consists of a hypervariable region with mainly hydrophobic, neutral residues [27]. The effect of ethanol concentration, therefore, would be minimal on the active site yet, over time, general capsid instability would occur, leading to inactivation. The findings of this study correlate well with those of Kampf *et al.* who showed no significant difference in FCV virucidal activity with varying concentrations of ethanol between 75 and 95% [9]. In contrast to FCV, the cell receptor binding motif of MNV consists of numerous hydrophilic residues, which would be affected by concentrations of ethanol ≥45%. In this study, the 62% ABHR reduced the MNV titre by nearly 2.5 $\log_{10}$ (99.7%) in as little as 15 seconds and by 20 seconds, the titre was reduced by over 3.0 $\log_{10}$ (>99.9%).

Of particular note is the lowering of virucidal activity with the increase in ethanol concentration (Fig. 2 & 3). Parke and Birch [28] investigated various concentrations of ethanol and found that optimal destabilization of water molecules (and thus hydrophilic amino acid residues) did not positively correlate with higher ethanol concentrations but peaked at or near 62% ethanol and lessened exponentially as the concentration increased. Thus, the effect of 75% or 80% ethanol would be significantly less than that of 62% ethanol at shorter periods of time. The data presented here follows with that of Gehrke et al [21] who demonstrated a similar difference of efficacy between 62% and higher concentrations of ethanol (as well as 1- and 2-propanol) with longer contact times of 0.5 and 1.0 minutes.

One limitation of this study was that the 62%-ethanol-based test substance was a commercial ABHR while the 75% and 80% solutions were non-commercial. However, as discussed above, the presented data focused on ethanol alone as the active ingredient and thus should not be extrapolated to other formulations that contain isopropanol, organic acids or other residual antimicrobial agents. That being stated, the dramatic difference in efficacy as it relates to contact time (Fig. 3) should not be overlooked.

The comparative data presented here using a standardized *in vivo* test protocol shows that MNV, a virus much closer to HuNoV in several respects, is more readily inactivated by ABHR in relatively short contact times. This suggests the need for a wider acceptance of MNV as a surrogate for HuNoV and eventual phase-out of FCV for the purpose. Health Canada's recent guidance document on human-use antiseptic drugs now recommends the use of MNV as a surrogate for HuNoV to generate data for product registration [29]. Any further discussion of the topic of surrogates in this regard should wait till one is able to routinely culture and assay the infectivity of HuNoV *in vitro*. Such a change may also help reverse the impression in the minds of many infection preventionists that ABHR are ineffective in dealing with HuNoV outbreaks, based on the available data using FCV as its surrogate.

This comparative *in vivo* study showed that at shorter contact times, MNV is less resistant to ethanol-based ABHR than FCV. Extending the contact time reduced the difference between the two viruses with 75% ethanol but not with 62% ethanol. These differences may be a result of the various physicochemical characteristics of FCV and MNV but that ethanol concentration and contact time do play a significant role in the performance of an ethanol-based ABHR.

Author Contributions

Conceived and designed the experiments: SAS JAT. Performed the experiments: MA. Analyzed the data: JAT SAS.

References

1. Patel MM, Widdowson MA, Glass RI, Akazawa K, Vinje J, et al. (2008) Systematic literature review of role of noroviruses in sporadic gastroenteritis. Emerging Infectious Diseases 14: 1224–1231.
2. Koopmans M (2009) Noroviruses in healthcare settings: a challenging problem. Journal of Hospital Infection 73: 331–337. DOI 10.1016/j.jhin.2009.06.028.
3. Gould D (2009) Management of Norovirus gastroenteritis in the community. Br J Community Nurs 14: 117, 119–117, 121.
4. Vivancos R, Keenan A, Sopwith W, Quigley C, Mutton K, et al. (2010) Management of an international outbreak of norovirus on board a cruise ship. International Journal of Infectious Diseases 14: E135. DOI 10.1016/j.ijid.2010.02.1783.
5. Hansen S, Stamm-Balderjahn S, Zuschneid I, Behnke M, Rüden H, et al. (2007) Closure of medical departments during nosocomial outbreaks: data from a systematic analysis of the literature. Journal of Hospital Infection 65: 348–353.
6. Kimura H (2010) A norovirus outbreak associated with environmental contamination at a hotel. Epidemiol Infect. pp 1–9. S0950268810000981 [pii];10.1017/S0950268810000981 [doi].
7. Lamhoujeb S, Fliss I, Ngazoa SE, Jean J (2008) Evaluation of the persistence of infectious human noroviruses on food surfaces by using real-time nucleic acid sequence-based amplification. Applied and Environmental Microbiology 74: 3349–3355.
8. D'Souza DH, Sair A, Williams K, Papafragkou E, Jean J, et al. (2006) Persistence of caliciviruses on environmental surfaces and their transfer to food. International Journal of Food Microbiology 108: 84–91.
9. Kampf G, Grotheer D, Steinmann J (2005) Efficacy of three ethanol-based hand rubs against feline calicivirus, a surrogate virus for norovirus. Journal of Hospital Infection 60: 144–149.
10. Whitehead K, McCue KA (2010) Virucidal efficacy of disinfectant actives against feline calicivirus, a surrogate forÂ norovirus, in a short contact time. American Journal of Infection Control 38: 26–30.
11. Cannon JL, Papafragkou E, Park GW, Osborne J, Jaykus LA, et al. (2006) Surrogates for the study of norovirus stability and inactivation in the environment: A comparison of murine norovirus and feline calicivirus. Journal of Food Protection 69: 2761–2765.
12. Wobus CE, Karst SM, Thackray LB, Chang KO, Sosnovtsev SV, et al. (2004) Replication of Norovirus in cell culture reveals a tropism for dendritic cells and macrophages. PLoS Biology 2.
13. Bae J, Schwab KJ (2008) Evaluation of murine norovirus, feline calicivirus, poliovirus, and MS2 as surrogates for human norovirus in a model of viral persistence in surface water and groundwater. Applied and Environmental Microbiology 74: 477–484. DOI 10.1128/AEM.02095-06.
14. D'Souza DH, Su XW (2010) Efficacy of Chemical Treatments Against Murine Norovirus, Feline Calicivirus, and MS2 Bacteriophage. Foodborne Pathogens and Disease 7: 319–326. DOI 10.1089/fpd.2009.0426.
15. Beekes M, Lemmer K, Thomzig A, Joncic M, Tintelnot K, et al. (2010) Fast, broad-range disinfection of bacteria, fungi, viruses and prions. Journal of General Virology 91: 580–589. DOI 10.1099/vir.0.016337-0.
16. Su XW, Howell AB, D'Souza DH (2010) The effect of cranberry juice and cranberry proanthocyanidins on the infectivity of human enteric viral surrogates. Food Microbiology 27: 535–540. DOI 10.1016/j.fm.2010.01.001.
17. ASTM International (2010) ASTM E1838 - 10 Standard Test Method for Determining the Virus-Eliminating Effectiveness of Hygienic Handwash and Handrub Agents Using the Fingerpads of Adults.
18. Bidawid S, Malik N, Adegbunrin O, Sattar SA, Farber JM (2003) A feline kidney cell line-based plaque assay for feline calicivirus, a surrogate for Norwalk virus. Journal of Virological Methods 107: 163–167. PII S0166-0934(02)00214-8.
19. Sattar SA, Ansari SA (2002) The fingerpad protocol to assess hygienic hand antiseptics against viruses. Journal of Virological Methods 103: 171–181.
20. Cheeseman KE, Denyer SP, Hosein IK, Williams GJ, Maillard JY (2009) Evaluation of the bactericidal efficacy of three different alcohol hand rubs against 57 clinical isolates of S-aureus. Journal of Hospital Infection 72: 319–325. DOI 10.1016/j.jhin.2009.04.018.
21. Gehrke C, Steinmann J, Goroncy-Bermes P (2004) Inactivation of feline calicivirus, a surrogate of norovirus (formerly Norwalk-like viruses), by different types of alcohol in vitro and in vivo. Journal of Hospital Infection 56: 49–55. DOI 10.1016/j.jhin.2003.08.019.
22. World Health Organization (2010) WHO Guidelines on Hand Hygiene in Health Care. Available: http://whqlibdoc.who.int/publications/2009/9789241597906_eng.pdf. Accessed 2011 Jan 26.
23. Sattar SA, Abebe M, Bueti AJ, Jampani H, Newman J, et al. (2000) Activity of an alcohol-based hand gel against human adeno-, rhino-, and rotaviruses using the fingerpad method. Infection Control and Hospital Epidemiology 21: 516–519.
24. Steinmann J, Nehrkorn R, Meyer A, Becker K (1995) Two in-vivo protocols for testing virucidal efficacy of handwashing and hand disinfection. Zentralblatt fur Hygiene und Umweltmedizin = International journal of hygiene and environmental medicine 196: 425–436.
25. Bidawid S, Malik N, Adegbunrin O, Sattar SA, Farber JM (2004) Norovirus cross-contamination during food handling and interruption of virus transfer by hand antisepsis: Experiments with feline calicivirus as a surrogate. Journal of Food Protection 67: 103–109.
26. Herskovits TT, Gadegbeku B, Jaillet H (1970) On the structural stability and solvent denaturation of proteins. I. Denaturation by the alcohols and glycols. Journal of Biological Chemistry 245: 2588–2598.
27. Geissler K, Schneider K, Truyen U (2002) Mapping neutralizing and non-neutralizing epitopes on the capsid protein of feline calicivirus. Journal of veterinary medicine B, Infectious diseases and veterinary public health 49.
28. Parke SA, Birch GG (1999) Solution properties of ethanol in water. Food Chemistry 67: 241–246.
29. Health Canada (2009) Guidance Document - Human-Use Antiseptic Drugs. Available: http://www.hc-sc.gc.ca/dhp-mps/prodpharma/applic-demande/guide-ld/antiseptic_guide_ld-eng.php. Accessed 2011 Jan 26.

Epidemiology of Pathogenic Enterobacteria in Humans, Livestock, and Peridomestic Rodents in Rural Madagascar

DeAnna C. Bublitz[1,2¤], Patricia C. Wright[1,3], Jonathan R. Bodager[4], Fidisoa T. Rasambainarivo[1], James B. Bliska[1,2], Thomas R. Gillespie[1,4,5]*

1 Centre ValBio, Ranomafana, Madagascar, **2** Department of Molecular Genetics and Microbiology, Center for Infectious Diseases, Stony Brook University, Stony Brook, New York, United States of America, **3** Department of Anthropology, Stony Brook University, Stony Brook, New York, United States of America, **4** Department of Environmental Health, Rollins School of Public Health, Emory University, Atlanta, Georgia, United States of America, **5** Department of Environmental Sciences and Program in Population Biology, Ecology, and Evolution, Emory University, Atlanta, Georgia, United States of America

Abstract

Background: Among the families of enteric bacteria are globally important diarrheal agents. Despite their potential for zoonotic and environmental transmission, few studies have examined the epidemiology of these pathogens in rural systems characterized by extensive overlap among humans, domesticated and peridomestic animals. We investigated patterns of infection with Enterotoxigenic *Escherichia coli*, *Shigella* spp., *Salmonella enterica*, *Vibrio cholerae*, and *Yersinia* spp. (*enterocolitica*, and *pseudotuberculosis*) in Southeastern Madagascar where the potential for the aforementioned interactions is high. In this pilot project we conducted surveys to examine behaviors potentially associated with risk of infection and if infection with specific enterobacteria species was associated with diarrheal disease.

Methodology/Principal Findings: PCR was conducted on DNA from human, livestock, and rodent fecal samples from three villages. Overall, human prevalence was highest (77%), followed by rodents (51%) and livestock (18%). Rodents were ~2.8 times more likely than livestock to carry one of the bacteria. The incidence of individual species varied between villages, with the observation that, *E. coli* and *Shigella* spp. were consistently associated with co-infections. As an aggregate, there was a significant risk of infection linked to a water source in one village. Individually, different pathogens were associated with certain behaviors, including: those who had used medication, experienced diarrhea in the past four weeks, or do not use toilets.

Conclusions/Significance: Different bacteria were associated with an elevated risk of infection for various human activities or characteristics. Certain bacteria may also predispose people to co-infections. These data suggest that a high potential for transmission among these groups, either directly or via contaminated water sources. As these bacteria were most prevalent in humans, it is possible that they are maintained in humans and that transmission to other species is infrequent. Further studies are needed to understand bacterial persistence, transmission dynamics, and associated consequences in this and similar systems.

Editor: Ulrike Gertrud Munderloh, University of Minnesota, United States of America

Funding: This study was supported by the Jim and Robin Herrnstein Foundation, Stony Brook University, and the Emory University Global Health Institute. Research reported in this publication that was performed by DeAnna Bublitz was supported by the National Institute of Allergy and Infectious Diseases of the National Institutes of Health under Award Number T32AI007539 (awarded to James Bliska). The content is solely the responsibility of the authors and does not necessarily represent the official views of the National Institutes of Health. The funders had no role in study design, data collection and analysis, decision to publish, or preparation of the manuscript.

Competing Interests: The authors have declared that no competing interests exist.

* Email: thomas.gillespie@emory.edu

¤ Current address: Host-Parasite Interactions Section, Laboratory of Intracellular Parasites, Rocky Mountain Laboratories, National Institute of Allergy and Infectious Diseases, Hamilton, Montana, United States of America

Introduction

Enteric diseases are a leading cause of illness and death in the developing world. Gastric infections and diarrhea are estimated to account for 2.2 million global mortalities annually. Diarrheal pathogens present an exceptional threat to children under 5, for whom nearly 15% of all deaths can be attributed to diarrhea, making it the second leading cause of death for infants worldwide [1,2]. Additionally, disease caused by these infections results in years of life lost due to malnutrition and stunted growth, both physical and cognitive [2]. These infections are especially prevalent in the developing world, particularly Africa, where infection-related diarrhea accounts for as much as 8.5% of all fatalities [3]. A recent 3-year study evaluating over 9000 children with moderate to severe diarrhea in Africa and Asia found that Enterotoxigenic *E. coli* and *Shigella* were two of the four most common causes of infection. *V. cholerae* was also identified as a significant cause of diarrhea in certain sites [4].

The source of these pathogens can be varied, though the interplay among humans, companion and food animals, and peridomestic animals is increasingly being recognized as a key interface for disease transmission [5–7]. As human populations grow they are increasingly pressed into higher density living. The same is true for the agriculture and livestock needed to support these communities. Moreover, in poorer communities there is a greater incidence of peridomestic rodents living in and around homes and food sources [8,9]. Residing in closer quarters creates a greater chance for the transmission of infectious diseases between humans, livestock, and rodents [5]. Numerous epidemics and pandemics have been linked to the cycle of transmission from livestock and humans including avian flu, Nipah virus, and swine flu [10–12]. Rodents present a similar risk as they can be the source of a wide range of diseases including tularemia, *Cryptosporidium* spp., *Campylobacter jejuni*, and hantavirus [7]. Furthermore, rodents are host to parasites such as ticks and fleas that can perpetuate the cycle of other pathogens like Lyme disease and plague [13,14]. Despite the high potential for zoonotic transmission, these interactions among humans, livestock, and peridomestic animals are still relatively understudied.

Madagascar is a nation of ~22 million people. While efforts have been made to improve living conditions for the people of Madagascar, only ~50% of the population is using improved water sources and less than 20% have access to improved sanitation facilities [15]. Diarrheal diseases cause approximately 37% of all infection and parasite-related deaths each year in this country [16]. A recent study investigating diarrheal disease in Madagascar found that nearly 50% of children under 5 tested positive for pathogenic intestinal microorganisms and roughly 10% of this age group died from diarrhea-related illness [15,17].

Much of the Malagasy population is rural and relies on livestock and rice farming for subsistence. Anthropogenic disturbance associated with agricultural practices and timber harvesting has led to nearly 90% of Madagascar's forest being lost [18,19]. Habitat loss and fragmentation can be devastating to biodiversity and endemic species but creates ideal spaces for invasive and generalist species such as introduced rodents [20–23]. Disruption of the natural environment coupled with high-density living presents an increased chance for contact with rodents and thus, the potential for disease transmission to both humans and livestock. Hantavirus, which can be transmitted as an aerosol from rodent urine, becomes more prevalent with habitat disturbance [7,21,22]. In regions where sanitation infrastructure is lacking, these interactions are all the more likely, exacerbating one's risk of infection with a zoonotic or waterborne pathogen [1,24]. In addition, zoonotic *Yersinia pestis*, the causative agent of plague, is endemic to Madagascar. It is estimated that 40% of the population is exposed to *Y. pestis*, which can be carried by rats and transmitted via aerosol or flea bites, resulting in severe and often fatal illness [25,26]. However, as this is not typically an enteric pathogen it is not covered in this study.

This pilot project was undertaken to look at the prevalence of five pathogenic enterobacteria: Enterotoxigenic *Escherichia coli* (ETEC), *Shigella* spp. (*flexneri* and *dysenteriae*), *Salmonella enterica*, *Vibrio cholerae*, and *Yersinia* spp. (*enterocolitica*, and *pseudotuberculosis*) in humans, livestock, and rodents. These groups were sampled from three villages near Ranomafana National Park: Ambatolahy (Amb), Ambodiaviavy (Avy), and Ankialo (Ank), in Southeastern Madagascar. The work herein estimates prevalence levels for these five bacteria in the above mentioned sample groups and looks at the relative risk association to various activities to identify potential sources or patterns of transmission. As humans interact with, and alter, their environment it becomes increasingly important to understand the risks in regards to pathogen transmission to and from all potential hosts and their environment. Our results highlight a little studied facet of disease ecology in Madagascar and suggest a relationship between humans, livestock, and rodents in propagating zoonotic and waterborne pathogens.

Methods

Ethics Statement

All protocols, including obtaining oral consent from participants, were reviewed and approved by the Ministry of Health of the government of Madagascar, the Stony Brook University Internal Review Board and Institutional Animal Care and Use Committee. As approved by the Stony Brook Internal Review Board, oral informed consent of participants was obtained prior to specimen collection and survey. In the case of minors, a parent or guardian provided informed consent. Given the low literacy rate of the population being studied, we opted for oral consent administered and recorded on the survey sheets by the native interpreter conducting the interview. All participants were anonymously given unique identifiers. Permits were not required for sample collection from the animals in this study. All cows and pigs sampled were handled according to the guidelines of the National Veterinary Services Laboratories (Publication N231597), USDA, Fort Collins, Colorado. Rodents were handled following protocols outlined by the CDC [27]. No endangered species were involved in this study.

Study Site

The study took place in and around Ranomafana National Park, Madagascar, (located 47°18′ 40 to 47°37′E and 21°2′ to 21°25′S) a 43,500 hectare World Heritage Site well known for its high levels of species endemism and diversity [28,29]. Three communities located on the edge of the park were selected as the focus of this study: Ambodiaviavy (Avy, population = 363), Ankialo (Ank, population = 361), and Ambatolahy (Amb, population = 256). The communities are located in different areas of the park and have distinct cultural practices. The study population included several peridomestic rodents (*Rattus rattus*, *Mus musculus*), bovine (*Bos indicus*), porcine (*Sus domesticus*), and humans.

Sample collection and surveys

In June and July 2011, household and individual surveys were administered in the three communities: Avy (n = 65, total households = 10), Ank (n = 70, total households = 10), and Amb (n = 47, households = 10). A cluster sampling method was used: in each village, ten households were selected and every person inhabiting a selected household was surveyed. Participants were chosen independent of age, sex, or symptoms, but some were selected based on livestock ownership. Surveys were comprehensive with inquiries of demographic information, health status, hygiene, medication usage, water usage, and exposure to livestock and wildlife (70 questions for individual survey and 40 variables for the household survey). Potential behaviors associated with risk for diarrheal disease and infection with enterobacteria were queried in both surveys. Trained local field assistants administered all surveys in the local language (Malagasy) in order to reduce survey bias. Data were recorded on paper forms, answers were converted from "Yes/Always," "Sometimes," or "No/Never," to a 2, 1, or 0, respectively. These numbers were entered into Microsoft Excel spreadsheets with the associated behavior, and reviewed for accuracy. Fisher's exact test using Prism 6 (Graphpad, La Jolla,

CA) was used to analyze associations and calculate confidence intervals (CI) and relative risk (RR) between survey responses and infection status.

All survey participants were asked to provide a fecal specimen for examination of diarrheal pathogens and 89% complied. Concurrently, domesticated animals of participants (bovine and porcine) were sampled and baited rodent live-traps were set inside participant homes overnight. The following morning, fecal specimens were collected from trapped peridomestic rodents. All of the traps were washed thoroughly with 10% bleach solution between uses. Human volunteers were instructed to wash their hands prior to collecting fecal samples in sealable plastic bags that were collected the same or the next day. Given that we did not have access to a clinic and were limited in time at each village, we cannot assure 100% sterile transfer of the samples from the participants into the bags. Fresh fecal matter from livestock was collected from the rectum using a non-sterile latex glove, or from the ground if defecation was observed. For the latter, only fecal material that had not directly been in contact with the ground was collected. All samples were moved to a field laboratory as soon as possible (Amb and Avy) or processed on site (Ank). Approximately one milliliter of feces from each sample was homogenized with an equal volume of RNAlater nucleic acid stabilizing buffer (Ambion, Life Technologies, Grand Island, NY) and stored at −20°C at CentreValBio until transport to the United States.

Molecular methods

Total nucleic acid was extracted from fecal specimens (n = 278) preserved in RNAlater using the FastDNA SPIN Kit for Soil (MP Biomedicals, LLC, Solon, OH), following the manufacturer-recommended procedures. Using PCR, we screened the samples for ETEC, *S. enterica*, *Shigella* spp. (*flexneri* and *dysenteriae*), *V. cholerae*, and *Yersinia* spp. We chose to amplify the gene *yadA* in *Yersinia* as it is similar in *enterocolitica*, and *pseduotuberculosis* species and could be used to screen for both simultaneously [30]. The *yadA* primers should generate a product of 849 bp with *Y. enterocolitica* serogroup 03/09 strains, a product of 759 bp ith *Y. enterocolitica* serogroup 08 strains, and 681 bp product with *Y. pseudotuberculosis* (including the positive control strain used). Likewise, the *invA* gene in *S. enterica* was used for its conserved nature across serovars [31]. A portion of the ipaH gene was amplified to detect *Shigella flexneri* and *dysenteriae*. For positive controls in the PCR reactions, *V. cholerae*, ETEC, and *S. flexneri* strains were obtained from American Type Culture Collection (ATCC, Manassas, VA). The 32777 strain in the Bliska Laboratory collection was used as a positive control for *Y. pseudotuberculosis*. The *S. enterica* serovar 14028 positive control strain was obtained from the laboratory of Dr. Adrianus van der Velden (Both: Stony Brook University, Stony Brook, NY). All positive control strains are listed in Table 1. Genomic DNA was isolated from each of the strains using a DNeasy kit (Qiagen, Valencia, CA) according to the manufacturer's protocol. All primers are listed in Table 1 and detect previously described genes for each bacterial species [26,31,32]. The primers were synthesized by Eurofilms MWG Operon (Stony Brook University, Stony Brook, NY). PCR was conducted on 2.0 µl of DNA sample using 0.5 µmol of each primer (Table 1) in 25 µl of Platinum PCR mix (Invitrogen, Life Technologies, Grand Island, NY). As a negative control, the same PCR reaction was run using water to confirm that there was no contamination of the reagents. Additionally, all of the primers were tested on all of the positive control strains to test for cross-reactivity and none was found. The amplification setting was as previously described; sensitivity of detection for each pathogen is listed in Table 1 [32].

Results

For this pilot study a cluster sampling method was used: in each village, ten households were selected and every person inhabiting a selected household was surveyed. Participants were chosen independent of age, sex, or symptoms. Participating households were selected at random except that preference was given to households owning livestock. Overall, 304 fecal samples were tested (humans = 163, cattle = 58, pigs = 18, and rodents = 65). Of the species sampled, humans had the highest overall prevalence of infection (77%, CI = 0.70–0.83), followed by rodents (51%, CI = 0.38–0.63), then livestock (18%, CI = 0.10–0.29) (Table 2). When looking at the prevalence of each pathogen individually, there was variability among villages. Among humans, *Shigella* spp. was the predominant pathogen detected in Amb (64%, CI = 0.48–0.77), while ETEC was the dominant bacterium found in human samples from Avy and Ank (69%, CI = 0.55–0.80 and 57%, CI = 0.43–0.70, respectively) (Table 3).

In regards to livestock, ETEC and *S. enterica* were the only enterobacteria detected in samples from Amb and Avy, while *Shigella* spp., *V. cholerae*, as well as the previous two, were found in samples from Ank (Table 3). These pathogens were more prevalent in pigs than cattle (67%, CI = 0.41–0.87 and 3%,

Table 1. Bacterial strains (positive controls), target genes, and primers* used in this study.

Genus and Species (ATCC #)	Target Gene	PCR primers (5′-3′)	Product Size	Sensitivity (cells)
Enterotoxigenic *E. coli* serotype O78:H11 (35401)	Enterotoxin (LT) gene	f - GAGACCGGTATTACAGAAATC r - GAGGTGCATGATGAATCCAG	117 bp	40
Shigella flexneri serotype 2b (12022)	*ipah*	f - CTTGACCGCCTTTCCGATAC r - CAGCCACCCTCTGAGAGTA	610 bp	5×10^4
Salmonella enterica serovar Typhimurium (14028)	*invA*	f - TATCGCCACGTTCGGGCAA r - TCGCACCGTCAAAGGAACC	275 bp	40
Vibrio cholerae (14035)	*ctxA*	f - GGCAGATTCTAGACCTCCT r - TCGATGATCTTGGAGCATTC	563 bp	40
Yersinia pseudotuburculosis serogroup O1 (32777)	*yadA*	f - CTTCAGATACTGGTGTCGCTGT r - ATGCCTGACTAGAGCGATATCC	681 bp (849[a], 751[b])	Unknown

*All primer sequences and sensitivities obtained from Wang et al. (1997) except *Yersinia* obtained from Thoerner et al. (2003).
[a]Product size with *Y. enterocolitica* serogroup 03 or 09 strains.
[b]Product size with *Y. enterocolitica* serogroup 08 strains.

Table 2. Prevalence of Enterobacteriaceae infection by subject and location.

Host	Location							
	Ambatolahy		Ambodiaviavy		Ankialo		All Villages	
	+/Total	Prevalence	+/Total	Prevalence	+/Total	Prevalence	+/Total	Prevalence
Human	43/47	0.91	42/58	0.72	41/58	0.71	126/163	0.77
Cattle	0/14	0.00	2/17	0.12	0/27	0	2/58	0.03
Pig	4/4	1.00	1/1	1.00	7/13	0.54	12/18	0.67
Rodent	12/33	0.36	10/14	0.71	11/18	0.61	33/65	0.51

CI = 0.004–0.12, respectively). Overall, few livestock tested positive for any of the target pathogens (Amb = 14%, Avy = 11%, Ank = 15%).

Except for *Yersinia*, all target species were detected in rodent samples, though *V. cholerae* was only found in rodent samples from Avy (Table 3). The occurrence of infection in rodents was 36% (CI = 0.20–0.55) in Amb, 71% (CI = 0.42–0.92) in Avy, and 61% (CI = 0.36–0.83) in Ank (Table 2). However, it should be noted that fewer rodents were sampled in either Avy or Ank versus Amb (n = 14, 18, and 33, respectively).

As depicted in Table 2, prevalence of enterobacteria infection was markedly higher for residents of Amb. This was linked to an increased risk association of having one or more of the pathogens for the residents of Amb vs. the residents of Avy or Ank (RR = 1.279, p = 0.0066) (Table 4). However, when broken down by pathogen, there was a reduced risk of *V. cholerae* and ETEC infection in Amb (*V. cholerae* RR = 0.0840, p = 0.0003; *E. coli* RR = 0.6762, p = 0.0229). Conversely, there was a higher risk of infection with these two pathogens in Avy (*V. cholerae* RR = 3.26, p = 0.0003; ETEC RR = 1.366, p = 0.0313). There was an elevated chance of *Shigella* spp.infection in Amb (RR = 1.575, p = 0.0092) compared to the other two villages, with a dramatically reduced risk in Ank (RR = 0.438, $p<0.0001$). Lastly, there was a higher prevalence of *Yersinia* spp. in humans from Amb versus Avy or Ank (RR = 2.241, p = 0.0344)(Table 4). All but one sample yielded a product of 681 bp in size indicating that *Y. pseudotuberculosis* is likely the species present. The one outlier was 759 bp suggesting infection with *Y. enterocolitica*.

Given that 77% of humans tested were found to be carrying at least one of these pathogens, we wanted to examine the prevalence of co-infections in this population. In Amb, none of the bacteria were significantly linked to one another while samples from Avy and Ank both showed patterns of co-infection (Table 5). In Avy, 86% of ETEC and 97% of *Shigella* spp. positive samples were also positive for one of the other bacteria tested, of which ETEC co-infection with *Shigella* spp was the most common (Prevalence = 75%, $p<0.0001$) (Table 5). While in Ank, *S. enterica* and *Shigella* spp. were both equally associated with co-infection with 100% of those infected with either pathogen testing positive for at least one other enterobacteria (p = 0.0029) and 60% of those were co-infections of *Shigella* spp. and *S. enterica* (p = 0.0011) (Table 5). *Shigella* spp. was also significantly linked to infection with *Yersinia* spp. in Ank (p = 0.0338). Overall, co-infections involving ETEC or *Shigella* spp. were most common at a prevalence of 74% and 91% respectively, across all three villages. ETEC co-infections with *Shigella*/EIEC was the most common with 55% of total ETEC infections co-occurring with *Shigella* spp. (p = 0.0276) (Table 5).

Broadly, none of the potential risk factors that we analyzed, including age, sex, working in fields, washing hands or boiling water, were significantly associated with an increased risk of infection in humans (Table 4). While there was no overall risk tied to fetching water from an open vs. a closed source in the three villages combined (RR = 0.8503, p = 0.1387), there was a substantial increase in risk of infection linked to collecting water from a closed source in Avy (RR = 2.174, p = 0.0041). Additionally, infection with ETEC was significantly linked to fetching water from a closed source (RR = 1.977, p = 0.0087). However, other activities, such as having experienced diarrhea within the four weeks prior to the survey, or tending livestock were not connected to an amplified risk of infection when all pathogens are considered as an aggregate (Table 4).

Certain factors and activities were associated with an elevated risk of infection when the pathogens are evaluated individually. There was an increased risk of *Shigella* spp. for individuals 15 years

Table 3. Incidence of each Enterobacteriaceae species in humans, livestock, and rodents by village.

Pathogen	Ambatolahy					
	Human		Livestock*		Rodent	
	+/Total	Prevalence	+/Total	Prevalence	+/Total	Prevalence
E. coli	20/47	0.43	4/29	0.14	10/33	0.30
Shigella spp.	30/47	0.64	0/29	0.00	4/33	0.12
S. enterica	15/47	0.32	0/29	0.00	6/33	0.18
V. cholerae	1/47	0.02	0/29	0.00	0/33	0.00
Yersinia spp.	13/47	0.28	0/29	0.00	0/33	0.00
	Ambodiaviavy					
	Human		Livestock*		Rodent	
	+/Total	Prevalence	+/Total	Prevalence	+/Total	Prevalence
E. coli	40/58	0.69	2/18	0.11	8/14	0.57
Shigella spp.	32/58	0.55	0/18	0.00	5/14	0.36
S. enterica	9/58	0.16	2/18	0.11	6/14	0.43
V. cholerae	10/58	0.17	0/18	0.00	2/14	0.14
Yersinia spp.	8/58	0.14	0/18	0.00	0/14	0.00
	Ankialo					
	Human		Livestock*		Rodent	
	+/Total	Prevalence	+/Total	Prevalence	+/Total	Prevalence
E. coli	33/58	0.57	6/40	0.15	8/18	0.44
Shigella spp.	15/58	0.26	6/40	0.15	10/18	0.56
S. enterica	15/58	0.26	6/40	0.15	5/18	0.28
V. cholerae	10/58	0.17	1/40	0.03	0/18	0.00
Yersinia spp.	6/58	0.10	0/40	0.00	0/18	0.00

*Cattle and pigs.

of age or under in Amb (RR = 1.655, p = 0.0355) while this group carried a greater risk of infection by ETEC in Avy (RR = 1.450, p = 0.0487) (Table 6). In Avy there was also a modest association between infection with ETEC and individuals who did not boil their water (RR = 1.447, p = 0.0487) as well as those who had used medication (RR = 1.826, p = 0.0348) or experienced diarrhea (RR = 1.513, p = 0.0438) in the past four weeks. Of those who had used medication, over 76% had used antibiotics (anti-bacterial, -protozoal, and – helmintic), 78% had used anti-inflammatories, and 52% had used both. There was a 3.8 and 4.5 times greater risk of infection with *V. cholerae* in Amb and Ank, respectively, for individuals who reported never using a toilet (Amb p = 0.022; Ank p = 0.0318). Lastly, when all three villages were combined, males were 2.14 times more likely to be infected with *S. enterica* (p-0.016). Additionally, people who never used a toilet carried a greater risk of infection with *Yersinia* spp. (RR = 3.575, p = 0.0013). Importantly, having suffered from diarrhea in the past four weeks was significantly associated with infection with *V. cholerae* (RR = 2.622, p = 0.0156) (Table 6).

Rodents tested had a greater risk of carrying one of these bacteria compared to livestock. With roughly equal numbers of samples, the RR of a rodent testing positive for one of the infectious agents was 2.756 times greater than that of the livestock tested (RR = .3628, p<0.0001). There was also a modest positive association between rodents in Amb and carrying at least one of the five pathogens as compared to rodents in Avy or Ank (RR = 0.5541, p = 0.0259). Additionally, there was no associated risk for humans having touched rodents by their tail (RR = 1.083, p = 0.4369) (Table 4). All of the significant findings have been summarized in Table 7.

Discussion

This study evaluated the prevalence of five pathogenic bacteria in humans, livestock, and rodents from three villages in Madagascar. Of the three sample groups, humans carried the highest prevalence (77%) followed by rodents (51%), and livestock (18%). The incidence of each pathogen varied from village to village with people from Amb carrying the greatest RR of infection (Table 4). Additionally, the distribution of the bacteria was different in livestock versus rodents with rodents testing positive for more of the pathogens and having a greater overall RR than livestock in all three villages (Table 4).

For many parts of the world, such as Madagascar, enteric pathogens are a major source of illness and death [1,2,15,17]. The impact of humans on their environment and the implications of those alterations on disease transmission are becoming more and more clear. Madagascar is an island with incredible species diversity across all taxa, of which a majority are endemic [33,34]. This country has also seen drastic changes to the original environment for agriculture and resource extraction, leading to fragmenting or clearing nearly 90% of the original forestland

Table 4. Risk factors for infection with Enterobacteriaceae in people living in villages in Southeast Madagascar.

			95% CI		
Variable	**n***	**RR**	**lower**	**upper**	**p**
Age (≤15)	162	1.079	0.898	1.297	0.486
Sex (male vs. female)	162	1.036	0.875	1.227	0.7103
Amb vs. Ank or Avy	**163**	**1.279**	**1.107**	**1.477**	**0.0066**
Avy vs. Amb or Ank	163	0.9052	0.7519	1.09	0.3292
Ank vs. Amb or Avy	163	0.8732	0.7221	1.056	0.1715
Amb vs. Ank or Avy *V. cholerae*	**163**	**0.0841**	**0.0118**	**0.5988**	**0.0003**
Amb vs. Ank or Avy *E. coli*	**163**	**0.6762**	**0.4716**	**0.9696**	**0.0229**
Amb vs. Ank or Avy *Shigella* spp.	**163**	**1.575**	**1.158**	**2.144**	**0.0092**
Amb vs. Ank or Avy *Yersinia* spp.	**163**	**2.241**	**1.144**	**4.389**	**0.0344**
Avy vs. Amb or Ank *V. cholerae*	**163**	**3.26**	**1.682**	**6.321**	**0.0003**
Avy vs. Amb or Ank *E. coli*	**163**	**1.366**	**1.057**	**1.766**	**0.0313**
Ank vs. Amb or Avy *Shigella* spp.	**163**	**0.438**	**0.2754**	**0.6966**	**<0.0001**
Collects water from an open source (vs. closed well or pump)	119	0.8503	0.6876	1.052	0.1387
Avy only - collects water from open source	**38**	**2.174**	**1.146**	**4.122**	**0.0041**
Boils water	163	0.9678	0.8197	1.143	0.7126
Washes hands prior to eating	163	0.9385	0.7664	1.149	0.8016
Uses a toilet	163	1.119	0.9441	1.327	0.449
Works in agricultural fields	153	0.9744	0.7503	1.266	1
Tends livestock	144	0.9198	0.7601	1.113	0.4386
Contact with rodents	151	1.083	0.911	1.288	0.4369
Experienced diarrhea (vs. no diarrhea) in past 4 Weeks	159	1.114	0.9155	1.357	0.4453
Experienced diarrhea with blood (vs. no blood) in past 4 weeks	25	0.7719	0.3409	1.748	0.4217
Used medicine (traditional or commercial) in past 4 Weeks	163	1.064	0.8684	1.303	0.5279
Rodents vs. livestock	**rodent-65 livestock-76**	**2.756**	**1.622**	**4.684**	**<0.0001**

*Total n varies due to incomplete notation on some surveys or respondents do not participate in the given activity (e.g. tend livestock).
Bold = statistically significant associations.

[18,19,34]. Overall, zoonotic pathogens account for nearly 61% of the organisms infectious to humans and 75% of emerging pathogens in the last decade [35]. While populations of humans, livestock, and rodents have been living together for thousands of years, these alterations to the landscape and ecology of Madagascar are an opportunity for new interactions between these populations, and potentially the transmission of zoonoses or waterborne pathogens.

This pilot study focused on the villages of Ambatolahy, Ambodiaviavy, and Ankialo near Ranomafana National Park in Southeastern Madagascar. Our results demonstrated that humans accounted for the greatest number of positive samples as compared to livestock or rodents (Table 2). Of the five pathogens tested, ETEC was the most prevalent in humans and livestock. When broken down by village, ETEC was also the dominant pathogen detected in human samples from Avy and Ank, while *Shigella* spp. was the predominant bacterium found in Amb (Table 3). It should be noted that Enteroinvasive *E. coli* (EIEC) strains can also have and express the toxin encoded by the ipaH gene. Having used the ipaH gene to screen for *Shigella* spp. it is also possible that the bacteria detected were EIEC. However, the disease caused by EIEC is nearly identical to Shigellosis and still presents an equal threat to the health of these communities [36]. This would be an important avenue to follow up on with sequencing of the samples to establish which species are present in these populations.

Globally, information about multiple enterobacteria infections is lacking, as such, this study also examined the prevalence of co-infections in humans. ETEC and *Shigella* spp. were predominantly associated with co-infections with 74% of ETEC and 91% of *Shigella* spp. infected samples testing positive for at least one other enterobacteria species (Table 5). These same pathogens were also the most prevalent individually in Amb and Avy while in Ank, *S. enterica* and *Shigella* spp. were present in equal amounts and both linked to co-infection in that village (Table 3, 5). Given that the numbers were identical for *S. enterica* and *Shigella* spp.in Ank, it was impossible to tease apart which might be the predisposing factor.

The percent of people infected with multiple pathogens was higher than reported rates from similar studies in Brazil and India [37–39]; however, the populations these previous studies sampled tended to be urban and in very different geographical locations than Madagascar. Co-infections in children under five in Madagascar were assessed in a recent report; however, they only documented co-infections between bacteria and parasites or viruses [17]. Given the paucity of data on rates of co-infection with multiple enterobacteria, it is difficult to say whether our data are within the expected range, and certainly this is an area needing further investigation. Furthermore, follow up work should be done to determine if the different co-infection profile of Ank is tied to its

Table 5. Prevalence of Enterobacteriaceae co-infections in humans from villages in Southeastern Madagascar.

	Ambodiaviavy			
	E. coli		*Shigella* **spp.**	
	Prevalence	**p**	**Prevalence**	**p**
Shigella **spp.**	0.75	<0.0001	N/A	N/A
S. enterica	0.23	0.0454	0.25	0.0333
V. cholerae	0.48	0.0022	0.56	<0.0001
Yersinia **spp.**	0.20	0.0484	0.25	0.0063
All enterics	0.86	<0.0001	0.97	<0.0001
	Ankialo			
	Shigella **spp.**		*S. enterica*	
	Prevalence	**p**	**Prevalence**	**p**
Shigella **spp.**	N/A	N/A	0.60	0.0011
S. enterica	0.60	0.0011	N/A	N/A
Yersinia **spp.**	0.27	0.0338	N/A	N/A
All enterics	1.00	0.0029	1.00	0.0029
	All Villages			
	E. coli		*Shigella* **spp.**	
	Prevalence	**p**	**Prevalence**	**p**
Shigella **spp.**	0.55	0.0276	N/A	N/A
S. enterica	0.30	0.0413	0.38	0.0001
V. cholerae	0.26	0.0148	0.31	0.0002
Yersinia **spp.**	N/A	N/A	0.25	0.0109
All enterics	0.74	0.0010	0.91	<0.0001

more remote location or other variations in behavior or activities from that of the people in Avy or Amb.

We attempted to identify potential risk factors amongst humans for infection with enteric pathogens. People in Amb were significantly more likely to be infected than people in Avy or Ank (Table 4). Water contamination is a notable source of these pathogens [1,40]. Given the high proportion of open water sources used by the subjects of this study, it was unexpected that there was no significant correlation between fetching water from a closed vs. an open source and their infection status (Table 4). Surprisingly, in the village of Avy, there was a substantial risk associated with people who fetched water from a closed source as opposed to the open sources and ETEC was implicated as the responsible agent (Table 4, 5). These data suggest that one or more of the pumps may be contaminated. It would be insightful to test the pump water directly and determine which families use which pump to see if there is a pattern of bacterial contamination and infection. This finding highlights the importance of these types of studies as follow-up analysis can be focused on areas of interest, such as these pumps.

In addition to the contaminated water source, there was a greater RR for infection with ETEC for people in Avy who reported not boiling their water (Table 5). Interestingly, people that reported always boiling their water before consumption were not at a reduced risk for infection by these bacteria (Table 4). There are several possible explanations. For one, there could be survey bias in that people felt pressure to report that they always boil water when in fact, they do not. This is a risk when having surveys administered in person rather than with complete anonymity. However, given the lower level of literacy and the need for explanation of certain questions, we felt the best way to conduct the surveys was with a native interpreter. Alternatively, coupled with the data from the open versus closed sources of water, this may not be a significant cause of disease transmission overall.

Other factors linked to infection were being under the age of 15 or male. People in Avy who had used medication, either traditional or commercial, in the past four weeks carried a greater risk of infection by ETEC. This finding could be due to several factors. There were a high number of people using either antibiotics (anti-bacterial, -protozoal, and- helmintic) or anti-inflammatories, often times both. It is possible that anti-inflammatory use may hinder the immune response making people susceptible to infection. Moreover, antibiotic misuse may mean a diagnosed infection was not cleared completely. These data could also be indicative of the more worrying trend of antibiotic-resistant bacteria which is well documented in developing nations, due in part to misuse of antibiotics [41,42]. Further studies are warranted to sequence the strains and whether genes associated with antibiotic resistance are present in these bacteria. Individuals who reported never using toilets had a greater RR of carrying either *V. cholerae* or *Yersinia* spp. Hygiene and sanitation are critical indicators of health [1,3,40]. Developing countries tend to have limited sanitation facilities and also have higher rates of infection with various enteric pathogens [40]. While Madagascar has made significant improvements in this area there is still work

Table 6. Risk factors for infection with individual Enterobacteriaceae species in people living in villages in Southeast Madagascar.

Ambatolahy						
				95% CI		
Variable	**Pathogen**	**n***	**RR**	**lower**	**upper**	**p**
Age (≤15)	*Shigella* spp.	47	1.655	1.031	2.658	0.0355
Does not use a toilet	*Yersinia* spp.	47	3.818	1.019	14.30	0.022
Ambodiaviavy						
				95% CI		
Variable	**Pathogen**	**n***	**RR**	**lower**	**upper**	**p**
Age (≤15)	*E. coli*	58	1.45	1.014	2.073	0.0487
Collects water from an closed source (pump, well)	*E. coli*	58	1.977	1.044	3.744	0.0087
Used medicine (traditional or commercial) in past 4 Weeks	*E. coli*	58	1.826	0.9169	3.637	0.0348
Does not boil water	*E. coli*	57	1.447	1.027	2.04	0.0478
Experienced diarrhea (vs. no diarrhea) in past 4 Weeks	*E. coli*	58	1.513	1.148	1.994	0.0438
Ankialo						
				95% CI		
Variable	**Pathogen**	**n***	**RR**	**lower**	**upper**	**p**
Does not use a toilet	*V. cholerae*	58	4.543	1.680	12.28	0.0318
All Villages						
				95% CI		
Variable	**Pathogen**	**n***	**RR**	**lower**	**upper**	**p**
Sex (male vs. female)	*S. enterica*	162	2.14	1.145	4.000	0.016
Uses a toilet	*Yersinia* spp.	163	3.575	1.868	6.843	0.0013
Experienced diarrhea (vs. no diarrhea) in past 4 Weeks	*V. cholerae*	163	2.622	1.393	4.934	0.0156

*Total n varies due to incomplete notation on some surveys or respondents do not participate in the given activity.

that needs to be done in providing facilities and changing behavior [15].

Lastly, in Avy, infection with ETEC was significantly associated with having suffered from diarrhea in the past 4 weeks. However, when all villages were factored together, *V. cholerae* was associated with participants having reported diarrhea in the past four weeks (Table 6). Both pathogens are known to cause diarrhea and depending on the study referenced, the location, and the population tested, both have been pointed to as leading causes of infection and disease [4,17,39]. Overall, a relatively low association of diarrhea with positive infection status is not surprising. Many of these pathogens can be carried in an asymptomatic state and people often suffer from diarrhea less upon subsequent infections with these enteric pathogens. Asymptomatic carriers can facilitate spread, especially in regions lacking adequate sanitation infrastructure. Meanwhile, repeated infections, especially in children have negative implications on their general health, growth and susceptibility to other infections [43–54]. Our study further confirms the role these pathogens play in causing disease in people and are perhaps where future attention should be focused as far as vaccine and treatment efforts.

All livestock species demonstrated relatively low prevalence of all five target pathogens, and there was no correlative risk for people who reported tending livestock vs. those who did not (Table 2 and 4). However, it should be noted that pigs carried a significantly higher risk of harboring one of these bacteria over cattle. This is especially pertinent as pigs have played a key role in other epidemics and pandemics, such as swine flu and Nipah virus [11,12].

While infection prevalence was relatively low for livestock, rodents had a nearly 2.8 times higher risk of carrying one of the pathogenic intestinal microorganisms over livestock. Moreover, rodents had the second highest overall prevalence at 51% (Table 2). Rodents are common in human and fragmented environments presenting a great opportunity for diseases to move between them, humans, and domestic animals [7,55]. Peridomestic rodents living in close quarters with human environments are known sources of various diseases including: hantavirus, *Salmonella* spp., *Campylobacter jejuni*, *Giardia* spp. and *Cryptosporidium* spp. [7] [21] However, there was no link between humans having reported touching rodents and an elevated risk of being infected. This could be due to underreporting of contact with rodents or contact people are unaware of, such as while sleeping or rodent fecal matter in their food. Given that *Yersinia pestis* is endemic to Madagascar, exposure to rodents and the fleas they carry is a serious risk for plague in addition to other diseases [25,26]. Enteric *Yersinia* spp. were detected in humans in all three villages; however, none of the cattle or pigs, the most likely source of enteric *Yersinia*, that we tested were found to carry the bacteria. The lack of positive livestock samples could indicate that there is another animal reservoir for enteric *Yersinia*. Regardless, there were positive samples, indicating that enteric *Yersinia* spp., especially *Y.*

Table 7. Summary of significant findings for infection with Enterobacteriaceae in human, livestock, and rodent populations.

Ambatolahy
Increased risk of *E. coli*, *Shigella* spp., *V. cholerae*, and *Yersinia* spp.
Increased risk for people 15 years or younger
Increased risk for people who did not use a toilet
Ambodiaviavy
Increased risk of *E. coli* and *V. cholerae*
Increased risk for people collecting water from an open source
Increased risk for people 15 years or younger
Increased risk for people who used medicine in past four weeks
Increased risk for people who did no boil their water
Increased risk for people who experienced diarrhea in past four weeks
Co-infection association between *E. coli* and *Shigella* spp.
Ankialo
Increased risk of *Shigella* spp.
Increased risk for people who did not use a toilet
Co-infection association between *S. enterica* and *Shigella* spp.
Co-infection association between *Shigella* spp. and *Yersinia* spp.
Additional risk factors (across all villages)
Higher prevalence of bacteria in rodents vs. livestock
Higher prevalence of bacteria in pigs vs. cattle
Males at higher risk for *S. enterica* than females
People who used a toilet at higher risk for *Yersinia* spp.
People who experienced diarrhea in past four weeks at higher risk for *V. cholerae*

pseudotuberculosis, persist in the human population in this region of Madagascar and make follow-up studies to sequence the present strains important.

There are many variables to consider when dissecting the lifecycle and transmission routes of a pathogen. As we expand our understanding of emerging infectious diseases it becomes increasingly clear that the way humans interact with their environment has profound effects on the dispersal of zoonotic pathogens [5,18,55–59]. This report points to areas for further study, namely water sources and human behavior that may account for the infection status of the human volunteers. Moreover, these data emphasize that humans, livestock, and rodents are all potential sources of pathogenic bacteria and as these groups interact more, the possibility for transmission increases, as does the likelihood of transmission to wildlife such as lemurs [18]. Understanding the host-origin and the subsequent dissemination of a disease at the human-livestock-wildlife interface can aid in combating the spread of these agents. Our work has shed light on the prevalence of various pathogenic bacteria in the human, livestock, and rodent populations in Southeastern Madagascar. More generally, this work has highlighted the complexity of these studies and that generalizations cannot always be drawn even from relatively related populations. What may be a risk factor in one village may not be for another nearby. It is important to take into account the individual as well as the population in studies such as these. Hopefully these findings will help in implementing preventative measures for people, their companion animals and livestock, and peridomestic rodents. More broadly, this work helps to expand our knowledge of disease transmission so that we can better combat these illnesses and enhance the quality of life for these people and others in similar settings.

Acknowledgments

We are grateful for logistical and infrastructural support from MICET, particularly director Benjamin Andriamihaja, the administration and support personnel of the Centre ValBio, Madagascar National Parks, Ian Fried, and Emilie Redwood. We would also like to thank Dr. Martha Furie and Dr. Jorge Benach for the generous use of their laboratory space at Stony Brook University and for helping to make this work possible.

Author Contributions

Conceived and designed the experiments: TRG PCW DCB. Performed the experiments: TRG DCB PCW JRB FTR JBB. Analyzed the data: TRG DCB. Contributed reagents/materials/analysis tools: TRG JBB PCW. Wrote the paper: TRG DCB JBB.

References

1. WHO/UNICEF (2000) Global Water Supply and Sanitation Assessment 2000 Report. Switzerland: WHO/UNICEF. Available: http://www.who.int/water_sanitation_health/monitoring/jmp2000.pdf. Accessed 2013 October 10.
2. Johansson EW, Wardlaw T (2009) Diarrhoea: Why children are still dying and what can be done. Switzerland: UNICEF and WHO. Available: http://www.who.int/maternal_child_adolescent/documents/9789241598415/en/. Accessed 2013 October 10.
3. Family and Community Health Unit, Water Sanitation and Health Unit, and WHO (2013) Water-related diseases. Available: http://www.who.int/water_sanitation_health/diseases/diarrhoea/en/. Accessed 2013 October 10.
4. Kotloff KL, Nataro JP, Blackwelder WC, Nasrin D, Farag TH, et al. (2013) Burden and aetiology of diarrhoeal disease in infants and young children in developing countries (the Global Enteric Multicenter Study, GEMS): a prospective, case-control study. Lancet 382: 209–222.
5. Daszak P, Cunningham AA, Hyatt AD (2000) Emerging infectious diseases of wildlife–threats to biodiversity and human health. Science 287: 443–449.
6. Rabinowitz P, Conti L (2013) Links among human health, animal health, and ecosystem health. Annu Rev Public Health 34: 189–204.
7. Meerburg BG, Singleton GR, Kijlstra A (2009) Rodent-borne diseases and their risks for public health. Crit Rev Microbiol 35: 221–270.
8. Calderon G, Pini N, Bolpe J, Levis S, Mills J, et al. (1999) Hantavirus reservoir hosts associated with peridomestic habitats in Argentina. Emerg Infect Dis 5: 792–797.
9. Katakweba AAS, Mulungu LS, Eiseb SJ, Mahlaba TaA, Makundi RH, et al. (2012) Prevalence of haemoparasites, leptospires and coccolbacilli with potential for human infection in the blood of rodents and shrews from selected localities in Tanzania, Namibia and Swaziland. African Zoology 47: 119–127.
10. Chen Y, Liang W, Yang S, Wu N, Gao H, et al. (2013) Human infections with the emerging avian influenza A H7N9 virus from wet market poultry: clinical analysis and characterisation of viral genome. Lancet 381: 1916–1925.
11. Daszak P, Zambrana-Torrelio C, Bogich TL, Fernandez M, Epstein JH, et al. (2013) Interdisciplinary approaches to understanding disease emergence: the past, present, and future drivers of Nipah virus emergence. Proc Natl Acad Sci U S A 110 Suppl 1: 3681–3688.
12. Garten RJ, Davis CT, Russell CA, Shu B, Lindstrom S, et al. (2009) Antigenic and genetic characteristics of swine-origin 2009 A(H1N1) influenza viruses circulating in humans. Science 325: 197–201.
13. Radolf JD, Caimano MJ, Stevenson B, Hu LT (2012) Of ticks, mice and men: understanding the dual-host lifestyle of Lyme disease spirochaetes. Nat Rev Microbiol 10: 87–99.
14. Chouikha I, Hinnebusch BJ (2012) Yersinia–flea interactions and the evolution of the arthropod-borne transmission route of plague. Curr Opin Microbiol 15: 239–246.
15. WHO/DFID-AHP (2013) Madagascar: health profile. Available: http://www.who.int/countries/mdg/en/. Accessed 2013 October 10.
16. World Health Organization DoMaHI (2011) Global Burden of Disease and Death Estimates. Available: www.who.int/gho/mortality_burden_disease/

global_burden_disease_death_estimates_sex_2008.xls. Accessed 2013 October 10.
17. Randremanana R, Randrianirina F, Gousseff M, Dubois N, Razafindratsimandresy R, et al. (2012) Case-control study of the etiology of infant diarrheal disease in 14 districts in Madagascar. PLoS One 7: e44533.
18. Junge RE, Barrett MA, Yoder AD (2011) Effects of anthropogenic disturbance on indri (Indri indri) health in Madagascar. Am J Primatol 73: 632–642.
19. Harper GJ, Steininger MK, Tucker CJ, Juhn D, Hawkins F (2007) Fifty years of deforestation and forest fragmentation in Madagascar. Env Conserv 34: 325–333.
20. With KA (2004) Assessing the risk of invasive spread in fragmented landscapes. Risk Anal 24: 803–815.
21. Dearing MD, Dizney L (2010) Ecology of hantavirus in a changing world. Ann N Y Acad Sci 1195: 99–112.
22. Mills JN (2006) Biodiversity loss and emerging infectious disease: An example from the rodent-borne hemorrhagic fevers. Biodiversity 7: 9–17.
23. Goodman SM (2003) Rattus on Madagascar and the dilemma of protecting the endemic rodent fauna. Conserv Bio 9: 450–453.
24. Laudisoit A, Leirs H, Makundi RH, Van Dongen S, Davis S, et al. (2007) Plague and the human flea, Tanzania. Emerg Infect Dis 13: 687–693.
25. Chanteau S, Ratsitorahina M, Rahalison L, Rasoamanana B, Chan F, et al. (2000) Current epidemiology of human plague in Madagascar. Microbes Infect 2: 25–31.
26. Hinnebusch BJ (2005) The evolution of flea-borne transmission in Yersinia pestis. Curr Issues Mol Biol 7: 197–212.
27. Mills JN, Childs JE, Ksiazek TG, Peters CJ (1995) Methods for trapping and sampling small mammals for virologic testing. Department of Health and Human Services, Public Health Service, CDC. Available: http://www.cdc.gov/hantavirus/pdf/rodent_manual.pdf. Accessed 2013 October 10.
28. Wright PC (1992) Primate Ecology, Rainforest Conservation, and Economic Development: Building a National Park in Madagascar. Evol Anthro 1: 25–33.
29. Wright PC (1997) The future of biodiversity in Madagascar: A view from Ranomafana National Park. In: Patterson B, Goodman, SM, editors.Natural Change and Human Impact in Madagascar.Washington D. C.: Smithsonian University Press. pp. 381.
30. Thoerner P, Bin Kingombe CI, Bogli-Stuber K, Bissig-Choisat B, Wassenaar TM, et al. (2003) PCR detection of virulence genes in Yersinia enterocolitica and Yersinia pseudotuberculosis and investigation of virulence gene distribution. Appl Environ Microbiol 69: 1810–1816.
31. Rahn K, De Grandis SA, Clarke RC, McEwen SA, Galan JE, et al. (1992) Amplification of an invA gene sequence of Salmonella typhimurium by polymerase chain reaction as a specific method of detection of Salmonella. Mol Cell Probes 6: 271–279.
32. Wang RF, Cao WW, Cerniglia CE (1997) A universal protocol for PCR detection of 13 species of foodborne pathogens in foods. J Appl Microbiol 83: 727–736.
33. IUCN (2009) IUCN statement on Madagascar. Available: http://www.iucn.org/?2995/IUCN-statement-on-Madagascar. Accessed 2013 October 10.
34. Ganzhorn JU, II LPP, Schatz GE, Sommer S (2001) The biodiversity of Madagascar: one of the world's hottest hotspots on its way out. Oryx 35: 346–348.
35. WHO/DFID-AHP (2006) The control of neglected zoonotic diseases. Switzerland: WHO/DFID-AHP. Available: http://www.who.int/zoonoses/Report_Sept06.pdf. Accessed 2013 October 10.
36. van den Beld MJ, Reubsaet FA (2012) Differentiation between Shigella, enteroinvasive Escherichia coli (EIEC) and noninvasive Escherichia coli. Eur J Clin Microbiol Infect Dis 31: 899–904.
37. Lindsay B, Ramamurthy T, Sen Gupta S, Takeda Y, Rajendran K, et al. (2011) Diarrheagenic pathogens in polymicrobial infections. Emerg Infect Dis 17: 606–611.
38. Gomes TA, Rassi V, MacDonald KL, Ramos SR, Trabulsi LR, et al. (1991) Enteropathogens associated with acute diarrheal disease in urban infants in Sao Paulo, Brazil. J Infect Dis 164: 331–337.
39. Nair GB, Ramamurthy T, Bhattacharya MK, Krishnan T, Ganguly S, et al. (2010) Emerging trends in the etiology of enteric pathogens as evidenced from an active surveillance of hospitalized diarrhoeal patients in Kolkata, India. Gut Pathog 2: 4.
40. Prüss-Üstün A, Bos R, Gore F, Bartram J (2008) Safer water, better health: costs, benefits and sustainability of interventions to protect and promote health. Geneva: World Health Organization. Available: http://www.who.int/water_sanitation_health/publications/safer_water/en/. Accessed 2013 October 10.
41. Okeke IN, Aboderin OA, Byarugaba DK, Ojo KK, Opintan JA (2007) Growing problem of multidrug-resistant enteric pathogens in Africa. Emerg Infect Dis 13: 1640–1646.
42. Hart CA, Kariuki S (1998) Antimicrobial resistance in developing countries. BMJ 317: 647–650.
43. Brunkard JM, Newton AE, Mintz E (2014) Cholera. In: CDC and Brunette GW, editors.CDC Health Information for International Travel 2014.New York, NY: Oxford University Press. pp. 158–160.
44. Bronze MS, Greenfield RA (2005) Biodefense: principles and pathogens. Wymondham, England: Horizon Bioscience.
45. Centers for Disease Control and Prevention (1982) Epidemiologic notes and reports outbreak of Yersinia enterocolitica – Washington state. Morbidity and Mortality Weekly Report.pp. 562–564.
46. Chapman PA, Siddons CA (1996) A comparison of immunomagnetic separation and direct culture for the isolation of verocytotoxin-producing Escherichia coli O157 from cases of bloody diarrhoea, non-bloody diarrhoea and asymptomatic contacts. J Med Microbiol 44: 267–271.
47. Cohen D, Block C, Green MS, Lowell G, Ofek I (1989) Immunoglobulin M, A, and G antibody response to lipopolysaccharide O antigen in symptomatic and asymptomatic Shigella infections. J Clin Microbiol 27: 162–167.
48. Gaudio PA, Sethabutr O, Echeverria P, Hoge CW (1997) Utility of a polymerase chain reaction diagnostic system in a study of the epidemiology of shigellosis among dysentery patients, family contacts, and well controls living in a shigellosis-endemic area. J Infect Dis 176: 1013–1018.
49. Gordon MA, Graham SM, Walsh AL, Wilson L, Phiri A, et al. (2008) Epidemics of invasive Salmonella enterica serovar enteritidis and S. enterica Serovar typhimurium infection associated with multidrug resistance among adults and children in Malawi. Clin Infect Dis 46: 963–969.
50. Harris JB, LaRocque RC, Chowdhury F, Khan AI, Logvinenko T, et al. (2008) Susceptibility to Vibrio cholerae infection in a cohort of household contacts of patients with cholera in Bangladesh. PLoS Negl Trop Dis 2: e221.
51. Nuorti JP, Niskanen T, Hallanvuo S, Mikkola J, Kela E, et al. (2004) A widespread outbreak of Yersinia pseudotuberculosis O:3 infection from iceberg lettuce. J Infect Dis 189: 766–774.
52. Perron GG, Quessy S, Letellier A, Bell G (2007) Genotypic diversity and antimicrobial resistance in asymptomatic Salmonella enterica serotype Typhimurium DT104. Infect Genet Evol 7: 223–228.
53. Qadri F, Saha A, Ahmed T, Al Tarique A, Begum YA, et al. (2007) Disease burden due to enterotoxigenic Escherichia coli in the first 2 years of life in an urban community in Bangladesh. Infect Immun 75: 3961–3968.
54. Qadri F, Svennerholm AM, Faruque AS, Sack RB (2005) Enterotoxigenic Escherichia coli in developing countries: epidemiology, microbiology, clinical features, treatment, and prevention. Clin Microbiol Rev 18: 465–483.
55. Lohmus M, Albihn A (2013) Gastrointestinal Pathogens in Rodents Overwintering in Human Facilities around Uppsala, Sweden. J Wildl Dis 49: 747–749.
56. Gillespie TR, Chapman CA, Grenier EC (2005) Effects of logging on gastrointestinal parasite infections and infection risk in African primates. J App Ecol 42: 699–707.
57. Gillespie TR, Greiner EC, Chapman CA (2005) Gastrointestinal parasites of the colobus monkeys of Uganda. J Parasitol 91: 569–573.
58. Hale CR, Scallan E, Cronquist AB, Dunn J, Smith K, et al. (2012) Estimates of enteric illness attributable to contact with animals and their environments in the United States. Clin Infect Dis 54 Suppl 5: S472–479.
59. Johnston AR, Gillespie TR, Rwego IB, McLachlan TL, Kent AD, et al. (2010) Molecular epidemiology of cross-species Giardia duodenalis transmission in western Uganda. PLoS Negl Trop Dis 4: e683.

Permissions

All chapters in this book were first published in PLOS ONE, by The Public Library of Science; hereby published with permission under the Creative Commons Attribution License or equivalent. Every chapter published in this book has been scrutinized by our experts. Their significance has been extensively debated. The topics covered herein carry significant findings which will fuel the growth of the discipline. They may even be implemented as practical applications or may be referred to as a beginning point for another development.

The contributors of this book come from diverse backgrounds, making this book a truly international effort. This book will bring forth new frontiers with its revolutionizing research information and detailed analysis of the nascent developments around the world.

We would like to thank all the contributing authors for lending their expertise to make the book truly unique. They have played a crucial role in the development of this book. Without their invaluable contributions this book wouldn't have been possible. They have made vital efforts to compile up to date information on the varied aspects of this subject to make this book a valuable addition to the collection of many professionals and students.

This book was conceptualized with the vision of imparting up-to-date information and advanced data in this field. To ensure the same, a matchless editorial board was set up. Every individual on the board went through rigorous rounds of assessment to prove their worth. After which they invested a large part of their time researching and compiling the most relevant data for our readers.

The editorial board has been involved in producing this book since its inception. They have spent rigorous hours researching and exploring the diverse topics which have resulted in the successful publishing of this book. They have passed on their knowledge of decades through this book. To expedite this challenging task, the publisher supported the team at every step. A small team of assistant editors was also appointed to further simplify the editing procedure and attain best results for the readers.

Apart from the editorial board, the designing team has also invested a significant amount of their time in understanding the subject and creating the most relevant covers. They scrutinized every image to scout for the most suitable representation of the subject and create an appropriate cover for the book.

The publishing team has been an ardent support to the editorial, designing and production team. Their endless efforts to recruit the best for this project, has resulted in the accomplishment of this book. They are a veteran in the field of academics and their pool of knowledge is as vast as their experience in printing. Their expertise and guidance has proved useful at every step. Their uncompromising quality standards have made this book an exceptional effort. Their encouragement from time to time has been an inspiration for everyone.

The publisher and the editorial board hope that this book will prove to be a valuable piece of knowledge for researchers, students, practitioners and scholars across the globe.

List of Contributors

Run Shi, Xia Yang, Lu Chen, Hong-tao Chang, Hong-ying Liu, Jun Zhao, Xin-wei Wang and Chuanqing Wang
College of Animal Science and Veterinary Medicine, Henan Agricultural University, Zhengzhou, People's Republic of China

François Dubos and Alain Martinot
Univ Lille Nord de France, UDSL, Lille, France
EA2694, Public Health, Epidemiology and Quality of Care, Lille, France
Paediatric Emergency and Infectious Diseases Unit, CHU Lille, Lille, France

Isabelle Pruvost
Univ Lille Nord de France, UDSL, Lille, France
Paediatric Emergency and Infectious Diseases Unit, CHU Lille, Lille, France

Alain Duhamel
Univ Lille Nord de France, UDSL, Lille, France,
EA2694, Public Health, Epidemiology and Quality of Care, Lille, France
Department of Biostatistics, CHU Lille, Lille, France

Emmanuel Chazard
Department of Biostatistics, CHU Lille, Lille, France

Valérie Hue
Paediatric Emergency and Infectious Diseases Unit, CHU Lille, Lille, France

Vipin Kumar Menon, Santosh George, Rajiv Sarkar and Gagandeep Kang
Department of Gastrointestinal Sciences, Christian Medical College, Vellore, India

Farah Aladin and Sameena Nawaz
Virus Reference Department, Centre for Infection, Health Protection Agency, London, United Kingdom

Ben Lopman
Division of Viral Diseases, National Center for Immunization and Respiratory Diseases, Centers for Disease Control and Prevention, Atlanta, Georgia, United States of America

James J. Gray
Norfolk and Norwich University Hospital Specialist Virology Centre, Microbiology Department, NRP Innovation Centre, Norwich, United Kingdom

Miren Iturriza Gomara
Department of Clinical Infection, Microbiology and Immunology, Institute of Infection and Global Health, University of Liverpool, Liverpool, United Kingdom

Yan Zhou
College of Life Sciences, Beijing Normal University, Beijing, China
National Institute of Biological Sciences, Beijing, China

Na Dong, Liyan Hu and Feng Shao
National Institute of Biological Sciences, Beijing, China

Sanjoy Kumer Dey and Chandan Kumar Shaha
Department of Neonatology, Bangabandhu Sheikh Mujib Medical University (BSMMU), Dhaka, Bangladesh

Mohammod Jobayer Chisti, Sumon Kumar Das, Farzana Ferdous, Fahmida Dil Farzana, Shahnawaz Ahmed, Mohammad Abdul Malek, Abu Syed Golam Faruque and Tahmeed Ahmed
Centre for Nutrition and Food Security (CNFS), International Centre for Diarrhoeal Disease Research, Bangladesh (icddr,b), Dhaka, Bangladesh

Mohammed Abdus Salam
Research Administration Services (RAS), icddr,b, Dhaka, Bangladesh

Muhammad Masroor Alam and Muhammad Naeem
Department of Biotechnology, Quaid-i-Azam University, Islamabad, Pakistan

Adnan Khurshid, Muhammad Suleman Rana, Shahzad Shaukat, Salmaan Sharif, Mehar Angez and Syed Sohail Zahoor Zaidi
Department of Virology, National Institute of Health, Islamabad, Pakistan

Maria Fiorentino and Alessio Fasano
Mucosal Immunology and Biology Research Center, Massachusetts General Hospital, Charlestown, Massachusetts, United States of America

Myron M. Levine and Marcelo B. Sztein.,
Center for Vaccine Development and the Departments of Pediatrics and Medicine, University of Maryland School of Medicine, Baltimore, Maryland, United States of America

Mostafizur Rahman, Rafiad Islam, Atanu Banik, M. Badrul Amin, Fatema Akter and Kaisar Ali Talukder
Centre for Food and Waterborne Diseases (CFWD), icddr,b, Dhaka, Bangladesh

Mohd S. Iqbal
Centre for Food and Waterborne Diseases (CFWD), icddr,b, Dhaka, Bangladesh
Centre for Control of Chronic Diseases (CCCD), icddr,b, Dhaka, Bangladesh

Terhi Uotila
Tampere University Hospital, Department of Internal Medicine, Tampere, Finland

Janne Laine
Tampere University Hospital, Department of Internal Medicine, Tampere, Finland
National Institute of Health and Welfare, Epidemiologic Surveillance and Response Unit, Helsinki, Finland

Markku Korpela
Tampere University Hospital, Department of Internal Medicine, Tampere, Finland
University of Tampere, School of Medicine, Tampere, Finland

Salla Toikkanen, Mikko J. Virtanen and Markku Kuusi
National Institute of Health and Welfare, Epidemiologic Surveillance and Response Unit, Helsinki, Finland

Jukka Lumio
University of Tampere, School of Medicine, Tampere, Finland

Eila Kujansuu
Nokia Health Centre, Nokia, Finland

Leigh A. Baxt and Marcia B. Goldberg
Department of Medicine, Massachusetts General Hospital, Cambridge, Massachusetts, United States of America
Department of Microbiology and Immunobiology, Harvard Medical School, Boston, Massachusetts, United States of America

Tianmu Chen, Ruchun Liu and Xixing Zhang
Office for Disease Control and Emergency Response, Changsha Center for Disease Control and Prevention, Changsha, The People's Republic of China

Ross Ka-kit Leung
Stanley Ho Centre for Emerging Infectious Diseases, The Chinese University of Hong Kong, Shatin, New Territories, Hong Kong SAR, The People's Republic of China

Zi Zhou
School of Public Health, Xiamen University, Xiamen, The People's Republic of China

Lijie Zhang
Chinese Field Epidemiology Training Program, Chinese Center for Disease Control and Prevention, Beijing, The People's Republic of China

Divya T. George, Carolyn A. Behm and Naresh K. Verma
Division of Biomedical Science and Biochemistry, Research School of Biology, The Australian National University, Canberra, Australia

David H. Hall and Ken C. Q. Nguyen
Center for C. elegans Anatomy, Department of Neuroscience, Albert Einstein College of Medicine, Bronx, New York, United States of America

Ulrike Mathesius
Division of Plant Science, Research School of Biology, The Australian National University, Canberra, Australia

Melanie Rug
Centre for Advanced Microscopy, The Australian National University, Canberra, Australia

Benjamin A. Cash
Center for Ocean-Land-Atmosphere Studies, Fairfax, Virginia, United States of America

Xavier Rodó
Institut Català de Ciències del Clima (IC3), Barcelona, Catalunya, Spain
Institució Catalana de Recerca i Estudis Avançats, Barcelona, Catalunya, Spain

Michael Emch
University of North Carolina Chapel Hill, Chapel Hill, North Carolina, United States of America

Md. Yunus and Abu S. G. Faruque
International Centre for Diarrheal Disease Research, Dhaka, Bangladesh

Mercedes Pascual
Department of Ecology and Evolutionary Biology University of Michigan, Ann Arbor, Michigan, United States of America
Howard Hughes Medical Institute, Chevy Chase, Maryland, United States of America

Divya T. George, Carolyn A. Behm and Naresh K. Verma
Division of Biomedical Science and Biochemistry, Research School of Biology, The Australian National University, Canberra, Australia

Ulrike Mathesius
Division of Plant Science, Research School of Biology, The Australian National University, Canberra, Australia

Salwa F. Ahmed, John D. Klena, Manal Mostafa and Peter J. Sebeny
United States Naval Medical Research Unit No.3, Cairo, Egypt

Jessica Dogantemur, Tracy Middleton and James Hanson
Incirlik Air Base, Incirlik, Turkey

Shuang Meng, Jianguo Xu, Yanwen Xiong and Changyun Ye
State Key Laboratory for Infectious Disease Prevention and Control, National Institute for Communicable Disease Control and Prevention, Chinese Center for Disease Control and Prevention, Changping, Beijing, People's Republic of China

Fan He
Zhejiang Provincial Center for Disease Control and Prevention, Hangzhou, People's Republic of China,

Ke Han
Guangdong Provincial Center for Disease Control and Prevention, Guangzhou, People's Republic of China

Lunguang Liu and Wei Sun
Sichuan Provincial Center for Disease Control and Prevention, Chengdu, People's Republic of China

Lijie Zhang, Baoping Zhu and Huilai Ma
Chinese Field Epidemiology Training Program, Chinese Center for Disease Control and Prevention, Beijing, People's Republic of China

Christina Faherty, Eileen M. Barry and James P. Nataro
Department of Medicine, Center for Vaccine Development, University of Maryland School of Medicine, Baltimore, Maryland, United States of America

Jill M. Harper, Terez Shea-Donohue and Alessio Fasano
Mucosal Biology Research Center, University of Maryland School of Medicine, Baltimore, Maryland, United States of America

James B. Kaper
Department of Microbiology and Immunology, University of Maryland School of Medicine, Baltimore, Maryland, United States of America

Jaana I. Halonen, Tuula Oksanen and Jaana Pentti
Finnish Institute of Occupational Health, Helsinki, Finland

Mika Kivimä ki
Finnish Institute of Occupational Health, Helsinki, Finland
Department of Epidemiology and Public Health, University College of London, London, United Kingdom

Jussi Vahtera
Finnish Institute of Occupational Health, Helsinki, Finland
Department of Public Health, University of Turku, and Turku University Hospital, Turku, Finland

Pekka Virtanen
Tampere School of Health Sciences, University of Tampere, Tampere, Finland

Mikko J. Virtanen
Epidemiologic Surveillance and Response Unit, National Institute for Health and Welfare, Helsinki, Finland

Mara Martinić, Anilei Hoare, Inés Contreras and Sergio A. Álvare
Departamento de Bioquímica y Biología Molecular, Facultad de Ciencias Químicas y Farmacéuticas, Universidad de Chile, Santiago, Chile

Victor E. Gonzaga, Mariana Ramos, Ryan C. Maves and Joel M. Montgomery
United States Naval Medical Research Unit Six (NAMRU-6), Lima, Peru

Randal Freeman
United States Army, El Paso, Texas, United States of America

Syed A. Sattar, Mohammad Ali and Jason A. Tetro
Center for Research on Environmental Microbiology (CREM), University of Ottawa, Ottawa, Ontario, Canada

Fidisoa T. Rasambainarivo
Centre ValBio, Ranomafana, Madagascar

DeAnna C. Bublitz and James B. Bliska
Centre ValBio, Ranomafana, Madagascar

Department of Molecular Genetics and Microbiology, Center for Infectious Diseases, Stony Brook University, Stony Brook, New York, United States of America

Patricia C. Wright
Centre ValBio, Ranomafana, Madagascar
Department of Anthropology, Stony Brook University, Stony Brook, New York, United States of America

Thomas R. Gillespie
Centre ValBio, Ranomafana, Madagascar
Department of Environmental Health, Rollins School of Public Health, Emory University, Atlanta, Georgia, United States of America
Department of Environmental Sciences and Program in Population Biology, Ecology, and Evolution, Emory University, Atlanta, Georgia, United States of America

Jonathan R. Bodager
Department of Environmental Health, Rollins School of Public Health, Emory University, Atlanta, Georgia, United States of America

Index